To Audrey

with best wishes,

[illegible]

Music, Medicine and Religion at the Ospedale di Santo Spirito in Rome

Music in Society and Culture

ISSN 2047-2773

This series brings history and musicology together in ways that will embed social and cultural questions into the very fabric of music-history writing. Music in *Society and Culture* approaches music not as a discipline, but as a subject that can be discussed in myriad ways. Those ways are cross-disciplinary, requiring a mastery of more than one mode of enquiry. This series therefore invites research on art and popular music in the Western tradition and in cross-cultural encounters involving Western music, from the early modern period to the twenty-first century. Books in the series will demonstrate how music operates within a particular historical, social, political or institutional context; how and why society and its constituent groups choose their music; how historical, cultural and musical change interrelate; and how, for whom and why music's value undergoes critical reassessment.

Proposals or queries should be sent in the first instance to the series editors or Boydell & Brewer at the addresses shown below.

Professor Vanessa Agnew, Technische Universität Dortmund,
Faculty of Cultural Studies, Room 3.211,
Emil-Figge-Straße 50, 44227 Dortmund, Germany
email: vanessa.agnew@tu-dortmund.de

Professor Katharine Ellis, Faculty of Music, University of Cambridge,
11 West Road, Cambridge, CB3 9DP, UK
email: kje32@cam.ac.uk

Professor Jonathan Glixon, University of Kentucky (emeritus)
email: jonathan.glixon@uky.edu

Boydell & Brewer, PO Box 9, Woodbridge, Suffolk, IP12 3DF, UK
email: editorial@boydell.co.uk

Previously published titles in the series are listed at the back of this volume.

MUSIC, MEDICINE AND RELIGION AT THE OSPEDALE DI SANTO SPIRITO IN ROME

1550–1750

Naomi J. Barker

THE BOYDELL PRESS

First published 2024
The Boydell Press, Woodbridge

ISBN 978-1-83765-065-1

The Boydell Press is an imprint of Boydell & Brewer Ltd
PO Box 9, Woodbridge, Suffolk IP12 3DF, UK
and of Boydell & Brewer Inc.
668 Mt. Hope Avenue, Rochester NY 14620-2731, USA
website: www.boydellandbrewer.com

A CIP record for this title is available
from the British Library

This publication is printed on acid-free paper

Contents

Illustrations

Plates

Figures

Tables

Music examples

Preface

This book started from a simple question: what was Frescobaldi doing working in a hospital? While attempting to find the answer by exploring the administrative archive of the Ospedale di Santo Spirito in Sassia, I discovered a wealth of material about this complex institution that employed some of the most respected physicians of the time and was a centre of medical education, while at the same time, was driven by religious conviction to care for social outcasts – unwanted babies, orphans and the sick poor. Crucially, it employed musicians and used music created by leading figures in Roman musical circles.

The variety and chronology of the sources that include the buildings themselves, administrative materials and an archive, albeit dispersed, of music manuscripts, renders a linear account of them difficult. Several key documents are reports written to satisfy papal authorities that are essentially reflective and backward-looking. Further, internal decrees were iterative and in force for long periods of time. Information extracted from such documents had to be mapped onto documents of a more mundane nature such as meeting minutes and financial documents that offered a more objective chronology. For this reason, the story of music in the Hospital has to some extent had to be told backwards.

The book is structured in two parts. The first provides a background to the institution and its foundation, exploring the relationship between religion and medicine and the role of music in both, while also outlining what was accepted as medical fact in the early modern world. The second part draws on the rich, but non-linear, archival material. Chapter 4 uses financial and documentary evidence to reflect on Bernadino da Cirillo's impact at the Hospital. Chapters 5 and 6 are broadly thematic, dealing with music in the church and the hospital wards respectively, while Chapter 7 is complementary to both Chapters 5 and 6, using iterations and revisions of a decree issued in 1644 to frame a broad chronological span from 1752 back to the late sixteenth century.

Acknowledgements

In writing this book I have racked up a debt of gratitude to many people. I am particularly indebted to Noel O'Regan for collegial exchanges of ideas and his detailed scrutiny of my text as it evolved. Thanks also to Helen Coffey, Silvia de Renzi, Rev. Philip Munch and David Rowland reading and commenting on draft chapters. Without their efforts the book would be much poorer. Any remaining errors are, of course, my own. I have also had a great deal of help with languages, and record here my thanks to Luca della Libera, Silvia de Renzi, Giovanna Gentile, Simone Longhi, David Noy and Shelagh Sneddon. Thanks too, to Tim Carter and Carrie Churnside who were brave enough to support my funding bids.

I was fortunate to enjoy the kindness and generosity of archivists and librarians who went the extra mile as institutions were reopening for study after the Covid-19 pandemic. Thank you to Dr Luca Cianfoni and Prof. Francesco Coviello at the Biblioteca del Conservatorio di Santa Cecilia, Rome; Dr Raymond Dittrich of the Bischöfliche Zentralbibliothek in Regensburg; Sophie Denham of the Museum of the Order of St John, London; Dottoressa Alessandra Facchinelli of the Biblioteca del Castello del Buonconsiglio, Trento; and Dottoressa Patrizia Ricca in the Biblioteca Lancisiana, Rome.

This project has been made possible by a series of awards. Grants from the Faculty of Arts and Social Sciences at the Open University, the British Academy (Small Research Grant, 2017–2018) and the Music and Letters Trust enabled the initial archival work on the career of Frescobaldi at the Ospedale di Santo Spirito. However, the book would not exist without the financial support of a Leverhulme Research Fellowship (2021–2022) that gave me the resources to spend time in the archives and crucially, the time away from normal duties to write.

The unsung heroes are my friends and family. My husband Chris has been a rock through it all, making me laugh every day even in tough times. The book may well have been written a lot quicker without him, but it wouldn't have been half as much fun. My father Peter Barker, who instilled in me a love of learning and championed my musical and academic endeavours, sadly passed away before the project was finished. It is to his memory that this book is dedicated.

Editorial Conventions and Notes

In English, the title of the institution would be 'Hospital of the Holy Ghost.' I will use the Italian form of the name, Hospital of Santo Spirito as there were (and are) various unrelated hospitals of the same name across Europe. Where the word 'Hospital' is capitalised, it refers to the institution as a whole, while 'hospital' with a lower-case 'h' indicates the hospital wards within the complex. The term 'Order' refers to the Hospital Order of religious men and women, living together in a community under specific regulations known as a Rule, in this case the Rule of the Order of Santo Spirito, while 'Confraternity' refers to the associated lay folk committed to pious works and communal prayer, but living in their own homes.

The commendatore of the Hospital of Santo Spirito, initially called the preceptor, was effectively the CEO of a large charitable organisation, overseeing all aspects of the institution. I will use the Italian term most commonly used in the archival sources of this period, that is, 'commendatore.' Where 'preceptor' is used, for example in quotations, it is an equivalent. Other key roles in the institution were the prior, the maestro di casa whose function was similar to a major-domo, and the school master, all of whom were answerable to the commendatore.

Discussions in this book that use financial records as the primary sources follow the simplest units of Roman currency in use c. 1600. Only two units are referred to in the financial documents – the larger unit is the scudo (assumed to be the silver scudo) and the smaller, the baiocco. The latter is usually referred to broadly as 'di moneta.' 100 baiocchi = 1 scudo d'argento.

Biblical quotes in English are from the New International Version. References to Psalms use the Vulgate numbering.

In short quotations from documentary sources the scribal abbreviations have been silently expanded, but original spellings and punctuation have been retained.

The music examples have been transcribed to present as literally as possible the material in the sources. However, some editorial discretion has been used to correct obvious mistakes and to provide missing accidentals. Bar lines are editorial as they are largely absent from vocal parts and sporadic in organ parts, where they are used with text incipits to mark crucial points of congruence with the voice rather than regular metrical divisions. Organ parts in the manuscript partbooks are usually referred to as 'basso ad organo' or 'bassus ad organum.' The use of figured bass is sparse, and the parts are clearly intended for accompaniment by a single instrument without reinforcement of the bass by a melodic instrument. Where an additional bass instrument is required, the term ripieno or concertato is used.

Abbreviations

D-Rp	Bischöfliche Zentralbibliothek, Regensburg
GB-En	National Library of Scotland, Edinburgh
GB-LBl	London, British library
GB-Lwl	Wellcome Library, London
I-Ras	Archivio di Stato di Roma[1]
I-Rc	Biblioteca Casanatense, Rome
I-Rla	Biblioteca Lancisiana, Rome
I-Rn	Biblioteca Nazionale, Rome
I-Rsc	Biblioteca del Conservatorio di Santa Cecilia, Rome
I-TRfeininger	Biblioteca Feininger, Castello del Buonconsiglio, Trento = TRf
I-Rvic	Archivio Diocesano di Roma (Archivio storico del vicariato di Roma)
V-CVaav	Archivio Apostolico Vaticano
V-CVbav	Biblioteca Apostolica Vaticana

1 The largest body of documents relating to the Hospital of Santo Spirito in Sassia is located in the Fondo dell'Ospedale di Santo Spirito held in the Archivio di Stato di Roma (I-Ras). For the purposes of this study, this source will be abbreviated to ASR OSS followed by the callmark of the item cited.

1

The Hospital of Santo Spirito: History, Architecture, Administration

In the third decade of the twenty-first century, visitors to Rome on a whistle-stop tour to take in the splendours of St Peter's Basilica are likely to miss the now unassuming-looking buildings comprising the Hospital of Santo Spirito in Sassia. The hospital, located just out of sight of the busy Via della Concilazione leading to Bernini's piazza, and a few minutes' walk from the Basilica, is still active today in a modern building adjacent to the fifteenth-century complex. It is an institution with a documented history dating back to 1198, though its origins as an ecclesiastical institution are even older.[1] The scope and function of what constituted a Hospital and similar charitable institutions at the time of the foundation of the Order of Santo Spirito and its hospital are, however, vastly different from their modern equivalents.

At the time of the Hospital's foundation and throughout the period with which this book is concerned, the separation of disciplines into science, religion, art and their subsidiary disciplines of biology, botany, music, philosophy and so on did not exist. A university-trained physician of the Renaissance would have had a thorough understanding of a wide range of topics embraced within 'natural philosophy', as well as music theory, rhetoric, logic and astronomy, all of which were included in grammar-school education. This study focuses in particular on the close relationship between religion and medicine – a relationship that is extremely complex, with roots reaching back to antiquity – and how music may be viewed as a point of triangulation between them.

1 The name of the Hospital, 'in Sassia' or 'in Saxia', is derived from the location in what was then the outskirts of the area around St Peter's known as the 'Schola Saxonum', an area occupied by an Anglo-Saxon Christian community founded in the eighth century by several kings from various parts of Britain: Cedwalla, king of the West Saxons (r. 685–688), Coenredo of Mercia (r. 704–709), Offa, king of the East Saxons (r. 757–796) and Ina, king of Wessex (r. 688–726). Prior to Christian occupation, the area was the site of a circus and gardens dating from the time of the emperor Nero. Archaeological details are given in Pietro De Angelis, *L'Ospedale di S. Spirito dalle origini al 1500*, 2 vols. Collana di studi storici sull'Ospedale di Santo Spirito in Saxia e sugli ospedali Romani (Rome, 1960; 1962), vol. 1, pp. 15–39 and 126–134. De Angelis's book remains the most detailed study of the history of the institution. As most secondary literature on the hospital is in Italian, this section makes available in English salient points from the work of De Angelis and others.

In pre-Christian and non-Western contexts, temples were (and are) places where the sick sought relief through rituals, and shamans functioned as mediators between the spirit world and physical world for guidance in curing diseases. We know from ancient literature that music played a part in these healing practices.[2] It should not be surprising that as Christian communities developed, their places of worship likewise became sanctuaries to which folk came to find cures for mental and physical illness.

Healing was a fundamental part of the activities of the followers of Jesus recounted in the New Testament and, according to the earliest defences of Christianity written by Justin Martyr, Tertullian, Origen and Irenaeus, continued in the Christian communities of late antiquity up until around the Council of Nicaea.[3] Christianity took over a number of elements of pagan healing cults, such as ceremonies of washing or purification and reclothing, sacrifice and prayers, as well as staff that included a chorus for singing ritual hymns.[4] Such sites often developed in the same location as pagan shrines and replaced them. The relationship between religious ritual and healing laid the foundation for the early history of the hospital, which was welded to the history of Christian communities in late antiquity. A hospital in the sense that we understand the word today, in its earliest manifestation, represents the unity of purpose of religion and medicine.

As music had for centuries played a part in temple rituals and in shamanistic practices, the triangular relationship of music, religion and medicine within the hospital as it later emerged was already established. The three disciplines have assumed different emphases at different times, and in different cultures, until medicine in the purely scientific sense became dominant. In this study, music, whether abstract and theoretical, or a sounding reality, offers a point of triangulation, relating to concepts of healing within both medicine and religion. The supremacy of medicine in the modern world has to a large extent sidelined holistic treatments and experimental therapies, and few medical faculties offer any training relating to spirituality, broadly conceived.[5] Although music ther-

2 Aristides, for example, provides some early evidence of the efficaciousness of music: '... while they were singing, there arose unnoticed a feeling of comfort, and sometimes everything which pained me went completely away.' *Aelius Aristides and the Sacred Tales*, ed. and trans. Charles A. Behr (Amsterdam, 1968), cited in Guenter B. Risse, *Mending Bodies, Saving Souls: A History of Hospitals* (New York & Oxford, 1999), p. 36.

3 For example, Justin Martyr, *The First Apology*, Origen, *Against Celsus*, Tertullian, *On the Resurrection of the Flesh*, Irenaeus, *Against Heresies*, cited in Morton T. Kelsey, *Healing and Christianity in Ancient Thought and Modern Times* (New York, 1973), pp. 33–38 and 142–144. Kelsey (p. 129) cites further examples drawn from Evelyn Frost, *Christian Healing: A Consideration of the Place of Spiritual Healing in the Church of Today in the Light of the Doctrine and Practice of the Ante-Nicene Church* (London, 1940).

4 Risse, *Mending Bodies*, p. 33.

5 The topic of educating medical practitioners with regard to religious practices is start-

apy is now recognised, the psychological and neurological understanding of its benefits are still little understood. It is only comparatively recently that the scientific investigation of music and emotion has emerged as a new development in medicine and psychology.

The early hospital

The birth of foundations recognisable as hospitals as we understand the term today, happened between 350–500 in the Eastern Roman Empire. In Christian Byzantium the duty to care for the weak and disadvantaged of any social level who could not care for themselves fell to the emerging churches. There is disagreement among scholars as to whether these early hospitals aimed to cure the sick, or only to care for them in their suffering, thus separating physical cure from the Christian acts of mercy. Descriptions of Basil of Caesarea's hospital, a series of buildings which Gregory of Nazianzus called the 'new city', situated on the edge of the city of Caesarea, epitomise these opposing views.[6]

Risse sees Basil's hospital as a monastic infirmary within a monastic charitable complex and Basil himself as an educated man with some knowledge of medicine, while Miller presents it as one of the first hospitals in which secular medicine is aligned with Christian monasticism and Basil as one of the physicians.[7] Porterfield acknowledges Basil's monastic experience in Egypt, Palestine and Syria, but suggests that his knowledge of Greek science, including the Hippocratic corpus, enabled him to recognise the failure of Christian ascetics to carry out the works of Christian philanthropy. Such opposing views seem inevitable as the early Christians themselves argued about whether secular medicine with its focus on the body could be aligned with Christian doctrine of abnegation of the body by following an ascetic life.[8] The latter position was bolstered by the lack of scriptural evidence of Jesus ever using any form of secular, physical medicine. A bone of contention in these disputes was the provision of medical care and curative therapies as opposed to care and comfort for those in distress.

Alongside Basil, Augustine of Hippo (d. 430) was an important influence in the development of monastic hospitals. In his Rule for monastic living, Augustine de-emphasised asceticism and underlined the need for interaction, love

ing to draw some scholarly attention, for example, Michael Balboni and John Peteet (eds), *Spirituality and Religion Within the Culture of Medicine: From Evidence to Practice* (New York, 2017), online edn.

6 Stephen M. Hildebrand, *Basil of Caesarea*, The Early Church Fathers (Abingdon, 2018), pp. 13–14.

7 Risse, *Mending Bodies*, pp. 76–77; Timothy S. Miller, *The Birth of the Hospital in the Byzantine Empire* (Baltimore and London, 1997 (1st edn 1985), p. 119.

8 Amanda Porterfield, *Healing in the History of Christianity* (Oxford, 2005), pp. 52–53.

and good works.[9] The monastic communities regulated under Augustine took on the resemblance of a family of no more than a dozen people all performing charitable acts as necessary for their own redemption.[10] Crucially, Augustine developed the idea of *Christus medicus* – Christ as the divine physician – who could cure the spiritual diseases which were believed to be the cause of bodily infirmities. As will be seen in the chapters below, this concept was central to the close relationship of medicine and religion in the early modern period. As the Hospital Order of Santo Spirito was ultimately placed under the umbrella of the Rule of Augustine, it was his ideal of monastic life that informed many later directives within the Hospital.

Until the mid-twelfth century hospitals developed largely in the eastern Mediterranean. Opinions as to why hospitals such as Santo Spirito emerged in Europe in the mid-twelfth century vary. There was certainly economic hardship triggered by failed harvests and famine that drove rural populations into urban areas, as well as gradual population growth and urbanisation. The initial response of the Church to poverty was to re-emphasise its own voluntary poverty, giving rise to new ascetic orders such as the Cistercians and Carthusians. The involuntary poor were a different challenge. New ideas emerging from the University of Paris, and the influential reformer Peter the Chanter (d. 1197) outlined the obligation of the entire Christian community towards the destitute.[11] These were to be fundamental in the foundation of new hospitals under Pope Innocent III who was deeply influenced by his time studying in Paris.

Keyvanian offers a different view, suggesting that it was an economic boom that fuelled early hospital construction projects in the mid-twelfth century, and that the care of the poor was not only an act of charity, but also a way of enhancing the political power of urban elites.[12] Cavallo further highlighted the financial advantages of charity, as the need for sick or injured workers to be quickly returned to the workforce had economic benefits to those who employed them, usually the wealthy and landowners.[13] Henderson, focusing on

9 *The Rule of St. Augustine with Commentary by Hugh of St. Victor*, trans. Dom Aloysius Smith, (n.d., n.p.).

10 John Henderson, *The Renaissance Hospital: Healing the Body and Healing the Soul* (New Haven, CT and London, 2006), p. 113; Risse, *Mending Bodies*, p. 92.

11 Attitudes towards poverty in the Middle Ages were complex. For example, those in distress, who were perceived as enjoying a status blessed by Jesus without having to voluntarily surrender their wealth, were regarded as the 'poor of Christ'. While charity to the poor was a Christian duty, there was much argument about what kind of poverty deserved aid. James William Brodman, *Charity and Religion in Medieval Europe* (Washington DC, 2009), p. 16; Risse, *Mending Bodies*, p. 92; Christopher F. Black, *Italian Confraternities in the Sixteenth Century* (Cambridge, 1989), pp. 130–137.

12 Carla Keyvanian, *Hospitals and Urbanism in Rome, 1200–1500* (Leiden and Boston, 2015), pp. 14–15.

13 Sandra Cavallo, 'The Motivations of Benefactors: An Overview of the Study of Charity', in Jonathan Barry and Colin Jones (eds), *Medicine and Charity before the Welfare State* (London and New York, 1991), pp. 46–62.

the medical conditions treated, has suggested that specific needs such as keeping infectious patients isolated and taking those with chronic conditions off the streets sparked the development of hospitals.[14] While medieval hospitals were commonly endowed and overseen by the Church, to view them as only providing care rather than physical cure is an oversimplification of the nature of these institutions.[15]

Innocent III and the foundation of the Order of Santo Spirito

By the time Guy (Guido) de Montpellier built a hospital in his home town of Montpellier and established the Hospital Order of Santo Spirito around 1174, Byzantine hospitals were institutions of some importance not just in Constantinople but in the major towns and cities of the Christian east. Soon after his election to the papacy, Pope Innocent III acknowledged the success of the Hospital Order of St John of Jerusalem by issuing a papal breve which protected the Order and gave them permission to build an oratory.[16] Shortly thereafter, in 1198, he issued a further Bull that confirmed the constitution of the Order of Santo Spirito, protecting its hospitals in Montpellier and several other locations. Notably, it explicitly outlined the purpose of the Order to charitably and mercifully care for the poor and the sick and also forbade professed members of the Order from leaving except to join a stricter Order.[17] The hospital in Rome was functioning by the time Innocent III entrusted property belonging to the church of Santa Maria in Sassia to it, in a Bull dated 1 December 1201, thus it was founded between 1198 and 1201.[18] What is clear from the papal Bulls of 1198 and 1201 is that the Order of Santo Spirito already had a network of charitable hospitals in Italy and France. This network would increase rapidly over the subsequent century. However, caution is required in lumping these institutions together, as there were many hospitals operating under the name of the Holy Spirit as well as unrelated confraternities of the same name, in cities such as Naples.[19]

Innocent III issued the first Bull indicating the official function of the Hospital in Rome in June 1204. This document outlines the acts of charity of the Hospital as the seven acts of mercy, or Misericordia: sheltering, clothing and

14 Henderson, *The Renaissance Hospital*, pp. 70–101.

15 Barry and James, *Medicine and Charity Before the Welfare State*, p. 2.

16 'Cum sitis operibus', 1 July 1198, cited in De Angelis, *L'Ospedale di S. Spirito dalle origini al 1500*, vol. 1, p. 208.

17 'Religiosam vitam', 25 November 1198, cited in De Angelis, *L'Ospedale di S. Spirito dalle origini al 1500*, vol. 1, p. 209.

18 All the Bulls relating to the establishment of the Order, the Hospital and the Confraternity in Rome and in other locations are transcribed in full in De Angelis, *L'Ospedale di S. Spirito dalle origini al 1500*, vol. 1, pp. 373–417.

19 Risse, *Mending Bodies*, p. 149; Black, *Italian Confraternities*, pp. 3, 51–52.

feeding the poor; tending to the sick; visiting those in prison; and burying the dead. These acts are made explicit through reference to Jesus's instruction in the Gospel of Matthew chapter 25 to feed the hungry, give drink to the thirsty, care for the poor, tend the sick, visit those in prison and to care for strangers, and they remained central to the Rule of the Order.[20] By implication they also aligned the founder of the Order with the characteristics of virtuous leadership. A confraternity of lay nobles and supporters was established around 1268 under Clement IV to financially support the work of the Order.[21] Around a decade later the Fourth Lateran Council decreed that all religious Orders must adopt either the Benedictine or Augustinian Rule.

Within the Order, the foundation of the Hospital is represented as an act of Christian charity on the part of Innocent III. He was apparently so moved by hearing about two drowned babies that had been pulled from the Tiber in a fisherman's net, that he immediately promised to build a hospital to house abandoned infants. The frescoes in the Sistine ward of the fifteenth-century building offer a visual account of the story. The repetition of this tale over time raises Innocent III to an almost mythical status and perpetuates an aura of saintliness around him. However, his role as founder needs some critical focus.

Born Lotario dei Segni, Innocent authored an influential treatise on the wretchedness of the human condition (*De miseria condicionis humanae*) in 1195, a work that was widely disseminated and remained popular down to the seventeenth century. In this work, Innocent demonstrated an understanding of the condition of poverty. While his ideas were not new, his rejection of traditional monastic contemplative asceticism and embrace of active charity expressed in works marked a shift in the way charity was enacted in growing urban communities.[22]

Whatever his views, Innocent III's construction of the Hospital of Santo Spirito was almost certainly also part of a strategic urban building programme. The dei Segni had emerged from the conflicts between baronial families in Rome and he needed to bolster his status. Rivalry and banditry made interesting partners to the apparently benevolent and charitable work of caring for the sick. The positioning of Innocent's great act of mercy, founding a hospital to save children and the poor, was no doubt also part of his programme of power building and had political motives too. At a time when the government of the city of Rome was unstable and at the mercy of baronial families, building a new hospital close to St Peter's indicated his intention to shift the power base of the pope away from the Lateran palace with its association with Constantine and Imperial Rome to a more defensible location.[23]

20 Matthew 25: 31–40. This text is foundational to the establishment of many charitable confraternities and is not unique to Santo Spirito.

21 Matizia Maroni Lumbroso and Antonio Martini, *Le confraternite romane nelle lore chiese*, (Rome, 1963) pp. 408–409.

22 Brodman, *Charity and Religion in Medieval Europe*, pp. 22–23.

23 Keyvanian, *Hospitals and Urbanism in Rome 1200–1500*, pp. 96, 201–287.

While Innocent III may have had strong opinions about charity, he had similarly strong views about the authority of Catholicism, and also instituted revisions to the Mass and Office as celebrated in the papal chapel.[24] These revisions may have had some effect on the way music was used in the Offices of the Order of Santo Spirito, but without graduals or antiphoners from the period, one can only speculate about the nature of the music in the earliest services of the Order.

Eugene IV and the Augustinians

Following the period of its institution and prominence in the thirteenth century, the fortunes of the Hospital mirrored that of the papacy. During the period of the schism and the Avignon papacy, the Hospital and the Order fell into decline and their buildings into disrepair. Pope Eugene IV (1431–1447) realised that the reinvigoration of the Hospital of Santo Spirito was central to rebuilding papal power in Rome. He overruled the right of the Order of Santo Spirito to elect its own leader and placed his nephew, Pietro Barbo, in control of the institution as its preceptor, a position later more commonly referred to as the commendatore.[25]

Eugene was a member of the Order of Augustinian Hermits. He established the Augustinian canons regular at the Lateran in 1446, and subsequently placed the Order of Santo Spirito under their rule. The Rule of Augustine thus became a crucial framework for the Rule and life of members of the Order of Santo Spirito. Eugene further signalled his intention to place the Hospital and Order of Santo Spirito at the heart of the papacy by taking on the role of commendatore himself in 1446. He also re-established the Confraternity of Santo Spirito, encouraging his bishops to garner support from their parishioners, whether rich or poor, for the work of the Order and also to support hospitals in their own communities.[26] He personally gave the Order 200 gold ducats and twelve

[24] For an analysis of Innocent III's character, see Barbara H. Rosenwein, *Generations of Feeling: A History of Emotion 600–1700* (Cambridge, 2016), p. 115.

[25] Barbo subsequently became cardinal (1440) and Pope Paul II (1464).

[26] The relationship between the Order and the Confraternity is difficult to unravel through the surviving documents. What is clear is that the Hospital of Santo Spirito is rather different from the confraternity hospitals described by Black, *Italian Confraternities in the Sixteenth Century*. The close involvement of the pope in its governance also sets it apart from the many lay confraternities operating across Italy established by artisans' guilds, pious aristocrats or rural parish worthies to address specific charitable needs. Many of these confraternities used music as part of their devotions. For music in Roman confraternities see especially Noel O'Regan, 'Music at Roman "Ospedali" in the Sixteenth Century', *Il Veltro*, XLVI:1–4 (2002), 251–260; *Institutional Patronage in Post-Tridentine Rome: Music at Santissima Trinità Dei Pellegrini 1550–1650*, (London, 1995).

of his cardinals followed his example. The members of the Confraternity signed the newly established *Liber fraternitatis*. His success at generating funds from royalty and nobility, men and women, as well as prominent lay folk is evident in the signatures in the book, which survives in the Biblioteca Lancisiana.[27]

What seems clear is that Eugene established the administrative model for the Hospital that never subsequently changed. As Eugene was born in Venice to the patrician Condulmer family, he would have been well aware of the Venetian confraternities or *scuole grandi*, their administrative structures and charitable work.[28] By placing the Order and Hospital under papal control, he separated it from other similar institutions. From Eugene IV onwards, the commendatore effectively became a papal appointment and was simultaneously preceptor of the Augustinian canons regular of the Order of Santo Spirito, with oversight of the running of the Hospital (including the orphanage, school, women's cloister etc.); manager of the priests responsible for the spiritual needs of the members as well as of the sick and other inhabitants of the Hospital; and governor of the Confraternity whose members were not just lay folk who served in the hospital but also fundraisers. He thus fulfilled duties overseeing both people and finances and was answerable to the pope.

Sixtus IV: rebuilding the Hospital edifice

While Eugene set the Hospital and Order of Santo Spirito on a secure financial and administrative footing, it was Pope Sixtus IV (r. 1471–1484) who physically rebuilt the Hospital. He initiated the project soon after his accession, thus making it one of the first of his architectural schemes in Rome. Sixtus was a great admirer of Innocent III and set about revitalising two of his creations – the Palatine chapel, now known as the Sistine chapel, and the Hospital of Santo Spirito. Although Sixtus was educated in the Paduan humanist tradition, he relied on other humanist scholars, especially Platina, who was to become the librarian of the Vatican library, to develop the visual and spatial rhetoric of his building projects: a rhetoric that would align the papacy with the centre of power through reference to Rome's past.[29]

27 The *Liber fraternitatis* is essentially a book of signatures of those who gave funds to the hospital. A compilation of the names is reproduced in De Angelis, *L'Ospedale di S. Spirito dalle origini al 1500*, vol. 2, pp. 76–80. A second wave of funding followed a further reinvigoration of the Confraternity from 1478. The signatories include around a dozen papal singers, vol. 2 pp. 125–126.

28 The Venetian *scuole* were essentially groups of lay people, initially of a specific trade or parish committed to pious, charitable work. Few had buildings of their own, and all were involved in the state occasions of the Republic. See Jonathan Glixon, *Honoring God and the City: Music at Venetian Confraternities, 1260–1807* (Oxford, 2003).

29 Eunice Howe, *Art and Culture at the Sistine court: Platina's 'Life of Sixtus IV' and the Frescoes of the Hospital of Santo Spirito* (Vatican City, 2005), p. 7.

The physical space of the fifteenth-century hospital complex was designed for specific purposes, and, besides the main hospital ward, comprised a number of other buildings, including a large building housing the foundlings and a separate space for noble patients. The living areas for unmarried women, orphans and the resident friars were situated around separate courtyards. Additional buildings to the south, between the immense hospital wards and the River Tiber, accommodated housing for women of the Order who worked as wet-nurses raising the foundlings, and separate living quarters for the hospital workers. All of these buildings are mentioned in the papal Bull of March 1478.[30]

The plan of the hospital was functional but also monumental. Situated on the main artery leading from the Ponte Sant'Angelo to the Vatican, with its eastern end directly abutting the entrance to the Borgo, it was not only in a dominant position, but it was also the largest edifice in the area, rivalling old St Peters, and the only hospital of its kind being endowed by the pope for public use.[31] The importance of the Hospital in Sixtus IV's political agenda is reflected in the frescoes of the Sistine chapel. On its north wall, Botticelli's 'Christ healing the leper' or 'The temptation of Christ' conflates the two biblical narratives, but depicts the eastern façade of the new ward of the Hospital of Santo Spirito in the background. The image represents papal authority to heal both sin and disease and, simultaneously, the Solomonic temple of Jerusalem which was believed to be a precursor of the triumphant Christian Church. The image of Jesus is rendered in Sixtus's heraldic colours of blue and gold, thus aligning Sixtus as pope as a direct descendent of Christ and St Peter. The figure of Moses on the opposite wall similarly depicts the Old Testament leader and law-maker in blue and gold. The images powerfully reinforce the message of papal primacy. This message was further enhanced by Leo X, who both confirmed Sixtus IV's Bull concerning the Hospital and commissioned a series of tapestry designs from Raphael. The tapestry that hung immediately below Botticelli's 'Christ healing the leper' depicted 'Peter healing the lame man at the gate of the temple' – a narrative that reinforced the message that the pope, as the descendant of Peter, had the authority to forgive sin and thus to heal sickness.[32]

At that time, the eight-sided Dome of the Rock in Jerusalem was popularly believed to be the Temple of Solomon, thus the octagonal drum of the Hospital was recognisable as a representation of it. However, in educated humanist circles, the temple was fully understood as rectangular and had certainly been thus understood by Innocent III who had calculated the biblical dimensions of the temple and had constructed the old Palatine chapel and the old hospital

[30] Eunice Howe, *The Hospital of Santo Spirito and Pope Sixtus IV*, PhD, Johns Hopkins University, 1977, *Outstanding Dissertations in the Fine Arts* (New York & London, 1978), p. 56.

[31] Howe, *The Hospital of Santo Spirito*, p. 57. Until the construction of the Via di Concilazione in the 1930s, it would have been one of the largest buildings in the immediate area.

[32] Keyvanian, *Hospitals and Urbanism in Rome 1200–1500*, pp. 347–349, 351.

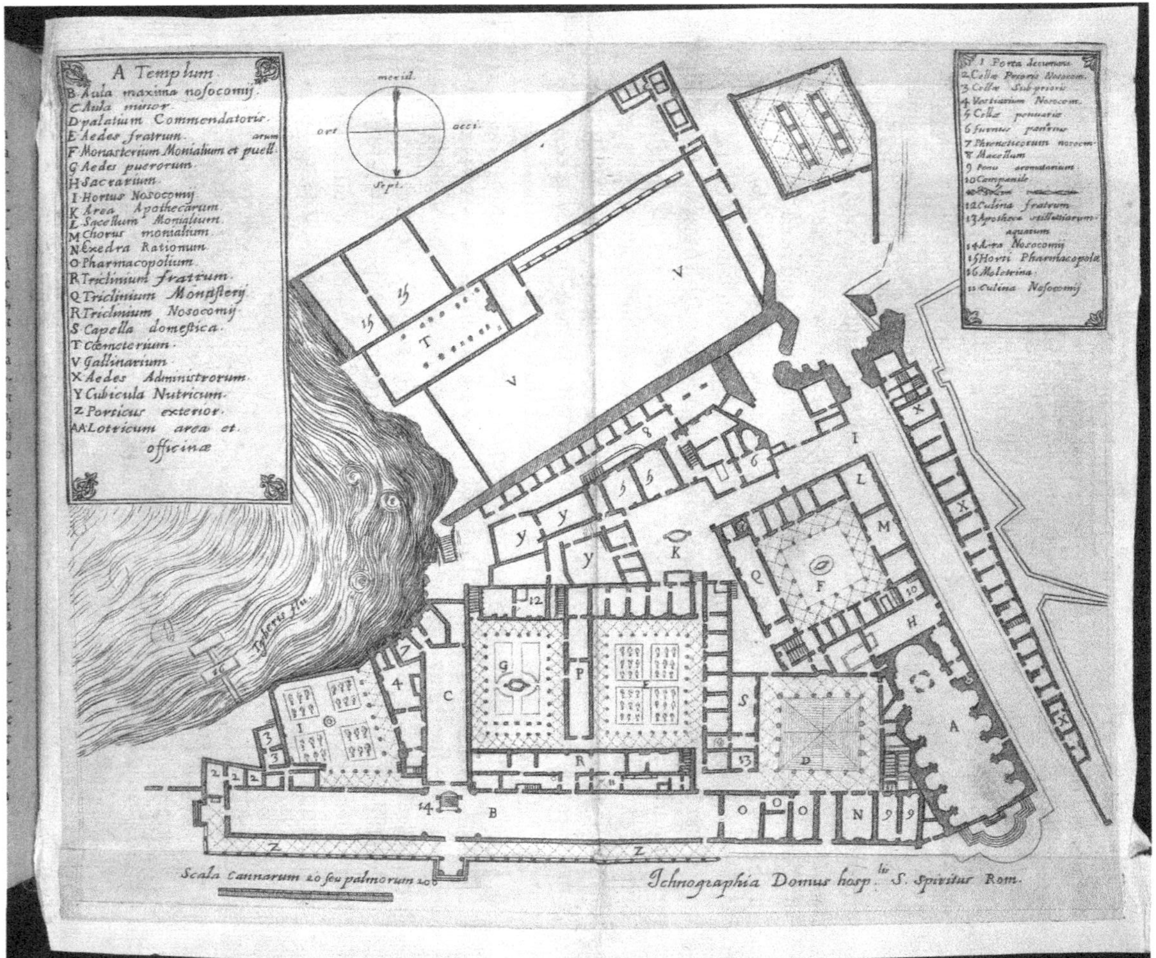

Plate 1.1 Hospital of Santo Spirito: ground plan. The location of the altar in the Sistine ward is at no. 14. Pierre Saulnier, *De capite sacri ordinis S. Spiritus dissertatio* (Lyon, 1649), plate opposite p. 18. London, British Library © The British Library Board, c.183.c.13.

building to mirror them. The hospital and chapel spaces would have been virtually identical at approximately thirteen metres wide, with a length three times its width (about forty metres). The foundations of the western end of the Sistine hospital are those of the original building. Sixtus IV simply extended the wards eastwards towards the River Tiber, adding the octagonal drum and lantern.[33]

The two wings of the ward stretch either side of the octagonal space surmounted by the drum and lantern – a striking external feature that, prior to the construction of the new basilica of St Peter's, would have dominated the urban space. The visitor entering from the street would move through a doorway, enriched by sculpted low-relief decoration, into this octagonal space to face the pillared and canopied altar, as this space also functioned as the hospital chapel. The vertical space of the drum is articulated by large windows that provide natural light. While apparently austere, the triforium is decorated with statues of apostles. Both the arched doorway and the altar are possibly by Andrea Bregno, who also worked on the Sistine chapel.[34] From this central space, the airy high-ceilinged wards stretched away to the right and to the left, lit by large windows set high in the walls conforming to medical thinking of the time regarding air and cleanliness. On the other axis it marked the transition from the street to the interior spaces of the cloisters occupied by the members of the Order.

Building design in the mid- to late fifteenth century was deeply influenced by the classical past, especially as transmitted in Leon Battista Alberti's treatise on architecture, *De re aedificatoria*. Alberti's theory of beauty of 'a harmony and concord of all the parts' depended on a mathematical system of harmonic proportions.[35] This reference to harmonic proportion was indebted to Vitruvius who suggested that an architect should understand the harmonic and mathematical theory of music.[36] Immediately following his recommendation concerning music theory, Vitruvius notes that an architect should also understand medicine, on account of the issues of climate that determine the healthiness or not of a site, for its water and air. This is a direct reference to the Hippocratic text 'On airs, waters and places', the principles of which remained in use in the Hippocratic-Galenic medicine predominant in the early modern period.

The design of the Hospital of Santo Spirito does seem to have been influenced by both Vitruvius and Hippocratic-Galenic concepts of airs.[37] The high

33 Keyvanian, *Hospitals and Urbanism in Rome 1200–1500*, p. 345.

34 De Angelis, *L'Ospedale di S. Spirito dalle origini al 1500*, vol. 2, pp 346–347, attributes the sculptural work to Bregno, citing Lavagnino, *Andrea Bregno e la sua Bottega* (1924). Howe regards the attribution to Bregno as 'tentative' and an alternative attribution to Sangallo as 'unsubstantiated'. Howe, *The Hospital of Santo Spirito*, p. 61.

35 Peter Murray, *The Architecture of the Italian Renaissance* (London, 1963), pp. 52–53.

36 Vitruvius, *The Ten Books on Architecture*, trans. and ed. Morris Hicky Morgan (New York, 1960; 1st edn, 1914), pp. 8–10.

37 Keyvanian has made a convincing argument that it was designed by Fra Giocondo da Verona on the basis of comparison with known designs as well as his treatise on

ceiling and windows opening at either end gave good ventilation. The high placement of the windows also maximised bed space. The Hospital was not unique in this respect as other European hospitals such as Notre Dame de Fontanilles, built in the 1290s, and the Hospital Maggiore in Milan evidence similar concerns about air and water.[38] Horden has suggested that medieval hospitals in general might be considered a non-natural environment in the Galenic sense. As the care that was provided was profoundly Galenic, it seems just as likely that their construction was carefully designed to reflect medical thinking of the time.[39] Although there is no evidence to suggest it was deliberate, the acoustic properties of hospital spaces and their suitability for hearing Mass celebrated in the chapel may also have been a consideration.

While clearly functional, the spaces of the wards were also decorated. A fresco frieze of scenes from the lives of Sixtus and Innocent III accompanied by texts adorn the walls high up under the windows, while lower down, there are niches containing sculptures and relief carvings of the papal insignia and heraldic imagery. The frescoes alone were a massive undertaking, comprising around 1,200m^2 of art work, completed by a team of artists.[40]

In 1527, about fifty years after the complex of the hospital and surrounding buildings were completed, both the church and the hospital suffered fire damage during the Sack of Rome. The roof of the hospital was repaired but the church had to be rebuilt. Under Paul III (r. 1534–1549) who once again wanted to use the prominence of the Hospital as a signal of papal power and intent, the new church building was designed and constructed by Antonio Sangallo the younger. Sangallo designed the church with a single nave and shallow

---

architectural inscriptions. Carla Keyvanian, 'Paduan Humanism in Sistine Rome: The Hospital of Santo Spirito in Sassia', unpublished conference paper, *Early Modern Rome IV*, Rome, 11–13 November 2021. Fra Giocondo had made extensive corrections to the first printed edition of Vitruvius's *Ten books on Architecture* that appeared in 1486, resulting in a new illustrated edition being printed in Venice in 1511. Ingrid D. Rowland, 'Vitruvius and his influence', in Roger B. Ulrich and Caroline K. Quenemoen (eds), *A Companion to Roman Architecture* (Oxford, 2014), pp. 412–425.

38 Lynn T. Courtnenay, 'The Hospital of Notre Dame de Fontanilles at Tonnerre: Medicine as *Misericordia*', in Barbara S. Bowers (ed), *The Medieval Hospital and Medical Practice* (Aldershot, 2007), pp. 77–106. The hospital of Notre Dame de Fontanilles has a similarly high ceiling (9m) and length (80m) and includes a canal and ditch system to provide fresh water, fed by the Fontanilles spring. The Ospedale Maggiore in Milan has an underground canal system for fresh water.

39 Peregrine Horden, 'A Non-natural Environment: Medicine Without Doctors and the Medieval European Hospital', in Bowers, *The Medieval Hospital and Medical Practice*, pp. 133–145.

40 For detailed study of the history, style and narratives of the frescoes, see Howe, *Art and Culture at the Sistine Court*; and Diana Bullen Presciutti, 'Dead Infants, Cruel Mothers and Heroic Popes: The Visual Rhetoric of Foundling Care at the Hospital of Santo Spirito Rome', *Renaissance Quarterly*, 64:3 (2011), 752–799.

side chapels: a style of church previously used for Orders and Confraternities as well as places of secular power. The façade too used an older style design, and was created from stucco and travertine that were cheaper alternatives to marble, in keeping with Paul III's attempts to create monuments that conveyed his attempts at economy.[41] The church was complete by 1548, and a new organ installed. The organ will be discussed in Chapter 6.

Evidence that the buildings needed further attention is found in Bernadino da Cirillo's account of the state of the institution written in 1571.[42] He oversaw the final stage of building the palazzo for the commendatore and administrators located between the hospital wards and the church. Further changes were made in the following century to improve the nuns' cloister. Decay over time, and modifications to reflect changing uses mean that the extant buildings, though externally substantially unchanged since the seventeenth century, are not exactly as Cirillo left them.[43] The gardens and monastic cemetery were lost to post-Napoleonic restructuring of the city, the construction of flood defences (1875–1910) and modern road systems in the 1930s. However, sections of the historical complex are still in use as part of a modern hospital that was built alongside the Sistine complex. There has thus been a continuously functioning hospital and church in this location for around eight hundred years. With a bit of historical imagination, one can build a picture of the spaces inhabited by the physicians and musicians who will feature in the later chapters of this book.

The Rule of Santo Spirito and care of the sick

The three popes who instigated the physical edifices of the Hospital of Santo Spirito were also those who shaped the governance of the institution. Although the Rule of the Order of Santo Spirito was apparently conceived by Guido de Montpelier, the earliest surviving copies of it date from the time of Eugene IV, by which date the Order was placed under the jurisdiction of the Augustinian canons regular.[44] The tone of documents outlining the history of the Hospital

41 For in-depth consideration of the architecture and construction of the church, see Louise Smith Bross, 'The Church of Santo Spirito in Sassia: A Study in the Development of Art, Architecture and Patronage in Counter-Reformation Rome' (unpublished PhD thesis, University of Chicago, 1994).

42 Bernadino da Cirillo, *Relatione della Fabrica e Casa di S. Spirito di Roma*, 1571. V-CVbav Ottob. Lat. 2473, ff. 179–204.

43 An extension of the ward towards the river was added in the eighteenth century, but subsequently removed and the façade rebuilt. Botticelli's painting in the Sistine chapel was used as a point of reference in the reconstruction process.

44 The earliest copy is located in the Biblioteca Vaticana, Fondo Borghese, Ms 292. A second later copy is held in the Archivio di Stato di Roma, ASR OSS 3193. This later copy includes an array of painted miniatures providing visual evidence of the life of

and the Order is often one of uncritical awe and reverence. For example, in his retelling of Saulnier's history, Dragondelli praises the Rule, describing its aim as one of perfect charity.[45] After comparing Guy de Montpellier to Moses, he goes on to cite the passage from the Gospel of Matthew that impelled the foundation of the Hospital as a Christian duty and which is cited at the start of the Rule: 'My God! How efficacious is this beginning, how powerful, certainly it is a firm foundation! With merit did St Basil say in his meditation on the final judgement that it is the pedagogy of mercy.'[46]

It is pertinent that Dragondelli indicates that the Rule retained what is good about other Rules, such as the habits and attitudes of the Rule of Augustine, but was adapted to work for different locations, conditions and dispositions of people who could embrace it.[47] He is clear to point out though, that from the time of Eugene IV, the Order had only one Rule and that was its own, although it was under the protection of the Augustinians.[48]

While mediaeval in origin, much of the Rule of the Order of Santo Spirito was not out of place in post-Tridentine Church politics. Misericordia, the seven acts of mercy described in Matthew chapter 25, was the driving force behind all charitable confraternities, though most focused on only one or two of them, such as ministering to prisoners or burying the dead.[49] Charitable care of the sick, orphans and widows was deemed a characteristic of the virtuous ruler, and had been since antiquity. For the Christian ruler, it was a necessity impelled by the Biblical model of Christ Jesus. Dragondelli's rhetoric presents the Rule of Santo Spirito and the charity it promotes as heroic. He devotes chapters of his book to elucidating the Misericordia as equivalent to sacrifice and martyrdom, as comparable to the sacraments, and to the theological virtues of prudence and justice. Misericordia is itself an act of prayer, and the gate of paradise.

---

the community. Available online http://www.cflr.beniculturali.it/Preziosi/preziosi.php?lar=1600&alt=900.

45 Dragondelli, *Trattato del sacro ordine di S. Spirito detto in Sassia ... del rev. Fra Pietro Saunier* (Rome, 1662), p. 32.

46 'Dio mio! Quante efficace e' questo innito, quanto possente, certo, e' fermo quel fondamento! Meritatemente dice San Basilio che la meditatione del giuditio finale, e' il pedagogo della pieta': Dragondelli, *Trattato*, p. 174.

47 Dragondelli, *Trattato*, p. 33.

48 'L'Ordine di S. Spirito fino del tempo di Papa Eugenio quarto è così più di 230 anni doppo la sua fondazione non haveva altra regola che la sua propria, senza trovarsi alcun' indizio della Regola di S. Agostino nell' ordine di S. Spirito': Dragondelli, *Trattato*, p. 38. Dragondelli may have been drawing on Borguarucci's 1623 account which uses almost exactly the same phrase. Domenico Borgarucci, *Relatione del modo; che si tiene da religione di S. Spirito nel governo dell'archihospitale apostolico di Santo Spirito in Sassia di Roma* (1623). GB-Lwl EPB 46633/B.

49 Black gives examples of different types of statutes based on the Misericordia. Black, *Italian Confraternities*, p. 63.

One might assume that as the Hospital Order of Santo Spirito was founded with the purpose of caring for the sick, the care of patients would feature as part of the Rule of the Order. This is of course the case. However, care of the sick is not the primary instruction, but might be interpreted as one that emerges from the commitment to charity and obedience. The first directive of the Rule is virtually identical to that of the Rule of Augustine, that no one dare call anything his own. All will have what they need, but possess everything in common, living in harmony with the community just as the disciples of Jesus were instructed.[50]

On receiving a patient at the hospital, the first duty of the carers was to see that they were attended by a priest. The patient was required to confess their sins and to reverently take Communion before being put to bed. The carers too were under strict instructions with regard to their behaviour towards the sick. A variety of instructions outline the charitable demeanour expected of a member of the Order and the dignity with which the sick and the poor should be treated. Daily observation of the Divine Offices and Mass were built into the routine and carers and patients alike were expected to participate. The priests were under orders to take Communion to the patients in their beds and instruction in Christian doctrine for the patients was of primary importance.[51]

Attention to the sacraments was a requirement, and in dealing with the sick, a form of celestial medicine. On this issue, Porterfield argues along the same lines as Kuhn that there was no real 'scientific revolution' but that the period of Christian reform in the late sixteenth and early seventeenth century, and shifts in medicine, were interrelated. Protestant reform turned the Christian to an internal, individualised relationship with God and away from the social, communal worship of saints and sacraments. As a result, Protestants turned away from charitable care of the sick and poor, while Catholic areas continued their support of hospitals as a means of enacting their devotion to Christ, ensuring the public devotion to human suffering continued as part of Catholic life.[52]

During this period, the fluid relationship between miracle and medicine apparent in medieval times continued and was as confused as the state of religion. The famous condemnations of Galileo and Bruno in the late sixteenth and early seventeenth centuries gave rise to the notion that the post-Tridentine Catholic Church sought to suppress science and medicine, particularly in Rome. However, the Vatican's relationships with the university, 'La Sapienza'; with scientific academies; as well as with its own communities with scientific interests such as the Jesuit Collegio Romano, have only comparatively recently

50 De Angelis, *L'Ospedale di S. Spirito dalle origini al 1500*, vol. 1, p. 247.

51 Regola VIII, cited in De Angelis, *L'Ospedale di S. Spirito dalle origini al 1500*, vol. 1, pp. 248–249. These rules are not dissimilar to the opening instructions to members of the Hospitaller Order of St John of Jerusalem. *Statuta ordinis domus hospitalis Hierusalem* (Rome, 1586).

52 Porterfield, *Healing in the History of Christianity*, p. 110.

been scrutinised, and we are a long way from really understanding the nuances of such interactions.[53] The Hospital of Santo Spirito is one such institution where the physicians were at the forefront of teaching medicine in the form of surgery and anatomy, but at the same time, the organisation was fundamentally tied to the Church through papal patronage.

The hunger for truth, order and clarity, and the quest for authenticity in religion and objectivity in science, co-existed.[54] Any assumption that prior to around 1900 hospitals were places that only offered nursing care and spiritual or moral support rather than supervised medical care, need to be set aside. The Hospital of Santo Spirito perhaps captures this paradox of inward introspection in terms of its religious practices and outward exploration of emerging scientific medicine. The lifestyle, philosophy and aesthetic of its governing Rule and the practices of the physicians within its walls reflect the confusing, interweaving polyphony of ideas of its time. It is to these interweaving strands that we now turn.

53 Maria Pia Donato and Jill Kraye (eds), *Conflicting Duties: Science, Medicine and Religion in Rome 1550–1750* (London and Turin, 2009), pp. 2–4.

54 Porterfield, *Healing in the History of Christianity*, pp. 114–116.

2

Music and Medicine in the Early Modern World

Little is known of the specific activities of the physicians at the Hospital of Santo Spirito. The administration of the Hospital was left in the hands of the Hospital Order of Santo Spirito and overseen by a man appointed by the pope for his administrative and religious capacities, not his medical knowledge. There are records of inspections of the dispensary, lists of the contents and costs of various ingredients for medicines and more general discussions of diet and cleanliness, but nothing has come to light that pertains to specific cases, treatments, or patient experiences.[1] This chapter outlines some of the concepts about health and the body that would have been shared by physicians, priests and musicians alike, and that are foundational to the investigations and analyses that follow.

During the period under consideration, there were four physicians employed in the hospital at any one time. These men were university-educated and therefore had a background in logic and natural philosophy as well as the medical theories of Hippocrates, Galen and Ibn Sina, known in the West as Avicenna. They worked alongside a team of barber-surgeons, lithotomists and apothecaries – occupations that were less strictly licensed. The nursing was done by friars of the Order and lay members of the Confraternity. While many eminent physicians were employed at the hospital, it must be remembered that treatment of the soul of the patient was a fundamental part of the regime of cure of the sick. Doctors worked alongside priests and chaplains and were expected to be good Christians. Whatever the scientific view of illness, and in the seventeenth century scientific views were shifting rapidly with each new discovery, prayer for the sick remained of fundamental importance, along with confession and the sacraments. This close relationship between religion and medicine became increasingly complex with growing anatomical knowledge and the shifting paradigms of the so-called 'scientific revolution'. Some of these complexities are illustrated by the processes for the beatification and canonisation of saints during which physicians were called upon to make judgements about apparent miracle cures.[2]

1 ASR-OSS 47, Virgilio Spada, *Stato della Casa dell'Archiospedale di S. Spirito di Roma l'anno 1661*, chapters 10–11; OSS 901, *Sacra visita, Atti diversi relazione 1592–1734*; OSS 78, *Congregationi: verbali delle deliberazioni 1644–1688*, etc.

2 This process was under scrutiny during and after the pontificate of Urban VIII (r. 1623–1644), but was put on a more 'scientific' footing by Benedict XIV. See Rebecca

While we have little or no evidence of the physicians' specific work in the hospital, many of the men employed there also held other positions: teaching at the university; as personal physicians to members of the aristocracy and high-ranking prelates; and in private medical practice. A number of them including Giulio Mancini (1559–1630) and Giovanni Maria Lancisi (1654–1720) became the private physician to the incumbent pope. Lancisi was in fact physician to three successive popes, Innocent XI, Clement XI and Innocent XII and worked closely with Cardinal Prospero Lambertini who was to become Pope Benedict XIV. Another, Paulo Zacchia (1584–1659) who wrote copiously, acted as an expert witness in legal cases, advising on such issues as primogeniture, paternity, mental disability, times and causes of death and so on, while Johann (Giovanni) Faber (1574–1629) was a consultant to the Congregation of the Index, making decisions about the potentially heretical nature of new medical books.[3]

The academic credentials of many physicians may have depended on books they wrote and had printed, but the everyday work of many of these men involved writing consilia, letters of consultation and exchanging observations with networks of colleagues.[4] The manuscript writings of Mancini are of considerable importance to this study, as he operated within a wide network of artists and musicians as well as the scientific community and the Vatican. Zacchia, though now regarded as the father of legal medicine on the basis of his published observations, also wrote a treatise in the vernacular on following a healthy diet during Lent and one on hypochondriac illness.[5] We can perhaps infer that his experience at the Hospital informed his views, especially regarding diet and religious observance as he would have had direct contact with the friars of the Order and perhaps also the enclosed women.

For all of the doctors at the hospital, we have to assume that their medical practice was based on the body of received knowledge transmitted during their studies, much of which still relied on ancient sources, generally written in

---

Messbarger, Christopher Johns and Philip Gavitt (eds), *Benedict XIV and the Enlightenment: Art, Science, and Spirituality* (Toronto, 2016).

3 Faber was also a professor of botany at La Sapienza and Curator of the Vatican botanic garden. He was asked by the Congregation of the Index to investigate and review Paracelsan books. Lyke de Vries & Leen Spruit, 'Paracelsus and Roman Censorship – Johannes Faber's 1616 Report in Context', *Intellectual History Review*, 28:2 (2018), 225–254. As a member of the Accademia dei Lincei, he was part of an intellectual network that included musicians.

4 Silvia de Renzi, 'A Career in Manuscripts: Genres and Purposes of a Physician's Writing in Rome, 1600–1630', *Italian Studies*, 66:2 (2011), 234–248.

5 Zacchia, *Il vitto quaresimale del Signor Paulo Zacchia* (Rome, 1655). Zacchia's Quaestiones medico-legales were published in numerous instalments from 1621. The first complete edition was published in 1661. Jacalyn Duffin, 'Questioning Medicine in Seventeenth-century Rome: The Consultations of Paulo Zacchia', *Canadian Bulletin of Medical History*, 28:1 (2011), 149–170.

Latin; and also that it would have related closely to printed advice about health and wellbeing found in health regimens aimed at ordinary people. Both academic learning and vernacular healthcare regimes drew on primary sources of medical knowledge dating back to pre-Christian and early Christian times in the shape of the Hippocratic writings and those of Galen of Pergamon (born 131 AD). Hippocratic-Galenic medicine was founded on a cosmology structured according to harmonic ratios and relied almost entirely on the understanding that the body and its healthy functioning depended on the correct balance of the humours. It is therefore also known as humoral medicine, and it remained central to the education and practice of physicians despite the rise of new anatomical investigations, for example by Vesalius.[6]

Humoral medicine

The theory of the humours was first laid out in a treatise, *The nature of man*, written by Polybus, a disciple of Hippocrates. The four natural humours, blood, phlegm, yellow bile and black bile, were the elements that governed the human body. Each of the humours was associated with combinations of two pairs of qualities – warm and cold and moist and dry. Thus, blood was warm and moist; yellow bile, warm and dry; black bile, cold and dry; and phlegm, cold and moist. Each humour was also associated with one of the four elements (air, fire, earth and water) and the four seasons which in turn were, from the Pythagoreans onwards, matched to the four ages of man: boyhood, youth, manhood and old age (see Figure 2.1). As well as regulating health, the humours also determined the temperament or personality of the individual.[7]

Although they were not visible, the humours were all based on visible substances such as blood, except black bile which represented a 'real composite of the human psyche'.[8] The physiological and psychological theory of the humours was based on assumption that consciousness was located within the viscera and that passions were formed in the spleen, liver, gall bladder and heart. The

[6] The transmission of ancient medical texts and of the rediscovery of Greek Galenic texts in the fifteenth century was complex and multi-faceted. See Richard J. Durling, 'A Chronological Census of Renaissance Editions and Translations of Galen', *Journal of the Warburg and Courtauld Institutes*, 24:3/4 (1961), 230–305; Donald F. Jackson, 'Greek Medicine in the Fifteenth Century', *Early Science and Medicine*, 17:4 (2012), 378–390.

[7] For Pythagoras as an early source on music therapy, see Martin West, 'Music Therapy in Antiquity', in Peregrine Horden (ed.), *Music as Medicine: The History of Music Therapy Since Antiquity* (Aldershot, 2000), pp. 54–56. For an overview of early modern humoral medicine see Nancy Siraisi, *Medieval and Early Renaissance Medicine: An Introduction to Knowledge and Practice* (Chicago, 1990).

[8] Noga Arikha, *Passions and Tempers: A History of the Humours* (New York and London, 2007), pp. 7–9.

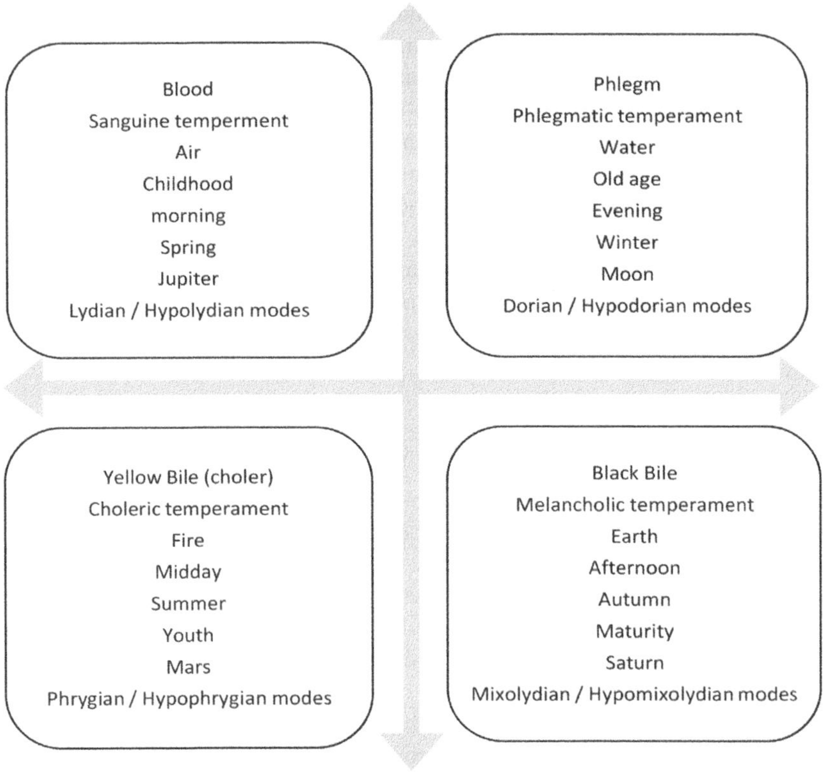

Figure 2.1 The humours and their associations.

passions were literally organic events – actions of the body that turned the soul inside-out – and listening to music was a visceral, bodily experience.[9]

After the fall of the Roman empire, ancient medical texts in the Hippocratic-Galenic tradition were preserved in the Near East and transmitted back to the West through Islamic sources. By the sixteenth century various compendia of Hippocratic-Galenic texts were available. Among the most popular was Galen's book on hygiene, *De sanitate tuende*, which was printed many times during the sixteenth century.[10]

Alongside the humours, which were defined as one of the naturals, or innate factors unique to the individual that governed the health and good function-

[9] Bettina Varwig, *Music in the Flesh: An Early Modern Musical Physiology* (Chicago, 2023) provides extensive documentation of the bodily experience of music, though largely from northern Europe.

[10] For a full list of printed editions of Galen's works, see Durling, 'A Chronological Census'.

ing of the body, were the non-naturals, or external factors that affected health. These would ultimately develop into the physical and psychological hygiene of more modern times. The non-naturals were air, exercise and rest, sleep and wakefulness, food and drink, excretion and retention and the passions or perturbations of the soul. Attention to the non-naturals was important in medical texts until well into the eighteenth century.

The management of the non-naturals to maintain health or to treat disease was, for centuries, the physician's main job. A fourth century Hippocratic text, *On airs, waters and places*, lays out the belief that the environment affected the humours and therefore the health of man. Further, Galen noted that a bad environment included the words and music that one listens to, and that a healer must understand these effects.[11] Horden has even argued that the physical structure of early hospital buildings should be considered a non-natural environment designed to maximise good air, water and wherever possible, geographical location.[12]

It is the passions or perturbations of the soul with which this study is most concerned. The term 'passion' and the related terms 'emotion', 'affect' and 'feeling' need some scrutiny in order to reimagine the framework of what today we would call the psychology of emotions. The regulation of the passions is the basis upon which music is drawn into both physical and spiritual healthcare, thus the depth and breadth of their application, and the ways in which they were controlled, need to be understood.

Passions of the soul

The problem of defining musical emotion has been explored at length by Michael Spitzer.[13] In essence, the word emotion is a modern one, and is derived from the original idea of 'motion towards'. An emotion moves, has a trajectory, but what emotion actually is is itself culturally constructed and, as Burke points out, only relatively recently has that even been acknowledged.[14] A passion on the other hand, was understood as literally passive and caused by something external, but that acted on the body in a visceral way such that the body might

11 West, 'Music Therapy in Antiquity', pp. 62–63.

12 Peregrine Horden, 'A Non-natural Environment: Medicine Without Doctors and the Medieval European Hospital', in Barbara S. Bowers (ed.), *The Medieval Hospital and Medical Practice* (Aldershot, 2007), pp. 133–145. It seems possible that the non-natural environment of the Hospital of Santo Spirito was enhanced by its architectural design which reflected harmonic proportions.

13 Michael Spitzer, *A History of Emotion in Western Music* (Oxford, 2020).

14 Peter Burke, 'Is there a Cultural History of Emotions?', in Penelope Gouk and Helen Hills (eds), *Representing Emotions: New Connections in the Histories of Art, Music and Medicine* (Aldershot, 2005), pp. 35–47.

respond in effects such as tears or smiles. The word 'perturbation' perhaps better describes that meaning. The two words 'passion' and 'emotion' reflect a shift in perception but essentially refer to the same phenomenon.

The way in which we use language to describe feelings or states of mind has also shifted over time. 'Melancholy' today suggests a very different state of mind to the one that Burton had in mind when writing his *Anatomy of Melancholy* first published in 1621, or that to which Playford and D'Urfey's song collection *Pills to Purge Melancholy* (1698) refers. We cannot assume that language used to describe feelings is unchanging. Today D'Urfey's title is more likely to bring to mind anti-depressant tablets than a collection of light-hearted songs and dances. The term 'melancholy', or 'melancholia', as understood at the time of Burton, D'Urfey and Playford, indicated various states of mental health that today would be recognised as ranging from depression to mania, though it could also simply mean crazy or nervous conduct. In the seventeenth century it was a common disease, with authors of medical treatises such as Melanchthon, Burton, Mercuriale, Chiodini and Du Laurens all remarking on the large number of cases of melancholia they had witnessed or treated.[15] The treatments they describe were all remarkably similar – diet and warm baths; purging induced by various medications or by bloodletting; and addressing the mental state of the patient through distracting conversation, exercise and music. The importance of music as an effective curative is noted by a number of English and Italian treatises.[16] Burton for example states that music is 'a roaring meg against melancholy to rear and revive the languishing soul', while Girolamo Cardano was a little more circumspect, noting that specific types of music were able to 'lighten the cares resulting from the misery of human misfortune', but that music generally afforded 'pleasure without detriment' and was 'beneficial to all'.[17]

15 There are some striking parallels between the 'epidemic' of melancholy in the seventeenth century – a period dominated by war and plague – and the spike in mental health problems in the post-Covid, modern world.

16 Stanley W. Jackson, *Melancholia and Depression: From Hippocratic Times to Modern Times* (New Haven, CT and London, 1986); Angus Gowland, 'The Problem of Early Modern Melancholy', *Past & Present*, 191 (2006), 77–120. Jackson and Gowland discuss many treatises including: Thomas Elyot, *The Castel of Helthe* (1530); Andrew Boorde, *The breviary of Helthe (*1547); Timothie Bright, *A Treatise of Melancholy* (1586); André Du Laurens, *A Discourse of the Preservation of Sight: of Melancholike Diseases, of Rheumes and of Old Age* (1599), trans. Richard Surphlet (London: 1599, STC 7304); Julius Caesar Claudinus (Chiodini), *Responsiones et consultationes medicinales* (1607), consultatio no 98.

17 Robert Burton, *Anatomy of Melancholy*, ed. Holbrook Jackson (New York, 2001), p. 115. A 'roaring meg' is a reference to a large cannon or other military ordnance. https://www.lexico.com/en/definition/roaring_meg; Girolamo Cardano, *De Subtilitate*, trans. Clement A. Miller; *Hieronymus Cardanus (1501–1576) Writings on Music* (n.p. 1973), pp. 198, 204.

Other related words have also changed meaning. Around the turn of the seventeenth century, discourse about music is full of references to its power to move the 'affetti'. The emotional impact of the 'new' music – monody and the recitational styles of the *dramma per musica* – is what separates it from the older styles. The term 'affetto' cannot be translated directly as 'affect' as its implications are different from the modern use of the word, which assumes a more representational form and distances emotion from any kind of transcendence.[18] The first edition of the *Vocabolario della Crusca* (1612) defines 'affetto' as 'passion of the soul, born of the desire for good and hatred of evil'.[19] This definition remains unchanged throughout the seventeenth century and implies emotional impact as having a spiritual or moral dimension.

To be healthy, the passions needed to be regulated, but different opinions as to the nature of the passions meant that there were diverse, often conflicting views as to how they should be controlled, and these opinions drew on prevailing medical and religious thinking. The Galenic view was that the passions were caused by material physiology rather than the intellect or reason. In contrast, the opinion based on Aristotle, Augustine and Aquinas posited that the passions were rebellious movements of the soul, reflecting conflict between the intellective and animal parts of the soul. A third stance was adopted by the Christian Stoic view that held that all passions were to be calmed through willpower in the quest for peace of mind. Faith and devotional practice were key to achieving comfort and acceptance. The emergence of the medieval Christian moral code of the seven deadly sins, all of which are also passions, invoked an even deeper connection between the passions (as sins) and morality.[20]

The importance of the passions to healthcare is reflected in a train of thought among physicians that psychological turmoil could cause illness and even death, derived from Galen's statements that 'every year we have cured a number of the sick, who have regained their health by no other means than the movement of their souls'.[21] This notion of sickness as somatic can be traced back to antiquity, but by the seventeenth century the role of the imagination, emotional upsets and the mental state more generally on physical health was implicitly understood in a number of contexts, but particularly in relation to the plague.[22] Various physicians advocated a holistic approach to

18 Spitzer, *A History of Emotion*, pp. 329–333.

19 'passione d'animo, nata dal disiderio del bene, e dall'odio del male': *Vocabolario della Crusca* (1612), qv. Affetto http://www.lessicografia.it/ (accessed 08/09/2021).

20 Stephen Gaukroger (ed.), *The Soft Underbelly of Reason: The Passions in the Seventeenth Century* (Abingdon, [1998] 2014), pp. 2–6.

21 Galen cited in Sheila Barker, 'Poussin, Plague, and Early Modern Medicine', *Art Bulletin*, 86:4 (2004), 659–689.

22 Burton devoted a whole chapter to the force of imagination, citing as an example the case of a man who died from fear under the mistaken assumption he had come into contact with someone suffering from the plague. Burton (ed. Jackson), *Anatomy of Melancholy*, p. 256.

healthcare advising that one should occupy oneself and keep the mind happy to avoid illness.[23]

The notion that holding terrible images in thought was deemed extremely dangerous to health was of particular significance to both Paracelsus, who spearheaded the move to chemical treatment of disease, and to Ficino. Although Paracelsian ideas were not widely circulated, they were certainly known by Johann Faber. Another strong advocate for the power of images on the body was Giulio Mancini. For him, the contemplation of art was a prophylactic and a restorative activity. These ideas of somatic illness and the role of art, music and literature in their cure, were deeply held and continued to influence artistic activities at least through the first half of the early seventeenth century. Even Kircher, that polymath whose musical exploits need little introduction, wrote a chapter discussing the question of the imagination in the onset of plague. Given that Kircher was also fascinated by tarantism – the use of music and dance to treat the bite of tarantula spiders – it is hardly surprising that he devoted his energies to this point, too. Modern studies have suggested that tarantism is entirely psychosomatic, which does raise some interesting questions as to whether these physicians may have had some insights into the psychological nature of illness that are only now being scientifically explored.[24]

Early modern music therapy

The passions of the soul, however they were theorised, and the power of music as an agent of change acting on them, are fundamental to understanding medical views of the health benefits of music. Belief in the therapeutic value of music has a long history reaching back into antiquity, the principles of which were transmitted to the medieval world by Boethius.[25] In the early modern period,

23 This idea was already current in the fourteenth century as evidenced by the protagonists in Boccaccio's *Decameron* who keep themselves occupied with music, dancing and storytelling; and advice from physicians such as, 'Do not occupy your mind with death, passion or with anything likely to sadden or grieve you, but give your thoughts over to delightful and pleasing things... And make use of songs and minstrelsy and other pleasurable tales without tiring yourselves out, and all the delightful things that bring anyone comfort'. Tomaso del Garbo, *Consiglio contro la pistolenza*, pp. 40–41, cited in Remi Chiu, *Plague and Music in the Renaissance* (Cambridge, 2017), p. 16. Pope Urban VIII even took part in occult rites, in which music may have been a part, during the plague outbreak of 1630. Peter Rietbergen, 'Urban VIII between White Magic and Black Magic, or: Holy and Unholy Power', in *Power and Religion in Baroque Rome: Barberini Cultural Policies* (Leiden, 2006), pp. 336–376.

24 Ernesto de Martino, *La terra del rimorso* (Milan, [1961] 2015); Jerry Daboo, *Ritual, Rapture and Remorse: A Study of Tarantism and 'Pizzica' in Salento* (Bern, 2010); Daniele Rota, *I Gesuiti e le tarantole* (Lucca, 2012).

25 Various aspects of the history of music therapy in the ancient world are discussed in: West, 'Music Therapy in Antiquity'; M. L. West, *Ancient Greek Music* (Oxford, 1992), pp. 246–253.

the efficacy of music as an important part of healthcare was widely understood across all levels of society. It is evident in the writings of learned physicians operating in academic networks, intellectual virtuosi circulating in aristocratic milieux as well as in popular health regimens used by the middle and lower classes. When Grazio Uberti described the sounds of music reaching a man lying in bed in pain and soothing him, or the sweet strains of music purging the tense atmosphere of a domestic row, he was articulating notions accepted as fact.[26]

One of the most widely disseminated vernacular books on maintaining health, *Il Tesoro della sanità* (1586) by the Roman doctor Castore Durante, included music and song as a way to achieve a healthy life through the happiness or *allegrezza* that it engendered.[27] Around a century earlier, Ficino had stressed the importance of delighting, comforting, fortifying and refreshing the spirits by delighting the senses, recommending music as one method for creating *allegrezza*. By the mid-seventeenth century, *allegrezza* was one of the most important elements of healthcare especially for those who wanted to care for their own health without recourse to a doctor.[28] A happy disposition was the foundation of good health, and the various means of maintaining happiness thus key preventive strategies. In the dedication to his *Arie devote* of 1608, Castore Durante's son, Ottavio, refers to his father's service in the Peretti household and the delight in which the dedicatee (now Cardinal Montalto), delighted in 'affective music'. Several of his instructions to the performer require the correct understanding of the affects in order for them to be embellished correctly and beautifully.[29]

26 'Ne mi sa difficile il credere questo, perché se ne vede l'esperienza trovasi un povero padre di famiglia in letto, pieno di travaglio; occorre, che si fa nel vicinato una bella serenata. Egli l'ode, è pur vero, che come tarantolato si consola al suono. Aviene in tempo notturno, che una famiglia stà sottosopra. Il marito grida con la moglie, un fratello con l'altro. Subito, che si sente una bella serenata, ogn'un corre alle fenestre; ogn'un s'affaccia. Cessano le risse domestiche': Grazio Uberti, *Contrasto musico* (Rome, 1630). Facsimile edition ed. Giancarlo Rostirolla (Lucca, 1991), p. 140.

27 'e sì come la virtù e la forza s'accrescono col cibo, col vino e con buoni odori, con tranquillità e allegrezza, e col lasciare le cose che attristano, e col conversar con gli amici; cosi parimenti conferisce ascoltare istorie grate, favole e ragionamenti piacevoli, con suoni e canti, e con dilettevoli lezione…': Castore Durante, *Il Tesoro della Sanità* (Rome, 1586) ed. Elena Camillo (Milan, 1982), p. 38.

28 Sandra Cavallo and Tessa Storey, *Healthy Living in Late Renaissance Italy* (Oxford, 2013), pp. 194–195.

29 'Sapendo quante diletto si prenda di diversa Virtù, e particolarmente della musica affettuoso, come ne fa chiaro testimonio il copioso numero de Virtuosi che tiene al suo servizio…' 'Knowing how much you delight in diverse virtues and particularly in affective music, as testified by the numerous virtuosi you hold in service …': Ottavio Durante, *Arie Devote* (Rome, 1608). For a full text of the preface see Jeffrey Kurtzman and Anne Schnoebelen, 'A Catalogue of Mass, Office and Holy Week Music Printed in Italy 1516–1770', *JSCM Instrumenta*, 2, 2014 (online).

For the illiterate, music was also the means of conveying medical knowledge in the form of broadsides sung and sold by the *cantastorie* and pedlars in urban marketplaces and piazzas.[30] The widespread acceptance of the beneficial power of music betrays its centuries-old roots in pre-Christian antiquity. If early modern writers needed a source to support their claim for music's efficacy, they had plenty to choose from, both in ancient Greek writings and, if a religious spin were needed, in the Judaic-Christian sources from the ancient Near East, some of which were incorporated in the Old Testament of the Bible.

With the rediscovery of Plato in the fifteenth century, thinkers tried to reconcile the ancient metaphysical philosophy, on which elements of medical understanding depended, with Christian doctrine. The resulting complex ebb and flow of ideas makes it difficult to separate the purely medical from the religious; and the speculative and philosophical from practice. Within this web, concepts of a music therapy, broadly conceived, follow two distinct but related paths: the astrological, drawing on Pythagorean and Platonic cosmology in which all the components of the universe are related to each other in harmonic proportions; and the ethical, based on Platonic and Aristotelian notions regarding the emotional content of music and its power to control mind and body, such as in *katharsis* for example.[31] Both try to explain in some way the transcendent qualities of music, drawing on and expanding ideas that reach back to antiquity. Music, because of its nature as something that was physically perceived, yet not tangible, was able to touch both body and soul, hence its potency. *Musica humana* was simply an echo of the far greater *musica mundana* of the cosmos.

From a music theoretical point of view, music's power lay in the ethical qualities encoded within it. The concept of musical ethos was well defined in ancient Greek music and is outlined in some detail in ancient texts on music theory. In music theoretical writings, musical ethos is inextricably linked to mode.[32]

30 Storey has identified broadside ballads that convey medical information about common ailments and universal conditions requiring care, such as pregnancy. Tessa Storey, '*La villanella della gravidanza:* Singing Medical Knowledge in Early Modern Rome', unpublished conference paper, *Early Modern Rome 4* (Rome: November 11–13, 2021).

31 Key passages describing the cosmos are in Plato, *Timaeus*, ed. and trans. Desmond Lee and Thomas Kjeller Johansen, 31a–37c, 47d–e, 87c–90d (London, 1965), pp. 21–22, 24–26, 38, 85–89. The use of music by legislators to control the population is described in *The Republic* 398c–402d, Plato, *Republic*, trans. Robin Waterfield (Oxford, 1994), pp. 95–101. For an extensive discussion of the relationship of music to both body and soul as it is discussed across Plato's writings, see Francesco Pelosi, *Plato on Music, Soul and Body*, trans. Sophie Henderson (Cambridge, 2010), esp. pp. 69–73; Jean Lombard, *Platone e la Medicina*, trans. M. A. Raggi ([Paris, 1999] Forlì, 2016); for *katharsis* see Aristotle, *Politics*, 1339a11–1342b34, cited in Andrew Barker, *Greek Musical Writings* (Cambridge, 1989) vol. I, p. 180.

32 It is beyond the scope of this book to discuss the complexities of Greek music theory. For detail and extracts see Barker, *Greek Musical Writings*; Thomas Matthieson, *Apollo's*

As noted in Figure 2.1, the modes in turn were associated with humours, temperaments and the cosmos. As these theoretical texts were rediscovered in the early modern period, notions of mode, and the ethos embedded within them, became a point of reference for music theory texts and, subsequently, critical evaluations of music, including those written by non-musicians, such as Bernardino da Cirillo, a sixteenth-century commendatore of the Hospital of Santo Spirito who is the focus of Chapter 4.

Ficino

One of the key transmitters of Platonic thought in the early modern period was the philosopher and physician Marsilio Ficino (1433–1499). In his various commentaries, especially those on Plato's *Timaeus* and the *Enneads* of Plotinus and in his own *Three books on life* (*De vita libri tres*), Ficino conveys a complex philosophy in which he tries to align Platonic philosophy with Christian doctrine. He follows Plato's crucial idea of music as able to reduce discordant conditions to concord, and with it, to draw the soul into union with the One, or the Good. In aligning his philosophy with Christian doctrine, he draws on Augustine, who had grappled with the Platonic notion of ascent to the divine.[33]

The final section of his commentary on Plato's *Symposium, Sopra lo amore* describes the four frenzies through which the soul ascends to union with God, the first of which is the poetic frenzy: 'its musical tones will arouse the parts that sleep; its harmonious sweetness will soothe the parts that are agitated; and lastly, its harmonization of divergent elements will drive out dissonant discord and temper the various parts of the Soul.'[34]

The notion of music as a form of medicine as well as a form of prayer informs much of Ficino's writing. His letters contain some of the most concise expressions of his thought. On the connection of music, medicine and theology he wrote:

> Do not be surprised, Francesco, that we combine medicine and the lyre with the study of theology. Since you are dedicated to philosophy, you must remember that within us nature has bonded body and spirit with the soul. The body is indeed healed by the remedies of medicine; but spirit, which is the airy vapour of our blood and the link between body and soul, is tempered

Lyre: Greek Music and Music Theory in Antiquity and the Middle Ages (Lincoln, NE and London, 1999).

33 Marsilio Ficino, *Commentary on Plotinus: vol 5 Ennead III, part 2 and Ennead IV*, ed. Stephen Gersh, I Tatti Renaissance Library (Cambridge, MA and London, 2018), pp. 216–218. In *City of God*, Augustine commented on the ancient Platonist rituals of 'theurgy', that is, rituals involving symbolic objects, prayers, chants, lights and thurification to channel the divine power to the officiant and participants.

34 Marsilio Ficino, *On the Nature of Love: Ficino on Plato's 'Symposium'*, trans. Arthur Farndell (London, 2016), p. 154.

> and nourished by airy smells, by sounds and by song. Finally, the soul, as it is divine, is purified by the divine mysteries of theology.[35]

A further letter to Antonio Canigiani develops the theme of music as a means of nourishing and changing the soul, drawing on a compendium of references to classical sources on the power of music, from Pythagoras and the Platonists, through the mythical characters of Orpheus and Amphion, to the biblical King David. However, for all the originality of Ficino's thought, he relates these correspondences to the accepted Galenic framework of medicine:

> For sound and song arise from consideration in the mind, the impulse of fantasy and the desire of the heart, and in disturbing the air and lending measure to it they vibrate the airy spirit of the listener, which is the link between body and soul. Thus, sound and song easily arouse the fantasy, affect the heart and reach inmost recess of the mind; they still, and also set in motion, the humours and the limbs of the body.[36]

Pulse, rhythm and proportional movement

Ficino the physician, like all doctors, had to rely on his own senses as diagnostic tools – looking at, listening to, touching and smelling the bodies and bodily fluids of his patients. Images of physicians, as exemplified by illustrations in the Statutes of the Hospital Order of St John, often capture the centrality of the senses in making diagnoses.[37] In Galenic medicine, the patient's pulse was a crucial element of diagnosis and a physician was required to develop acute sensitivity to minute deviations in pulse. Pulse was described as dense, low, light and so on. A faster or more forceful pulse indicated fever, seen as an increase in internal heat associated with the element of fire, while a slower pulse resulted as fever abated or was a symptom of some other ailment. Beyond simple awareness of the speed of the pulse, there was a long tradition that held that pulse was musical and contained within it harmonic proportions, although the proportions identified by Galen are not in themselves musical (5:2, 7:2, 9:2 etc.). The belief was transmitted from ancient medical sources via Islamic medical writers, notably Avicenna, and by Boethius, whose books were standard texts in the Latin schools of the Middle Ages.[38]

35 Ficino to Francesco Musano of Iesi, *The Letters of Marsilio Ficino, vol 1*. Translated from the Latin by members of the Language department of the School of Economic Science, London (London, 1975), pp. 39–40 (letter 5).

36 *The Letters of Marsilio Ficino, vol 1*, p. 142 (letter 92).

37 *Statuta ordinis domus hospitalis Hierusalem* (Rome, 1556), p. 30.

38 For transmission of ancient musical texts to the Renaissance and beyond, see Claude V. Palisca, *Humanism in Italian Renaissance Musical Thought* (New Haven, CT and London, 1985) and *Studies in the History of Italian Music and Music Theory* (Oxford, 1994). Among the most influential scholars who adopted the idea of a music of pulse

The idea of actually measuring proportion in the pulse in medieval medical texts derives primarily from sources written in Arabic, especially Avicenna. These describe ten genera for categorising pulse, with a number of different conditions that might cause them.[39] By the fourteenth and fifteenth centuries, medical concepts of the music of pulse appear in numerous Italian texts and were widely accepted.[40] The belief that consonance and harmonic proportions were inherent in pulse that was part of Ficino's ethical-astrological concept of music as therapy is thus not as eccentric as it might appear, but was a refinement of a long tradition. Indeed, even as late as 1829, René Laennec described heartbeats heard through his stethoscope in musical terms.[41] For Ficino, musical pulses were to be 'well-tempered' and music was the ideal corrective to 'temper' a pulse that was too fast or too slow.[42] Ficino attempted to identify specific numeric proportions in a healthy pulse and outlines them as 2:1, 3:2 and 4:3. Ficino related these to the density of the blood and the proportions of the humours within it, thus the correct proportions of blood to phlegm 2:1, of blood to yellow or red bile 1:4 and blood to black bile 1:8.[43]

Pulse was also not an exclusively medical issue. Augustine's treatise on music is almost entirely preoccupied with proportion and measure in the correct chanting or recitation of text. For Augustine the rhythms of pulse and breathing were operations of the soul, and number and proportion are inherent in the soul.[44] Cassiodorus too saw pulse associated with rhythm as evidence of the power of harmony. Correct singing of chant would have expressed correct rhythmic proportions and aligned the one singing with the spiritual – a concept closely related to the pre-Christian notion of alignment with the proportions of the cosmos and its celestial harmony.

was Pietro d'Abano (1250–1315) who Palisca identifies as one of the earliest musical humanists. Parallel to his medical studies, Pietro studied vibrating strings and also tried to understand principles of consonance and dissonance.

39 On the importance of music in Islamic writings, see Charles Burnett, 'European Knowledge of Arabic Texts Referring to Music: Some New Material', *Early Music History* (1993), 1–17; and '"Spiritual Medicine": Music and Healing in Islam and its Influence in the West', in Penelope Gouk (ed.), *Musical Healing in Cultural Contexts* (Aldershot, 2000), pp. 85–91; Nancy Siraisi, 'The Music of Pulse in the Writings of Italian Academic Physicians (Fourteenth and Fifteenth Centuries)', *Speculum*, 50:4 (1975), 689–710, esp. p. 697.

40 Siraisi, 'The Music of Pulse', p. 702.

41 Concetta Pennuto, 'Pulsations du Corps en Medicine: Sentre et Mesurer par la Musique', *Histoire, Médecine et Santé*, 11 (2017) online.

42 Jacomien Prins, 'The Music of Pulse in Marsilio Ficino's Timaeus Commentary', in Karl A. E. Enenkel (ed.), *Blood, Sweat and Tears: The Changing Concepts of Physiology from Antiquity into Early Modern Europe* (Leiden, 2012) pp. 393–413.

43 Prins, 'The Music of Pulse', p. 405.

44 Siraisi, 'The Music of Pulse', p. 702.

How physicians accurately measured pulse, and by extension, how musicians conceived of pulse in a period prior to the invention of accurate timepieces is worth consideration not just in terms of healthcare, but also with regard to how it might impact our understanding of performance practice. The understanding of pulse, comprised of alternating moments of movement and rest relating to the diastole and systole – the rest and stroke – of the heatbeat, was deeply reliant on the Aristotelian definition of time as a quality of motion, 'a number of motion in respect of before or after.'[45] Stillness was comprised within this conception of time, 'Since time is the measure of motion, it will be the measure of rest too – indirectly. For all rest is in time.' For Aristotle time was 'not described as fast or slow, but as many or few and as long or short.'[46]

From the earliest printed treatises in the early decades of the sixteenth century, through until at least the mid-seventeenth century, music theoretical definitions of beat (tactus, battuta) were profoundly Aristotelian and betray a common knowledge of medical theories of pulse.[47] Zarlino, for example, draws on the medical authority of Galen, Paulus Aegineta and Avicenna in his description of what he calls the measure, that is the pair of downward and upward movements, and explicitly connects the concept to the diastole and systole of the heart. While Ficino presents a complex view of the music of pulse, Zarlino renders the idea understandable to the musician. Zarlino writes:

> '... since medical authorities say that the pulsebeat may be either equal or unequal, musical rhythm results from the kind of equality and inequality found in quick and slow notes. Thus rhythm is born, and from it the many-proportioned movements contained in the multiplex, superparticular, and other genres of ratios.[48]

The relationship between mode, time and prolation (*modus, tempus* and *prolatio*) was thus fixed by ratio and proportion.

While the movement of the hand in determining the measure of music may have been real (in an ensemble performance) or imagined (a solo performer), correct proportional divisions of time could also regulate actual physical movement in dance and gymnastics. Aristocratic training in fencing and the correct use of the sword was related to both. The pairing of music and gymnastics as a means of regulating an ideal society was supported by the authority of Plato, but for one not engaged in military activity, walking was considered suitable exercise, so long as it was undertaken correctly. These activities were deemed

45 Aristotle, *Physics*, trans. R. P. Hardie and R. K. Gaye, Book 4, Part 11, http://classics.mit.edu/Aristotle/physics.4.iv.html (accessed 18/01/2022).

46 Aristotle, *Physics*, book 4, part 12, http://classics.mit.edu/Aristotle/physics.4.iv.html (accessed 18/01/2022).

47 For further discussion of early modern theoretical concepts and practical aspects of time and pulse, see Roger Matthew Grant, *Beating Time and Measuring Music in the Early Modern Era* (Oxford, 2014), especially chapters 1–3.

48 Zarlino, *The Art of Counterpoint: Part III of Le Istitutione Harmoniche 1558*, trans. Guy A. Marco and Claude V. Palisca (New Haven, CT and London, 1968), pp. 117–118.

appropriate for gentlemanly exercise by sixteenth- and seventeenth-century physicians including Girolamo Cardano and Giulio Mancini.[49]

In a manuscript volume which survives in the Vatican library, alongside Mancini's better-known writings on art, there is a treatise on dance that also touches on music and gymnastics. His conception of dance relies on the fundamentals of proportion and the Aristotelian concept of time as motion.[50] The nobility of dance lies in its imitation of the harmonious and proportionate movement of the heavens, and the movements of the body are ordered in relation to the proportion of the music. In the rhythm and proportions of dance, the body itself reflects cosmic harmony. Mancini's brief consideration of music refers to Galen, noting that the music one listens to, whether good or bad, can influence health.[51]

Mancini's descriptions of certain dances relate to how the movements imitate bodily actions. The galliard for example imitates the movement of a youth demonstrating his robustness and mobility. He does not mention the speed of the dance (and thus its music) in terms of tempo. Of course, music for dance in its nature has rhythmic features that are audibly more distinct, and, in terms of practice, the tactus of the music has to relate to the physical movement of the body, and is thus directly related to pulse. While Mancini's treatise is little known, his ideas were hardly unique. The ability of music, separate from text, to regulate aspects of the human body is equally evident in sixteenth- and seventeenth-century manuals on fencing, gymnastics and horsemanship.[52]

Listening and hearing

While physicians were reliant on the senses for diagnosis and treatment, their understanding of the workings of the senses remained largely Aristotelian.[53] Aristotle argued that while sight was more important for survival and to provide the basic necessities of life, hearing was superior for developing intelli-

49 Frances Gage, 'Exercise for Mind and Body: Giulio Mancini, Collecting, and the Beholding of Landscape Painting in the Seventeenth Century, *Renaissance Quarterly*, 61:4 (2008), 1167–1207.

50 Giulio Mancini, *Dell' Origine et nobilità dell ballo*, Biblioteca Apostolica Vaticana, Barb.Lat 4315, f157r–157v, available at https://digi.vatlib.it/view/MSS_Barb.lat.4315 (location 162 of film).

51 Mancini, *Dell'Origine*, Barb.Lat 4315, f 190.

52 For example Cesare Fiaschi, *Trattato dell'imbrigliare, manegiare et ferrare cavalli…* (Bologna, 1556), book 2, p. 88. This trend is not restricted to Italy. For the influence of Pythagorean harmonic proportions in French society, see Kate van Orden, *Music, Discipline and Arms in Early Modern France* (Chicago, 2005), chapter 2.

53 Stephen Pender, 'Medicine and the Senses: Physicians, Sensation and the Soul', in Herman Roodenburg (ed.), *A Cultural History of the Senses in the Renaissance* (London and New York, 2014), pp. 127–147.

gence. The perception of sound was connected to the element of air, the medium through which it travelled.[54] Ficino followed the traditional view that the sense organs consisted of the same substance as what is sensed, thus if there was sufficient air in the sense of hearing, the sound could travel unhampered through the body and thereby influence the soul.[55] In the sixteenth century Girolamo Cardano argued for the primacy of hearing on the grounds that it was more subtle than any other sense because it alone is concerned with motion. Sounds in motion act on the animal spirits in the ear, which in turn act on internal spirits in the body. Music affects the passions because it transmits movement.[56]

The belief that the anatomical process of hearing was a channel fundamentally connected to the passions of the soul in some way, and to the physical response of the pulse can be assumed.[57] However, the understanding of the anatomy of the ear and of the physical process of hearing is different to listening, the attitude of focusing on sound in order to understand something about what is conveyed by the sense of hearing. Listening, like so many human activities, is socially constructed, including listening to music. By comparing the aural affective connotations of harmonic intervals in the music cited by Zarlino and Vicentino, McKinney has shown that even comparatively close contemporaries had a different perception of the sonic affective qualities of the same interval.[58]

The religious, medical, social and political environments all play a part in conditioning responses to music. The chain from philosophical and abstract conceptions of music, to the physically heard sound (however that process was understood) to the socially conditioned responses to music, is what makes the study of music in relation to a religious-medical community particularly complex. As Becker has noted, given communities will behave in particular ways in response to music as they occur within complex systems of thought and behaviour.[59] She suggests adopting Bourdieu's term 'habitus' – an alternative

54 Aristotle, *On Sense and the Sensible*, part 1, trans. J. I. Beare.

55 Prins, 'The Music of Pulse', p. 404.

56 Jacomien Prins, 'Girolamo Cardano and Julius Caesar Scaliger in Debate about Nature's Musical Secrets', *Journal of the History of Ideas*, 78:2 (2017), 169–189.

57 There are some key studies that have attempted to integrate musical and medical thought, but not musical practice. See especially Penelope Gouk, 'Raising Spirits and Restoring Souls: Early Modern Medical Explanations for Music's Affects', in Viet Erlmann (ed.), *Hearing Cultures: Essays on Sound, Listening and Modernity* (Oxford and New York, 2004), pp. 87–105; and 'Sister Disciplines? Music and Medicine in Historical Perspective', in Gouk (ed.), *Musical Healing in Cultural Contexts*, pp. 171–196.

58 Timothy R. McKinney, 'Hearing in the Sixth Sense', *The Musical Quarterly*, 82:3/4 (1998), 517–536.

59 Judith Becker, 'Anthropological Perspectives on Music and Emotion', in Patrik N. Juslin and John A. Sloboda, *Music and Emotion: Theory and Research* (Oxford, 2001), pp. 135–160, esp. pp. 137–138.

to 'culture' – to describe attitudes to listening. The habitus of listening encompasses the interrelatedness of the perception of musical emotion and learned interactions with our surroundings.

The habitus of listening includes the emotional community in which the activity occurs. Hence, in mid-sixteenth and seventeenth-century Rome, particular communities might be seen as developing their own listening habitus. Just as Dell'Antonio identified a particular listening habitus within the elite communities of the Barberini circle in his study of spiritual listening, so too the Hospital of Santo Spirito might similarly be described as an emotional community with its own listening habitus.[60] With the interweaving strands of intellectual thought that drew on medical knowledge and a specific physiological understanding of how the ear perceived sound, as well as religious views on correct listening derived from the teachings of the Church Fathers and Augustine in particular, modes of listening or the habitus of listening of this community is likely to have been different from that of the elite curial courts of the same city.

Vestiges of the Santo Spirito listening habitus emerge in some surviving documents. While scribal conventions are of course evident, as are traces of the rhetorical 'discourse about' reminiscent of the curial elites discussed by Dell'Antonio, there are perhaps some more specifically nuanced aspects. Words such as 'comfort', 'relieve', 'recreate' for example straddle the medical and religious environments, while within the discussion of Church music, the vocabulary and frame of reference for listening is the wider controversy around religious reform, and reference is made frequently to 'devotion' and 'piety'. To borrow Carolyn Abbate's terms, the 'drastic' approach to the effects of music rather than the gnostic 'objective' or critical approach appears to dominate.[61] In terms of music as a means of eliciting a change in the body or mind of the listener, the drastic must of necessity prevail if it is to be an effective treatment. For it to act as a curative of either body or soul, it must move the humours and therefore affect the passions, in whatever sense they are constructed.

In the Hospital of Santo Spirito, as a religious community as well as a place of medical scholarship and care, the undercurrent of Tridentine and post-Tridentine discourse and ultimately reform will have been a factor in how music was perceived and used. The intellectual discussion of the passions in relation to music is however very different from the practice of music. Evidence in text sources helps us to trace scholarly, perhaps elitist views of music and

60 Dell'Antonio describes their practice as a 'discourse about' in which the marker of an elite thinker was the way in which he could listen to and describe music without using the language of the professional musician, which resulted in a particular type of rhetoric. Andrew Dell'Antonio, *Listening as Spiritual Practice in Early Modern Italy* (Berkeley and Los Angeles, CA, 2011), pp. 7–9. For extended discussion on how emotional communities functioned, see Barbara H. Rosenwein, *Generations of Feeling: A History of Emotion 600–1700* (Cambridge, 2016).

61 Carolyn Abbate, 'Music: Drastic or Gnostic?', *Critical Inquiry*, 30:3 (2004), 505–536.

emotion. It is far harder to evaluate sources that only suggest, make oblique references to or describe something observed, especially if that something is as intangible as sound. How early modern musicians understood physiological aspects of the sense of hearing and of sound perception, and the way in which that understanding may have affected their compositional endeavours, is a topic that is largely untouched by music historians. Indeed, the study of the history of the senses and of sense perception is a comparatively recent phenomenon.[62]

It is only by establishing a strong foundation of known and accepted attitudes and assumptions that one can begin to explore musical practices in the Hospital of Santo Spirito. That exploration will inevitably be incomplete as we can never bring back the huge range of unwritten musical practices that we know existed from documentary evidence. The extent to which music conceived for this space and this community, whether secular or sacred, instrumental or vocal, invoked the power of harmony and thus had an additional dimension and purpose – to regulate and control the body by means of pulse and simultaneously influence the humours via the mind or soul – will be the focus of later chapters.

62 Robert Jütte, *A History of the Senses from Antiquity to Cyberspace,* trans. James Lynn (Cambridge, 2005).

3

The Harmonious Soul

Music and the passions were of as much interest to religious thinkers as they were to physicians. In his eloquent reflections on the nature of spirituality and music, Cobusson speaks of music as occupying a liminal space in which all assured and secure structures and boundaries of our existence are undermined. It is neither subject nor object but an 'inbetweenness' connecting body and soul, the divine and the human; a threshold that by definition is neither one thing nor the other, and therein lies its power or efficacy.[1] The proximity of body, mind and soul is reflected in religious writings concerning the passions and music's capacity to act on them. These concerns are already evident in the late antique sources documenting the history of the Christian Church in the east and in the west.

Music in the Christian liturgy in the form of recitation, chanting and singing evolved in the same Christian societies of late antiquity responsible for the emergence of the hospital. The divisions between Christians who chose isolation in desert communities to focus on their own spirituality and those who set up monasteries in urban areas to minister to the local population are reflected in different rules of monastic living, expressed most clearly by the enclosed work of prayer of the Benedictines and the community-focused Augustinians. Viewed in this way, monasteries and hospitals are twins. The historical development of the hospital runs parallel with the development of the monastic Offices, and this close relationship between religion and medicine is entwined with music. Those ministering to the sick were also committed to a life of constant prayer and psalm singing.

The passions in religious thought

Late antique sources written by the Church Fathers active in the fourth century, such as Jerome, Basil of Caesarea, Augustine and Gregory of Nyssa were core to early modern religious education and therefore to the men who ran and worked in the Hospital of Santo Spirito. Many of these antique sources mention music in general terms, and psalmody in particular, and it is clear that the psalms, unlike readings, were sung. These sources also note the regularity of singing

1 Marcel Cobussen, *Thresholds: Rethinking Spirituality through Music* (Aldershot, 2008), especially pp. 45, 61.

and its beauty, demonstrating an appreciation of the rhetorical power of psalmody and the ability of psalm singing to control the passions.[2]

Even in these early Christian texts, the Hippocratic-Galenic understanding of the passions and music's capacity to act on them is evident. For example, Basil's homily on Psalm 1 identifies the psalms as tools for teaching, for helping ordinary folk towards Christian behaviour and comportment, including self-control, dignity, endurance and wisdom. He notes that the book of Psalms:

> ... heals the old hurts of souls, and brings about recovery where the wound is fresh. It wins the part that is sick and preserves that which is sound. As far as lies within its power, it destroys the passions which lord it in this life in the souls of men. And all this it effects with a musical persuasiveness and with a gratification that induces wise and wholesome reflexion.[3]

The implication of psalm singing as a means of healing is significant, as of course, it was Basil's great hospital at Caesarea that became the model for urban hospitals elsewhere in the eastern Mediterranean.

Basil was not alone in his concern about controlling the passions. The tension between what is sung and how it is sung is a recurring theme – psalm singing is spiritually beneficial, but simultaneously open to abuse through the temptation of seductive melody. Possibly the most influential texts on this matter are those of Augustine. Trained in the Greek classical tradition, Augustine was particularly influenced by the writings of Plato, Cicero and the Stoics. Just as Plato understood music to be a powerful means of education as well as a danger to the morals of the unwary, so Augustine was aware of the dual nature of music. For him, the text was of primary importance, but he confesses to being distracted by the beauty of the song, and to enjoying the music, not just the meaning conveyed by the sung words.[4] The emotions music conjured up were worrying, as he understood emotions to be morally ambiguous. It was the will that was the moral determinant. For example, a bad person could rejoice at an enemy's death. Joy, a 'good' emotion, is inverted where the will is evil.[5] How-

2 For detailed study and transcription of relevant antique sources relating to the emergence of liturgical music, see Christopher Page, *The Christian West and its Singers: The First Thousand Years* (New Haven, CT and London, 2010). For transcriptions of the early sources, see especially pp. 72–87; James McKinnon, 'Desert Monasticism and the later Fourth-century Psalmodic Movement', *Music and Letters*, 75:4 (1994), 505–521; Joseph Dyer, 'The Desert, the City and Psalmody in the Late Fourth Century', in Sean Gallagher et al (eds), *Western Plainchant in the First Millennium: Studies in the Medieval Liturgy and its Music* (Aldershot, 2003), pp. 11–43.

3 Philip Schaff (ed.), *St. Basil: Letters and Select Works*, Nicene and Post-Nicene Fathers, Series 2 vol 8, https://ccel.org/ccel/schaff/npnf208/npnf208.vi.ii.iii.html (accessed 08/10/2021).

4 *Saint Augustine: Confessions*, ed. and trans. R. S. Pine-Coffin, Book X, chapter 33 (London, 1961), pp. 238–239.

5 Barbara H. Rosenwein, *Generations of Feeling: A History of Emotions, 600–1700*, (Cambridge, 2016), p. 64.

ever, he refused to ban music in church as he realised how it could help those of weaker faith to more devotion, just as it had helped him recover his faith in his early days as a Christian.

A variety of early modern sources refer to music's benefits on the one hand, and its capacity to distract and tempt humanity away from virtue on the other. Although working for a different Order of Hospitallers, that of St John of Jerusalem, Sabba di Castiglione articulates the view of the Christian hospitaller unequivocally, that secular music draws one away from the contemplation of the divine and should therefore be shunned in favour of hymns and psalms.[6] The arguments for and against music could be equally bolstered by the great authorities of antiquity, but the overriding concern was for the correct spiritual passions to be evoked in the listener.

The medieval establishment by Gregory the Great of seven deadly sins, all of which were also passions, muddied the waters of the two passions transmitted by Boethius from the Aristotelian tradition – sorrow and joy. Sorrow *(tristitia)* had a positive and a negative aspect. As sorrow for wrongdoing transformed into repentance, it was a virtue, but as an expression of worldly distress it was a negative and led to death. *Tristitia* was also the medieval term for a condition closely related to melancholia, called acedia, first identified by John Cassian as an affliction of monks. The symptoms were feelings of restlessness, of not being spiritually fruitful, a desire for company or pursuit of diversionary activities that would distract him from his spiritual purpose. Acedia as a cardinal sin demanded confession, but confession was a form of healing for it. Confession and penitence thus became 'medicine for the soul'.[7]

The two passions, sorrow and joy, represent the extreme ends of a continuum between which the fluctuations seemed to represent all the vicissitudes of life. Christian thinkers saw parallels in scriptural references to music as an agent that enabled the passage from mourning to joy. Even the founder of the Hospital of Santo Spirito, Pope Innocent III dei Segni, provides an example of how sorrow intrudes into worldly joy, as the final scriptural quotations in his *De miseria* are from Job 21:12–13: 'They take the timbrel and the harp and rejoice at the sound of the organ. They spend their days in wealth, and in a moment they go down to hell'. This is followed by Job's response regarding the fate of his children: 'my harp is turned to mourning, my organ into the voice of those who weep' (Job 30:31). The explicit mention of music as indicative of specific states of mind, of sorrow and joy, is suggestive of commonplaces about the transformative power of music.[8]

6 Sabba di Castiglione, *Ricordi di Frate Sabba di Castiglione* (Bologna, 1549), Riccordo LXXII.

7 Stanley W. Jackson, *Melancholia and Depression: from Hippocratic Times to Modern Times* (New Haven, CT and London, 1986), pp. 67–69.

8 Thomas Connolly, *Mourning into Joy: Music, Raphael, and Saint Cecilia* (New Haven, CT and London, 1994), pp. 3, 156–157.

For Thomas Aquinas, music was the art most closely associated with aesthetic pleasure, and thus important for creating the right frame of mind for devotion in the listener. In his *Summa theologica* Aquinas considers the question 'whether God should be praised with song' and concludes that song is of benefit in inciting those of weaker faith to devotion.[9] Aquinas drew his notions of musical arousal of emotion from Aristotle's *De Anima* and Plato's *Republic*, but he made a clear distinction between music for moral education and 'theatrical' music. For him, *tristitia* was one of the basic passions. Paired with joy (*gaudium*), *tristitia* was the reaction of man's sensitive nature in withdrawing from evil. Acedia on the other hand was the sorrow or aversion one feels against spiritual good, and clearly a sin.

Transcendent song

The passions, especially those aroused by music, are clearly regarded as ambiguous in religious writings. The role of music in religious, spiritual and mystical experience is a trope that flows through hagiographies. Whether expressed as joy in the biblical sense or the more extreme ecstasy or rapture that is recounted in overtly sensual or sexual terms to describe the spiritual union with Christ, these passions are all commonly described as accompanied by music.[10]

Augustine's contemporary in the Western church, St John Cassian (d. c. 433) describes a kind of ecstasy ignited by psalm singing that suggests that it was something done with intense feeling.

> Sometimes when we have been singing, the verse of some psalm has offered the occasion for fiery prayer. Now and then the melodious modulation of a brother's voice [*canora fraterna vocis modulatio*] has excited the insensible minds to intense prayer. We know as well that the distinction and gravity of the cantor [*distinctionem gravitatemque psallentis*] have contributed a great deal to the fervour of those in attendance.[11]

9 'the praise of the voice is necessary in order to arouse man's devotion towards God. Wherefore whatever is useful in conducing to this result is becomingly adopted in the divine praises. Now it is evident that the human soul is moved in various ways according to various melodies of sound, as the Philosopher states (Polit. viii, 5), and also Boethius (*De Musica*, prologue). 'Hence the use of music in the divine praises is a salutary institution, that the souls of the faint-hearted may be the more incited to devotion': Thomas Aquinas, *Summa Theologica*, trans. The Fathers of the English Dominican Province, 2-2, Q91 (Cincinnati, 1947).

10 Spiritual ecstasy and rapture triggered by music is explored in a number of late seventeenth century oratorios. See Holly Roberts, 'Ecstatic Devotion and Erotic Death in Seventeenth- and Eighteenth-century Iconography, Operas and Oratorios' (unpublished PhD thesis, University of Oregon, 2020).

11 John Cassian, *Conlationes* 9.26.1–2 cited in Peter Jeffery, 'Monastic Reading and the

It was this kind of mystical experience that Cassian refers to as *excessus mentis*, or fiery prayer to which medieval religious men and women aspired, and it was evidently a deeply powerful religious experience associated with singing. Far from being rote and routine, the proper performance of the psalms meant for the singer to feel the same emotions the Psalmist felt, and to personalise one's love, fear, desire toward God through the medium of chant or song. Cassian suggests that we know God, love God and experience God when our experience and that of the Psalmist come together.[12]

Other descriptions of the rapturous experience of the divine in early monastic literature are similarly accompanied by images of fire or light.[13]. This transformation of the inner being in which God lives in the mind of man – the transformative 'fiery prayer' – is the last stage of three leading towards a deep, spiritual experience.[14] It is usually a short-lived experience of 'pure prayer' that might be termed 'mystical'. The nature of these experiences varies, but they are united by descriptions of a kind of union with the transcendental, principally identified as love, and are similar to the ideas expressed in Plato's *Symposium*, especially as transmitted by Ficino.[15]

The notion of 'singing in the heart' is often mentioned in accounts of religious experiences such as those of St Cecilia. This phrase has a biblical source but is also found in writings of the early Christian tradition. The heart was metaphorically the centre of the spiritual senses – a parallel of the five physical senses that encapsulated implications of changes of emotion and thought (as in the modern phrase 'a change of heart'). The Rule of Benedict for example opens with an injunction to 'listen with the ear of the heart'.[16]

Another means of accessing correct spiritual emotions was conceived by the medieval philosopher and theologian Jean Gerson (1363–1429). He distinguished between the audible song of the mouth and the silent song of the heart. Using hexachord theory, he articulated a way in which each note stood

Emerging Roman Chant Repertory', in Sean Gallagher et al (eds), *Western Plainchant in the first Millennium: Studies in the Medieval Liturgy and its Music* (Ashgate, 2003), p. 58.

12 Amy Hollywood, 'Song Experience, and the Book in Benedictine Monasticism', in Amy Hollywood and Patricia Z. Beckman (eds), *The Cambridge Companion to Christian Mysticism* (Cambridge, 2021), pp. 59–79, esp. p. 66.

13 The imagery of fire and light relates to biblical accounts of the presence of the Holy Spirit in Baptism (Matthew 3:11) and at Pentecost (Acts 2: 1–3).

14 The three stages are *anachoresis* (seeking the place of God), *prosoche* (struggle with the self) and *proseuche* (dwelling in the place of God). Douglas Burton-Christie, 'Early Monasticism', in Hollywood and Beckman (eds), *The Cambridge Companion to Christian Mysticism*, pp. 37–58, esp. p. 43.

15 Connolly, *Mourning into Joy*, p. 61.

16 Timothy Fry, OSB (ed.), *The Rule of St. Benedict in English* (Collegeville, MN, 1982) p. 15.

for a vowel sound that was connected to a passion on which the singer might contemplate. The basis of his thought was that the syllable was a symbol of an emotion through which the heart moved to reach union with the divine. By contemplating the meaning behind each syllable, the singer could move from merely physical sound to a deep spiritual experience that resulted in change.[17]

Spiritual change, the change of heart from sorrow to joy and the fluctuations between those two passions is central to Gerson's musical analogies. Gerson's thought was transmitted in Italian by the preacher Pietro da Lucca, in his *Regule della vita spirituale* and *L'arte del ben pensare.* The latter was first printed in Bologna in 1523 but reprinted many times at least until 1592.[18] Perhaps more significantly though is that his idea of the ascent of the soul has many parallels with so many other more influential texts: Augustine, Plato and the Christian Neo-Platonic writings of Ficino. They epitomise how the passions, however conceived, dominate intellectual endeavours for over a thousand years and have to be taken as a given when evaluating musical affects and effects within an early modern context.[19]

The capacity of music, particularly in the form of psalm singing, to both express and evoke emotion is a recurring theme that is deeply connected to concepts of healing and central to the investigation of music at the Hospital of Santo Spirito in the early modern period. The constant reminders to the members of the Order 'to be often in the choir' is perhaps some indication that a heightened religious experience, perhaps triggered by singing, would better enable them to carry out their duties in caring for the sick.[20]

Music and the foundation of the Hospital of Santo Spirito

The foundation of the Order of Santo Spirito was deeply informed by early Christian practices as transmitted by the Church Fathers. The patristic writings also shaped the thinking of later governors of the Hospital, including notions about music and worship. The earliest monastic Rules indicate psalm singing, whether responsorial or antiphonal, but what music sounded like at the time of the establishment of the Hospital and Order of Santo Spirito in the 1180s is harder to establish.[21] The earliest notated chant had already appeared two

[17] Joyce L. Irwin, 'The Mystical Music of Jean Gerson', *Early Music History: Studies in Medieval and Early Modern Music*, 1 (1981), 187–201.

[18] *L'arte del ben pensare e contemplare la passione del nostro signore Jesu Cristo* (Bologna, Girolamo di Benetti, 1523; Venice, Francesco de' Francheschi Senese, 1592) and *Regule della vita spirituale* (Bologna, 1526).

[19] Connolly, *Mourning into Joy*, pp. 145–146, and Rosenwein, *Generations of Feeling*, p. 237.

[20] This instruction also has a biblical origin in 1 Thessalonians: 5:16: 'Pray without ceasing'.

[21] The Rule of St Benedict and the so-called Rule of the Master which has a provenance from the area around Rome both date from around the sixth century when times for prayer were organised and some of the specific content outlined.

centuries earlier. It is impossible to know if, by the late twelfth century the Order relied on this already well-developed repertory, or adopted the simple polyphony that was emerging in northern France, along with new genres such as the motet. To get a sense of the early repertoire of the Hospital, we have to rely on information from other more general sources about twelfth- and thirteenth-century liturgical music in both southern France (Montpellier) and Rome supported by what we can glean from surviving notated music.

What we do know is that by the time Guy de Montpellier established the Order of Santo Spirito in his home town in the last quarter of the twelfth century, the texts of a Roman (as opposed to Eastern) liturgy had been established. However, there was a significant variety of chant used in churches and monasteries across Europe so ascertaining what kind of singing he may have envisaged for members of his Order would be pure speculation. Benedictine houses tended to follow localised traditions unlike the newly formed Cistercian Order which had laid down exemplars of practice in the twelfth century.[22] If the Hospital and its church in Montpellier followed Frankish norms, chant would have been of the Gregorian type first notated in the ninth century, rather than Old Roman chant which was probably a later development. In Rome where the Hospital of Santo Spirito in Sassia was constructed a stone's throw from old St Peter's, chant was probably in the Old Roman style, which persisted there into the thirteenth century. One surviving fragment of chant will be discussed below.

The medieval Rule of the Order of Santo Spirito remained unchanged throughout the early modern period. However, in the sixteenth and seventeenth centuries, obedience to the Rule was observed in parallel with newer Tridentine initiatives. As will be seen in Chapters 5 and 7, by the mid-seventeenth century, the broader intellectual religious notions that had informed the foundational activities of the community were impacted by Tridentine reforms that increasingly attempted to control both liturgical practices (including music) and the care of the sick. Localised variants and the intellectual and artistic creativity that flourished up to around the third decade of the seventeenth century were gradually supressed. Ultimately the professional musicians who served the Hospital were dispensed with altogether in the eighteenth century.

For the Order of Santo Spirito and the place of music within the Hospital, the patristic writings of Augustine, Ambrose, Gregory and Basil are an important point of reference. Music, and in particular psalmody in the Hospital Order of Santo Spirito will almost certainly have had the additional purpose of 'care of the soul.' Its medieval foundation followed an existing tradition not just of social care within Christian communities but also of song as part of spiritual discipline. The accounts of Saulnier and Dragondelli indicate that the lifestyle of the Christians of late antiquity was known to the founder of the Rule of Santo Spirito and books by Augustine, Ambrose and others were definitely

22 David Hiley, *Gregorian Chant* (Cambridge, 2009), p. 155.

in the library of the Hospital by the mid-sixteenth century.[23] The patristic writings would also have been central to the education of the elite churchmen who were to take the role of preceptor or commendatore during the late sixteenth and seventeenth centuries. The Hospital, although a leading centre for medical science and intellectual endeavour on the one hand, was on the other, also a centre of devout religious practice, adhering to monastic tenets and obedience to the authority of the pope and the various officials of the Catholic Church.

As noted in Chapter 1, Innocent III, who established the Hospital of Santo Spirito in Rome, was also the author of an influential treatise in which citations of psalms and of other scriptural texts concerning music feature prominently. Innocent's treatise was not unique but reflects wider medieval thinking in which there was a re-emergence of ascetism and imitation of desert monasticism with its focus on recitation of the Psalter, the imitation of David as the humble shepherd exalted to be king, who subsequently sins, is humbled, falls from grace, repents and is restored. David the songwriter, the healer, the penitent, is viewed as the model. The psalms as the direct expression of spiritual progress are the object of contemplation.

It is perhaps significant that Pope Innocent III was also responsible for a revision of the Mass and Office in the Papal chapel in 1213–1216. Subsequent revisions continued to the middle of the century with Nicholas III (1277–1280) ordering the destruction of any books that did not conform to the revisions.[24] It would seem to be a reasonable assumption, given the close relationship between Innocent III and the Order of Santo Spirito, that the so-called Roman-Franciscan revised versions of missals, breviaries, graduals and antiphoners would have been used for their services at the time of its foundation.

Psalmody and the Rule of Santo Spirito

There is little specific mention of the divine Offices or how they are to be observed in the Rule of the Order of Santo Spirito, let alone singing. In this respect it was similar to the statutes of the military Hospitaller Order of St John of Jerusalem, which stipulates only that the Offices should be observed, and not how this is to be done.[25] However, it is clear that daily observation of the Offices

23 Commendatore Bernardino da Cirillo noted that such books should be available for ornament and for the convenience of the many in the house who had need to see various doctrines. 'per ornamento e per commodita di molti che nelli casi occurreti volessino vedere varie dottrine': I-Rla Ms 388, *Epistolario di Bernardino Cirillo*, fol. 31v letter 11. Books by the Church Fathers are also mentioned by Saulnier, *De Capite Sacri Ordinis Sancti Spiritus Dissertatio* (Lyon, 1649) and Dragondelli, *Trattato del Sacro Ordine di S. Spirito detto in Sassia ... del rev. Fra Pietro Saunier* (Rome, 1662), p. 33.

24 Hiley, *Gregorian Chant*, p. 157.

25 *Statuta ordinis domus Hospitalis Hierusalem* (Rome, 1586).

was required as per the Rule of Augustine.[26] The Augustinian Rule requires the monk to be attentive to prayer 'at fixed times and appointed hours'. There is also a requirement not to sing anything other than what has been ordained to be sung, and at the same time that when psalms and hymns are sung to 'let the heart ponder what the mouth utters'.[27]

Within the Rule of Santo Spirito, one can glean from places where psalmody or sung prayers are mentioned that there is an assumption of familiarity with the daily cycle of services. At a time when the lives of entire communities, whether urban or rural, were governed by the sound of church bells ringing the hours, it seems a safe assumption that anyone seeking to join the Order would already be well aware of the 'Opus Dei' – the great work of prayer – that underpinned a monastic lifestyle, albeit a somewhat more flexible one, dictated by the needs of the community under its care.

Rule XXVIII instructs the friars to go to the church on rising in the morning to listen to Matins and 'Ore' – prayers of the Blessed Virgin – standing or genuflecting if able to. Then seated, they are required to listen to the psalms and lessons to which they sing the responses. At the 'Gloria patri' they are to stand and bow their heads to the altar. Lay brothers, instead of going to church for Matins, must recite the 'Pater noster' thirteen times, then a further seven times for prayers of the Blessed Virgin and nine times for Vespers.[28] Aside from instructing lay brothers to recite the Lord's Prayer instead of the Offices, there is no mention as to how these Offices are to be carried out. Like the Rule of Augustine, this element remains flexible and subject to the need of the localised Christian community. Knowledge of the Benedictine and Augustinian practices would have been so well known that such details needed no further commentary.

The instruction that friars listen to the psalms and sing the responses raises questions about performance and listening practice. The instruction implies that a person or body of people were doing the singing while the rest listened. While it might mean even at this early period that there was a choir set apart from the rest of the friars, it is more likely that one person was designated as a cantor to lead the services for the day. Later documents suggest that there was a weekly rota, as the term 'hebdomadary'(*hebdomadario*) is used, indicating an individual chaplain or cantor who is responsible for leading services for a week, presumably on a rotational basis. The responses would have been short

26 Domenico Borgarucci, *Relatione del modo; che si tiene da religione di S. Spirito nel governo dell'Archihospitale Apostolico di Santo Spirito in Sassia di Roma*, 1623. GB-Lwl EPB 46633/B.

27 *The Rule of St. Augustine with Commentary by Hugh of St. Victor*, trans. Dom Aloysius Smith (n.d., n.p.), part 2.

28 Pietro De Angelis, *L'Ospedale di S. Spirito dalle origini al 1500*, 2 vols. Collana di studi storici sull'Ospedale di Santo Spirito in Saxia e sugli Ospedali Romani (Rome, 1960; 1962), vol 1. p. 256.

enough to be easily remembered, but it is likely that professed friars of the Order would have memorised at least the most frequently used and important chants.[29] By the sixteenth century, the friars who were also singers are marked out as different, as they are paid for their services and their names survive in the financial records.

One of the functions of the Hospital was the care of orphans, some of whom may have been earmarked for profession into the Order rather than apprenticeship to a trade, and were therefore taught to sing at a level beyond the simple Catechism provided for all children. At the time the Rule was written, society was still dominated by oral-aural modes of transmission. Listening and memory were fundamental to education and knowledge acquisition. The friars, by listening to the psalms, were probably actively engaged in following the text and its melodic rise and fall, in order to be able to respond correctly.

While instructions about the daily cycle of Offices are not laid out specifically in the Rule of Santo Spirito, there are rules that give musical details and indications that psalmody was central to the daily life of the Order.[30] Perhaps unsurprisingly, instructions for the observation of Pentecost in Rule CIX feature considerable detail, but much of it is to do with the administration of the Order. It was at Pentecost that the running of the House was reviewed by the Chapter, elections to the roles of Prior, Chamberlain and Treasurer carried out, and all were reminded of the Rule to which they had committed themselves, their charitable duties and so on. The hymn 'Veni creator spiritus', proper to the feast of Pentecost, featured at the start of proceedings. The many mentions of this hymn in various documents indicate its importance to the Hospital, and in the crowded streets at times of multiple processions, it would have been the 'sound mark' of the Order. As will be seen in Chapter 5, the musical embellishment of this feast continued to be of importance at least until the early eighteenth century. Similarly, rules for behaviour in the refectory contain a lot of information about psalms and prayers, especially those for Holy Week.

The Rule concerning the profession and acceptance of novices, Rule LXIX, gives further text incipits from which musical detail may be inferred, at least at the level of chant. After having made their vows and been given clothing by the maestro da casa, the novices kiss the cross, and prostrate themselves. The hymn 'Veni creator spiritus' is then sung by all the friars. While the initiates remain prone before the cross, a series of psalms and prayers are sung

29 For a detailed consideration of the memory skills prior to widespread literacy, see Mary Carruthers, *The Book of Memory: A Study of Memory in Medieval Culture* (Cambridge, 2008).

30 The charter document of the hospital of Notre Dame des Fontanilles in Tonnerre, although somewhat later (1293) offers a parallel example. It stipulates the number of daily Masses and the canonical hours, noting that the chanting must be in a loud voice so as to be heard in the infirmary, indicating that liturgical music was evidently thought to play a significant role in the patients' well-being. Rosenwein, *Generations of Feeling*, p. 64.

including Psalm 66,[31] 'Deus misereatur nostri' with the 'Gloria patri,' which is followed by the 'Kyrie eleison' and the Lord's Prayer up to the last line, 'Et ne nos'; then a series of psalms and responses: Psalm 85, 'Salvum fac servum tuum, Mitte ei domine'; Psalm 60, 'Esto ei (nobis) Domine turris fortitudinis'; Psalm 102, 'Domine exaudi orationem meam'; and closing with the traditional blessing and response, 'Dominus vobiscum, Et cum spirito tuo.' The community of the Order then accepted the novice according to the next instruction in the Rule (Rule LXX). This too includes details about specific psalms and prayers to be sung or recited by the prior on behalf of the friars. These include 'Levavi oculos' (Psalm 120), 'De profundis' (Psalm 129) and 'Ecce quam bonum' (Psalm 132), followed by a sequence starting with a further Kyrie, that repeats much of the previous section of the ceremony.[32]

A single manuscript fascicle in a miscellaneous bundle of documents in the Hospital archive preserves what appears to be an order of service for the profession of novices.[33] It follows exactly the detail in Rule LXIX. Although the document bears no date, it appears to be eighteenth century. The series of texts stipulated for the ceremony of profession matches the sequence of items for the Fourth Sunday (Feria 4) of Lent. It could be that novices made their profession on that particular day, and therefore the texts simply coincide, but there is an interesting textual concordance between these texts in the Rule, and a Parisian missal dating from the thirteenth century held in the Bibliothèque nationale de France.[34] The fact that this missal is contemporary with the foundation of the Order by a Frenchman does raise the possibility that the early liturgical practices of the Order may have followed a French model.

Aside from the Rule, early documents from which one might deduce elements of musical practice in the Order are scanty. A fifteenth-century manuscript described as a martyrology in the catalogue of the Hospital archive but is, more correctly, a *Liber annualium*, is possibly the closest we can get. This manuscript is a complex one as it was continually added to over several centuries, with the deaths of various officials, governors of the Hospital and local personages of note all being annotated in the appropriate places in the calendar. Along with the expected calendar of saints, martyrs, popes, clerics and distinguished members of the Order who are to be remembered in prayers for the dead, there is also an extract from a medical treatise, formulas for absolution and various other fragmentary texts, as well as two pages of chant notated in the opening pages.[35]

31 Psalm texts are given here with the Vulgate numbering.

32 De Angelis, *L'Ospedale di S. Spirito dalle origini al 1500*, vol. 1, pp. 267–268.

33 ASR-OSS 1296, separate unnumbered fascicle with a red and gold cover.

34 https://cantus.uwaterloo.ca/node/690754 and https://gallica.bnf.fr/ark:/12148/btv1b6000450z/f73.

35 ASR-OSS 72. For a discussion of the content of this manuscript, see Angelo Restaino, 'Il Liber Annualium e la memoria cultuale dell'Ordine,' in Letizia Leli (ed.), *Vivere la*

These chant settings start with 'Isti sunt agni novelli qui', usually associated with Saturday 'in Albis', the Saturday after Easter. The chant on the bottom three staves of the first page is a setting of the text 'Crucifixum in carne laudemus', proper to Easter and the Octave of Easter.[36] The second page of music starts with 'Regina celi [coeli] laetare' – a Marian text but also one that is associated with the Octave of Easter. This is followed by 'Christus resurgans ex mortuis', also proper to Easter and the Octave of Easter. It is perhaps significant that there are concordances with all of these texts in a single manuscript with a provenance extremely close to Santo Spirito, San Pietro B. 79 which dates from the twelfth century.[37] While the melody of 'Regina coeli' is similar to the Old Roman Chant melody used for this text in San Pietro B.79 and in many other concordances listed on the Cantus database for settings of this text,[38] the melody of 'Crucifixum in carne laudemus' is different from that in San Pietro B. 79.[39] These chants are probably in the book to indicate that they are to be used as part of the general Requiem Mass for the saints, martyrs and departed worthies that would probably have taken place annually, in all likelihood close to Easter given the texts used.

Prior to the Council of Trent and the reforms subsequently made to the liturgy, the Order had its own particular way of celebrating the Offices. The evidence for this is an inventory dating from 1535 that lists an old breviary according to the use of Santo Spirito, now lost.[40] A useful comparator is a surviving sixteenth-century breviary according to the use of the Order of St John of Jerusalem. This pocket-sized print contains all the texts of each ferial and feast day in order, but with a more extended celebration of feasts important to the Order, such as the feast of St John the Baptist (24 June).[41] A breviary according to the use of the Order of Santo Spirito is likely to have been similar except for the particular celebrations of feast days special to the Order, such as Pentecost, St Thecla (to whom the church for the women was dedicated) and specific Roman saints.

The gradual increase in more sophisticated music making at the Hospital during the sixteenth and seventeenth centuries seems to indicate a shift from a medieval monastic round of Offices consisting of chant and recitation to an approach in which certain Offices and feasts were prioritised and more elaborate musical settings used: the more important the feast, the richer the musical

---

Misericordia nel trecento: le miniature del Liber Regulae dell'ospedale romano di Santo Spirito in Sassia (Rome, 2018), pp. 129–131.

36 I-Rvat SP B.79 https://cantus.uwaterloo.ca/source/123661 (accessed 07/12/2021).

37 https://cantus.uwaterloo.ca/chant/671278 (accessed 07/12/2021).

38 US-Cai 1911.142b https://cantus.uwaterloo.ca/chant/672398 (accessed 07/12/2021).

39 I-Rvat SP B.79 https://cantus.uwaterloo.ca/source/123661 (accessed 07/12/2021).

40 ASR-OSS 231 Instrumenti 38v-39v.

41 *Breviarium secundum usum Ordinis Sancti Johannis Hierosolymitani* (Lyon, 1518).

adornment. The musical activity of the professional choir and the surviving musical sources will be examined more fully in Chapter 5.

A thread of documentation noting the need for devout attention to the daily Offices stretches from the earliest records through to the eighteenth century and beyond. While the Hospital complex may have been a busy place with orphans to be cared for, children to be taught in the school and the sick to be tended, the activity must have been accompanied by the almost continuous round of Offices and Masses. The sounds of prayer, chant and bells would have been part of the sonic landscape.

Later evidence of psalmody in the Hospital of Santo Spirito

Although not following such a strict monastic regime as the Benedictines, the Order of Santo Spirito nevertheless had psalmody at the heart of its daily Offices. As will be seen in Chapter 5, attention to the ferial Offices became even more important following the reforms of the Council of Trent. Successive governors encouraged members of the Order to apply themselves to the psalms with appropriate devotion. In 1611 the then commendatore, Pietro Campori, issued a series of instructions on the correct observation of the Offices and Masses in which he gives instruction to 'sing psalms with devotion and reverence'.[42] The use of psalm as a verb, literally 'psalming', echoes much earlier uses of the word in patristic writings. Campori was to some extent echoing instructions issued by his predecessor Giovanni Battista Ruini who issued a similar plea for devout observation and obedience in 1585.[43]

One of the most frequently copied documents in the Hospital archive is Virgilio Spada's instructions to the master of the novices and the rules for novices and spiritual exercises that accompany them. Although they were originally part of his *Stato della Casa* written in 1660, they were published well into the nineteenth century.[44] Spada's report is a crucial source of information about all aspects of the Hospital, as will be seen in the later chapters of this book.

42 'salmeggiando con devozione e reveranze e nel religione': ASR OSS 1299 *Ordine per la Chiesa, p.o di novembre 1611 da Mons. Campori.*

43 ASR-OSS 120 f147v–148r. It may be significant that these instructions start to appear around the time that the Council of Trent emphasised moral and spiritual catechism, linking prayer and biblical exegesis and the role of secular clergy in preaching. The evidence of printed sermons in the vernacular suggests that the psalms were of primary importance. Elise Boillet, 'Vernacular Sermons on the Psalms Printed in Sixteenth-century Italy: An Interface between Oral and Written Cultures', in Stefano Dall'Aglio, Brian Richardson and Massimo Rospocher (eds), *Voices and Texts in Early Modern Italian Society* (London and New York, 2017), pp. 200–211.

44 ASR-OSS 47. Virgilio Spada, *Stato della Casa dell'Archiospedale of Santo Spirito di Roma l'anno 1661; Notificazione sopra li dieci capitoli di avvertimenti di Monsignor Spada per li novizi dell'ordine dei canonici regolari di S. Spirito* (Rome, 1815).

Spada opens his discourse by citing both the Bible and the Rule of the Order, making a comparison between the modern novitiate and the young David – obedient, listening, punctual.

> 'Take these ten loaves of bread and run to your brothers in their camp' 1st Kings chapter 17. This order was given to the young David by his father Jesse when his other older sons found themselves in the camp with King Saul fighting against the Philistines. David obeyed with solicitous obedience to his father's command, going to the camp and doing his duty to his brothers as much as he had to.[45]

The requirement for obedience from novices is hardly surprising as it was an element of all monastic life, but the specific invocation of David seems to suggest an underlying aspect that is not directly voiced, and that is the charitable purpose of the Order in the care of the sick. In the Old Testament narratives David is a healer-king, simultaneously heroic and compassionate; a singer-poet and a leader. Perhaps most significantly he was also the ancestor of Jesus, whose consummate ability to heal signalled his divinity and leadership within his community.[46] Hence the strength of belief in the efficacy of singing the psalms. Novices entering the Order after around 1585 would have had a further reminder of this in the form of a fresco in the church of the royal author of the psalms singing to his harp.

Following his opening salvo in which the novice is shown in no uncertain terms who his role model should be, Spada's instructions to novices further serve to illustrate the primary focus on religious devotion in relation to care of the sick. The demand to be often in the choir is second only to the requirement not to leave the house without permission and come immediately before instructions regarding work in the hospital. While the choir was a physical space in the church, it seems clear from the context of further instruction to sing the psalms devoutly that he means not just being in the location but also singing.

> Active life without the contemplative one is like a body with no soul. That is why our founder wanted to bind each other together in his institute; so that

45 The Latin quote is a corrupt version of the Vulgate, not 1 Kings but 1 Samuel 17:17–18. 'Dixit autem Isai ad David filium suum: Accipe fratribus tuis ephi polentæ, et decem panes istos, et curre in castra ad fratres tuos, et decem formellas casei has deferes ad tribunum: et fratres tuos visitabis, si recte agant': ('Now Jesse said to his son David, "Take this ephah of roasted grain and these ten loaves of bread for your brothers and hurry to their camp. Take along these ten cheeses to the commander of their unit. See how your brothers are and bring back some assurance from them."') The remainder of the original reads, 'Tal Ordine fu dato al giovinetto David dal suo padre Isai allora che gl'altri figliuoli maggiori si trovavano nel campo con il Re Saul guerreggiando contro i filistei. Obbedì David con sollecita puntualità al paterno commando, andossene [andarsene] al campo, compi co' fratelli quanto doveva': ASR-OSS 47. Spada, 'Brevi regoli o capi di avvertimento per li novizii...' in *Stato della Casa,* f192.

46 The genealogy of Jesus is given in Matthew 1:1–16, a lineage confirmed in Luke 2:4.

> with the active one we committed ourselves to our fellow creatures, and with the contemplative one we committed ourselves to God through service of his church, being engaged in sacred functions, and in Divine Office, singing psalms, and singing to the Lord, about which Saint Bernard said: 'Whoever faithfully and with an intent mind sings the psalms, is in a way associated with the angels of God: because in his singing he adores Him inwardly, whom the angels glorify in heaven.'[47] Our novices therefore, in order to have such blessed comfort, will not fail to attend the choir at the appointed time, however, those who will be priests, or are going to take Orders, therefore with modesty and care, will recite the Divine Office; and should some of them be busy with some occupation, he must inform his Master, not to lose the merit of obedience. And they will not leave the choir, even if called, without informing the Prior.[48]

Spada's juxtaposition of the active and contemplative life echoes a common humanist, even Neo-Platonic view. In so doing he cements his own position in favour of music as an essential part of the daily life of the Hospital, directing the mind, even if the body is busy. Singing in the choir reinvigorates those who committed to actively serving the sick and the poor.

The focus on devout psalming that is documented over a sustained period of time leaves no doubt that the intention, at least in the earlier iterations, reflects a desire of the Order to align themselves with those promoted by the Church Fathers. The ideals however seem to have been eroded over time. In the next chapter, a key text concerning Church music in the sixteenth century penned by a commendatore of the Hospital of Santo Spirito is the vehicle for exploring music within the hospital community in greater depth.

47 The quote is from Bernard of Clairvaux, *Liber de Bono Vivendi ad Sororem*, cap LII, De Psalmis & Hymnis, *Opera omnia* (Paris, 1839), vol. 2. p. 346.

48 'La vita attiva senza la Contemplativa è come un corpo senza anima. Di qui è che il nostro fondatore nel suo instituto volle unire insieme l'una coll'altra; acciò con l'attiva ci impiegassimo in beneficio degl'Infermi nostri prossimi, e con la contemplativa portassimo in Dio per mezzo del servigio della sua Chiesa, occupandoci nelle sacre funtioni, e ne' Divini officij, salmeggiando, e cantando al Signore, del che disse San Bernardo: quicumque fideliter, et intenta menta psalmos decantat, quodammodo Angelis Dei sociatur: quia pro modulo suo illum laudat interius, quem Angeli glorificant in Caelis. Li nostri novitij dunque per haver così beato il confortio non mancheranno di frequentare il Choro nel tempo destinato; quelli però, che saranno sacerdoti, o iniziati negli ordini, accio con modestia, et attentione recitino li Divini offitij: e se alcuno di loro fosse trattenuto da qualche occupatione ne faccia avisato il Maestro, per non perdere il merito della obbedienza. Né dal Choro partiranno anche essendo chiamati senza farne segno al Priore': ASR-OSS 47 Spada, *Stato della Casa*, p. 302.

4

Bernardino da Cirillo: the Impact of Humanism and Reform

Bernardino da Cirillo is known to musicologists as the author of a letter that has featured in studies on the reform of liturgical music following the Council of Trent.[1] While the letter is significant in the context of Tridentine musical reform, existing musicological readings, to some extent, reflect a binary perception of religious thought of the sixteenth century, positioning it in relation to the Reformation versus Counter-Reformation, or humanist versus Catholic. Its position as a critique of polyphonic Church music is emphasised as a significant precursor or influence on Tridentine reform, especially with regard to the networks within Church hierarchies to which Cirillo was connected that might have been sympathetic to musical reform.

Cirillo was a key figure in the history of the Hospital of Santo Spirito. His tenure as commendatore of the Hospital (1556–1575) was one of the longest and most stable periods of leadership in the institution, and coincided with the period in which some of the significant changes instigated by the Council of Trent were enacted. It is surprising therefore that the music emanating from

1 Lewis Lockwood incorrectly refers to him as Bishop Cirillo Franco, a mistaken identity arising from a 'Defence of modern music against the views of Bishop Cirilo Franco', ostensibly by John IV of Portugal and published in 1649. The Defence was translated into Italian. Lewis H. Lockwood, 'Vincenzo Ruffo and Musical Reform after the Council of Trent', *The Musical Quarterly*, 43:3 (1957), 342–371. Lockwood provides an almost complete translation in the Norton Critical Score, Lewis Lockwood (ed.), *Giovanni Pierluigi da Palestrina, Pope Marcellus Mass* (New York, 1975). The details of Cirillo's networks and the identity of the recipient are explored in Claude V. Palisca, 'Bernardino da Cirillo's Critique of Polyphonic Church Music of 1549: Its Background and Resonance', in Jessie Ann Owens and M. A. Cummings (eds), *Music in Renaissance Cities and Courts: Studies in Honor of Lewis Lockwood* (Warren, MI, 1997), pp. 282–292; 'The Humanist Reaction to Polyphony', in Palisca (ed.), *Music and Ideas in the Sixteenth and Seventeenth Centuries* (Champaign, IL, 2006). More recently a new critical reading of the various versions of the letter is given in Chiara Bertoglio, *Reforming Music: Music and the Religious Reformations of the Sixteenth Century* (Berlin and Boston, 2018) and Chiara Bertoglio, 'Cats, Bulls and Donkeys: Bernardino Cirillo on 16th-Century Church Music', *Early Music*, 45:4 (2017). Bertoglio's transcription and translation in the latter collates the available printed and manuscript versions of the letter, and is therefore recommended as a point of reference for this chapter.

and performed in the Hospital of Santo Spirito, an organisation over which he had charge for a significant period, and where he could dictate roles and expectations of music and musicians, has never been fully explored. Further, the letter has never been situated within the context of Cirillo's other writings nor a broader view of his aesthetic considered.

Cirillo in the context of early modern Catholicism

Cirillo's early career no doubt shaped his views about music. He was born in Aquila in 1500 to a family of humble background but was able to pursue his studies thanks to the financial support of a local merchant.[2] The death of both his parents left him to care for his family, forcing him to change career path to pursue the priesthood, obtaining a chaplaincy with a small stipend. In spite of the change of direction in his career, he continued to immerse himself in reading philosophy – Plato, Plotinus, Ficino, Pico della Mirandola and so on. Thanks to the income from his benefices, he was able to return to his studies in Rome and graduated 'decretorum doctor' in 1526. He became archpriest of the Santa Casa di Loreto in 1535 where he stayed for eighteen years. The election of Giovanni Pietro Carafa to the papacy in 1555 as Paul IV opened the way for the appointment of Carlo Carafa as cardinal in the same year. The Carafa family had connections with Aquila, as the pope's mother came from that town. Cirillo was invited to Rome to take up a position in the Cancelleria Apostolica. He subsequently became canon of Santa Maria Maggiore and then in 1556 was nominated by Paul IV to take the position of commendatore at the Hospital of Santo Spirito.

His leadership at Santo Spirito was closely scrutinised by Apostolic Visitations. In 1571, for example, he submitted a report that outlined the poor state of some of the structures and the restorations and improvements he had instructed to be carried out.[3] On his directive, unsafe structures were demolished and rebuilt, the Sistine wards were renovated and work was started on constructing the palazzo to house the commendatore and administrative offices.[4] Cirillo emerged from the Apostolic scrutiny unscathed, continuing in the post until his death in June 1575. He was buried in the church of S. Spirito and

[2] According to his own account, by the age of fourteen he 'took the clerical habit and tonsure and went to study law.' *Epistolario all'Aquila* I p. 393, cited in http://www.treccani.it/enciclopedia/bernardino-cirillo_(Dizionario-Biografico)/ (accessed 07/02/2020).

[3] V-CVbav Ottob. Lat. 2473, fols.179–204, *Relatione della fabrica e casa di S. Spirito di Roma* (1571).

[4] A chronological list of Cirillo's building work is provided in Flavia Colonna, *L'Ospedale di Santo Spirito a Roma: lo sviluppo dell'assistenza e le trasformazioni architettonico-funzionali* (Rome, 2009), pp. 143–147.

his name added to the martyrology of the Order of Santo Spirito for constant prayer and memorial.[5]

Although his career path took him into the Church, Cirillo was at heart a man of letters whose early humanist studies had a significant impact on his life. As O'Malley, Fillipi and others have shown, humanism was not anti-Catholic nor anti-religious.[6] Humanist scholarship included new investigations of the Church Fathers and their relationship to classical antiquity. The subjects of Cirillo's writings bear out a dual interest in classical philosophy and the early Church, especially in Christian Neo-Platonism. Cirillo was a prolific letter writer, and it is from these that we know that he wrote a number of books that have not survived, including one on the mystic theology of the Christian Neo-Platonist Dionysius the Aeropagite (also known as Pseudo-Dionysius), a reduction in verse of Pico della Mirandola's *De ente et uno*, plays on the story of Job and *Pianto della Virgine*, moral tracts and eulogies for famous men.[7]

Given that training for the priesthood would have been based on scholastic theology, it seems likely that Cirillo's interest in Pseudo-Dionysius, at least initially, would have been filtered through the writings of Thomas Aquinas. Aquinas' *Commentary on the Divine Names* and the early treatise *De pulchro et bono*, attributed to him, but likely to be by Albertus Magnus, on the beautiful and good were influenced by commentaries on Pseudo-Dionysius. These texts suggest that Aquinas held the opinion that beauty was a transcendental, that is, a constant property of being, characterised by clarity, integrity and proportion.[8] In the real universe all beauty is good: 'Beauty, like the good, is grounded upon form, but form is the reason why something has actuality, so is good for its own sake'.[9] In his *Summa Theologica* Aquinas deals more with the psychological and subjective aspects of beauty. Cirillo's distinct desire for clarity and fitness for purpose comes from Aquinas.

Cirillo's interest in Pseudo-Dionysius and early Christianity would also have intersected with the interests of his friend Fillipo Neri. Neri's Oratorians were among those investigating the early history of the Church as part of the reform

5 ASR-OSS 72, fol. 53.

6 J. W. O'Malley, 'Early Modern Catholicism: The State of Research', in D. V. Fillipi and M. Noone (eds), *Listening to Early Modern Catholicism* (Leiden, 2017), pp. 21–34; and O'Malley, *Trent and all that: Renaming Catholicism in the Early Modern Era* (Cambridge, MA, 2000).

7 Cirillo's treatise on the shrine of the Madonna of Loreto has survived. *Trattato sopra l'historia della santa chiesa et casa della gloriosa Madonna Maria Vergine di Loreto* (Venice, 1572). Although written in 1540, *Annali della città dell'Aquila con l'historia del suo tempo* was not published until 1570 (in Rome). Collections of letters survive in Aquila, Florence, Milan and in Rome in the Biblioteca Lancisiana. http://www.treccani.it/enciclopedia/bernardino-cirillo_(Dizionario-Biografico)/ (accessed 19/07/2017).

8 Umberto Eco, *The Aesthetics of Thomas Aquinas*, trans. Hugh Bredin ([Milan, 1970] n.p., 1988), p. 46.

9 Eco, *The Aesthetics of Thomas Aquinas*, p. 47.

movement. Oratorian Cesare Baronio's *Annales ecclesiastici* was one of the first major publications of early Church history and resulted in the Oratory becoming a centre for the study of the history of the Church – a history that set Catholicism apart from the Protestant movement, and endowed it with an inescapable ancestry that bolstered its authority. Rediscovery of the simple gatherings of early Christians in the catacombs provided an impetus to the style of worship observed by Neri's followers.[10]

Beyond the writings of the Church Fathers, Cirillo's humanist studies included philosophical texts from Plotinus and Plato to the more recent works of Ficino and Pico della Mirandola. While the only source he actually names in the 1549 letter is Plato's *Laws*, which he uses to underline the correct separation of musical genres for specific purposes, his identification of four modes rather than Plato's two is drawn from Aristotle's *Politics*. The additional descriptions of the affective character of the modes come from later sources such as Cassiodorus's *Variae epistolae* and were well known.[11]

Cirillo's wish that musicians would try to recover the art of antiquity in their profession in the way that sculptors, painters and architects had done; and his observation that all sciences had been 'brought back to purity' by going back to ideals of the past, seems less a desire for reform than to revive practices of the past that he deemed more effective and affective. The emotive power of music is absolutely central to the message of the letter, and is underlined by the rhetorical structure and persuasive 'tricks' he employs.

The letter of 1549

Cirillo's letter was printed by Aldo Manuzio without the author's permission and it survives in more than one version. The date of the letter according to the printed version was February 1549, but it was not published until 1564.[12] The manuscript copy in the Biblioteca Lancisiana is apparently of a later date than that assigned to it in the printed version, but is part of a large collection of Cirillo's letters. Palisca suggests that the manuscript is either an unreliable copy or a draft.[13] The survival rate of so many letters, normally ephemeral documents,

10 Anne Piéjus, 'Artistic Revival and Conquest of the Soul in Early Modern Rome', in Fillipi and Noone (eds), *Listening to Early Modern Catholicism*, pp. 149–172. Piéjus identifies the author of *Roma sotterranea* as Tommaso, but it was Antonio who was the author (see p. 152).

11 Palisca identified these sources and also noted the Cirillo used Ficino's translation of the *Laws*. Palisca, 'Bernardino da Cirillo's Critique', p. 288.

12 'Lettere volgari di diversi nobilissimi huomini et eccellentisimi ingegni, scritte in diverse materie' (Venice: [Aldo Manuzio] 1564), vol 3, fols 114r–118v; I-Rla Ms 338 (fols 7–10).

13 Palisca, 'Bernardino da Cirillo's Critique', p 284.

written by Cirillo, is evidence of a substantial corpus of correspondence. He was clearly a man who wrote to a wide variety of people on a diverse array of topics, but also retained copies for himself. His was an organised mind, with control over a great deal of information.

The addressee of the letter is Ugolino Gualteruzzi, although the copy in the Biblioteca Lancisiana is addressed to Ugolino Guastenezzo. As Gualteruzzi's father Carlo was one of the leaders of the reform movement in Rome, Palisca understood the letter to be a critique of polyphonic Church music of the mid-sixteenth century targeted at a network of men in a position to influence musical reforms. Its contents have resonances with other observations of Church music made by Erasmus, Cornelius Agrippa and Jacopo Sadoleto.[14] Chiara Bertoglio has more recently considered the letter within the wider context of reform in Church music and has suggested that it is not just about the music. She argues that Cirillo's positioning was also a critique about the outward splendour of the Church that had lost what mattered about spiritual things. In the same way as music should look to ancient models, the Church 'should and could recover the wisdom of old and thus hopefully reach new heights in its own art of sanctity'.[15] Further, she claims that within Cirillo's clever use of imagery, there is a hidden criticism of Pope Julius II.[16]

Bertoglio adds to the argument that Cirillo's views were critical in shaping the reform of Church music as carried out by Annibale Zoilo and Palestrina by suggesting that another of his letters, addressed to 'Messer Anibal', may well have been directed to Zoilo. In it, Cirillo refers back to his letter on Church music addressed to Gualteruzzi, stating that it was written twenty-five years previously.[17] He notes with pleasure that he was sent a Mass that conformed to what he was looking for because it showed the degree to which music could attract good Christians to devotion. Bertoglio's proposition seems highly likely, as the Zoilo family had close connections with the Hospital of Santo Spirito. Annibale's brother, Giovanni Domenico, was the maestro da casa (major-domo), and his son Cesare was to become one of the longest serving maestri di cappella there, from c. 1610.[18] Neither Bertoglio nor Lockwood mention a further letter

14 Palisca, 'Bernardino da Cirillo's Critique', p. 283.

15 Bertoglio, *Reforming Music*, pp. 161–163.

16 Bertoglio, 'Cats, Bulls and Donkeys', pp. 562–563.

17 On this basis Lockwood dates the letter to c. 1575. Given that Cirillo died in June 1575, I would suggest that Cirillo's statement that the letter was written twenty-five years previously is probably an approximate memory of an elderly man and a more cautious dating of between 1570–1575 should be adopted. The letter was published in Italian in De Angelis, *Musica e musicisti nell'arcispedale di Santo Spirito in Saxia dal quattrocento allo'ottocento* (Rome, 1950), pp. 44–45. Lockwood gives a partial translation in *Giovanni Pierluigi da Palestrina, Pope Marcellus Mass*, pp. 26–27.

18 In April 1578, following the death of Giovanni Domenico, Annibale was paid 34 scudi as he was deemed his heir, Giovanni Domenico having apparently died without testament. ASR-OSS 1904, *Copie di mandati* 1578 item 665.

also addressed to 'Annibale carissimo' preserved in the Lancisiana. This letter too refers to the music of the ancients and its power specifically to move the soul, and reads as an afterthought or postscript to a letter sent previously to the same addressee. In this third letter, Cirillo notes that he had forgotten to mention the specific example of Terpander, the famous singer from Lesbos who with his music and singing had calmed and rendered peaceful a rebellious crowd, such was the force and efficacy of music of that time.[19] The attention in all three letters on the effects of music on the human psyche places Cirillo's thought neatly within the framework of medical thinking about the agency of the passions of the soul, as well as within religious views on the matter.

One aspect of Cirillo's 1549 letter that has not been addressed in existing studies is how its structure relates to its content and potentially indicates how it was intended to be read. The form of the letter is a testament to Cirillo's humanist education and learning as it follows, with almost textbook precision, the structure of a classical oration as expounded by Cicero and Quintillian among others.[20] Bearing in mind the strong oral-aural traditions that continued throughout the early modern period, this letter may have been written deliberately in a way that lent itself to being read aloud. It is clear that Cirillo intended its contents to be passed on to others, and that may well have been by reading aloud. The letter assumes a considerable amount of knowledge about music of the time as well as knowledge of classical sources, making it suitable to be read to an educated audience, or indeed, from the point of view of the publisher, to be placed in a collection of letters that would appeal to a certain market of educated book collectors. The clarity of its structure and argument may well have been a reason for its inclusion in a collection of printed letters. Whether shared by audible or silent reading, Cirillo articulates his argument in a way that would be unambiguously understood by his audience, inviting him (or her) to come to the same conclusion through techniques of persuasion.

19 'Annibale Carissimo scordai dirve ne nell'altra mia che essendo nata gran' briga et seditione tra sacedemonii sicome referisce sui da Ebreo ricorso all' oracolo che havesse a farse accio venisse sedato tal tumulto e dissidio: fu alor' risposto che chiamassero un cantore dell'Isola di Lesbo: et fu chiamato un trapandro di quell' Isola il quale con la sua musica et col suo canto rese si dolci et placabili li animi de sacedemonii che subbito hor ridusse a pace et Concordia rimossa ogni seditione. Questa era la forza et efficacia grande dell'arte musica a quelli tempi. Piacciane de aggiungere questo esempio agli altri che già ne scrisse': I-Rla Ms 342 *Epistolario di Bernardino da Cirillo*, fol. 58r–58v, letter 142.

20 Key classical texts on rhetoric included: Cicero, *De Oratore* (2 vols), trans. E. W. Sutton, Loeb Classical Library (Cambridge, MA, 1976 (1st edn 1942); Quintillian, *The Orator's education* (*Institutio oratoria*), 3 vols, trans. Donald A. Russell, Loeb Classical Library (Cambridge, MA, 2001); Pseudo-Cicero, *Ad Herennium*, trans. Henry Caplan, Loeb Classical Library (Cambridge, MA, 1989 (1st edn 1954). For a general background on the importance of rhetoric in the early modern world, see especially Brian Vickers, *In Defence of Rhetoric* (Oxford, 1988).

Following a textbook exordium, Cirillo states his case about the efficacy of the music of the ancient Greeks in moving the passions of the soul in a classic *expositio*. Although the only source acknowledged by Cirillo comes later in the letter, by placing this point in such a prominent position within the rhetorical structure, he indicates that it is key to the argument that follows. Having made his point about the power of ancient music, Cirillo immediately contrasts it with the weakness of modern Church music. It is worth noting that he does not criticise the music he identifies from the viewpoint of an aesthetic judgement of absolute beauty, but because it is inappropriate for its purpose and fails to move the affections. He continues by praising secular dance music, which he claims is effective and therefore good because at the sound of a pavane or galliard, the 'good women' all start to move.

Although reaching back to antiquity to bolster his argument, Cirillo's aesthetic judgement betrays the filter of Thomist scholastic views. For Aquinas, beauty consists in integrity or perfection, proportion and clarity, but ultimately these are measured against fitness for purpose. There is no suggestion that Cirillo was concerned that an emotional response to the sensuousness of the music was a problem, which is what bothered Augustine. Instead, he bemoans the lack of any response to the music, that it doesn't move the affections or inspire devotion.

Having presented his argument against modern Church music, Cirillo then outlines what he sees as desirable in Church music, followed by a clarification of what he is not arguing for. These paragraphs present a synthesis of his understanding of the classical sources as well as the contemporary situation. Once again, the touchstone is the way in which music affects the passions of the soul. First, he wants musical settings of texts that draw on the power of modal affects to move the listener to piety. Then he rejects the complexities of the chromatic and diatonic harmonies that he claims were abandoned by the ancients. The rejection of diatonic harmonies seems out of place here, and it seems likely that he may have misunderstood the three ancient genera – the diatonic, chromatic and enharmonic – and intended to reject the complex enharmonic rather than diatonic music.

At the point at which Cirillo appears to be reaching a conclusion, but which is not yet at the end of the letter, he finally makes his request to the recipient clear, articulating the actions he wishes him to take, first to talk to good musicians and second to make the letter's contents known to a third person. By echoing the self-deprecating tone of the exordium, Cirillo asserts his subservience to Gualteruzzi, placing him in the position to choose to act on his suggestions or not. It is here that Cirillo names the person who he really wants the letter to go to – Signor Beccadello, who Palisca identified as Lodovico Beccadelli (1501–1577).[21] Only after identifying Beccadelli does he emphatically convey

[21] Palisca, 'Bernardino da Cirillo's Critique', p. 286. Beccadelli was a friend of Ugolino Gualteruzzi's father, Carlo, and a secretary to the Council of Trent.

his goal to 'let our church with its deeds move to religion and piety', underlining it with further reference to ancient authority. Only now does he identify a classical source – Plato's *Laws* – and presents a paraphrase of a section of that work. If generic references to the music of the ancients were not sufficient to sway his reader, the 'big guns' in the form of a highly esteemed ancient text would drive his point home.

The peroration reverts to a lighter tone, referring to an Arcadelt madrigal, which offers another fixed chronological point of reference for the music to which Cirillo refers.[22] It also provides further evidence that Cirillo was not against either modern music, or secular music, but wanted the affective and effective qualities of that music to be put to greater purpose. The positioning of the most crucial points of the letter inside a carefully fashioned frame in which Cirillo denies his expertise in the topic but at the same time uses well-known classical sources to bolster his point of view makes his argument powerful and impersonal. His rhetorical skill focuses the argument: to replace complicated, corrupt Church music with music that moves the affects for the sake of the spiritual health of the Church.

The rhetorical gesture suggesting inadequacy in the opening statement, and the invitation to the reader to 'read in it more than he can write' positions the writer in such a way as to excuse 'clumsiness' of thought and express 'subservience' to the reader. While it suggests a difference in status between sender and recipient, the writer is artfully aware of making his intention understood without violating those social boundaries. Cirillo's self-deprecating statement about his position as 'a layman and an ignoramus' with regard to music places the onus on the recipient to understand his point. It is evident from the range of Cirillo's commentary though, that while he may not have been a practising musician, his thinking on the subject is well-developed and coherent, and his reader would no doubt have realised this.

Cirillo's opening gambit is to suggest that he has been thinking about the topic for some years but has been unable to articulate his thoughts. If we take this statement literally, it would suggest that the document outlines a position that the author has developed over a period of years prior to 1549. Towards the end of the letter, Cirillo says that 'it is twenty years since these ideas entered [his] brain'. This time frame is posited in passages directly addressed to the reader; thus, the recipient is expected to understand exactly the kind of music targeted. If we assume that the date assigned to the letter in the printed version

22 The madrigal 'Chi mi tiene il mio ben' does not exist, but Calcagno suggests that Cirillo probably confused the text with 'Ahimé dov'è il ben viso' from Arcadelt's *Primo libro di madrigali à 4*, printed in Venice in 1539, the last line of which reads *Dov'è il ben mio che più non mi risponde*. Mauro Calcagno, *From Madrigal to Opera: Monteverdi's Staging of the Self* (Berkeley, Los Angeles, CA, and London, 2012), p. 120. Calcagno's argument is that Cirillo unconsciously perceived what he calls subject-effects communicated through specific musical techniques that were foundational for Monteverdi's style.

is correct, the music which triggered his criticism is that of the period of his youth, c. 1500–c. 1545. However, the two letters addressed to 'Messer Annibal' in the early 1570s suggests that the power of music, and more particularly the right kind of music, was an issue that continued to concern him, even towards the end of his life.

The significance of the passions

Bertoglio's view, that Cirillo's focus in the letter on the emotional effects of music relates to a bigger picture about Church reform, is further bolstered if the connections between the passions and health are taken into consideration. As noted in Chapter 2, music was deemed a powerful means of healing that induced movement of the bodily humours though movement of the passions of the soul. This notion seems to lie at the heart of much of Cirillo's text. While Cirillo does not engage directly with notions of cure of body or soul, the status of music as a curative was so well known that it did not need to be spelled out. Understood in this way, Church music that moves the passions as advocated by Cirillo was medicine for the soul – the means through which erring, sinful humanity could be returned to piety and devotion and thus to spiritual health that in turn would cure the body.

Comparing the results of modern studies of emotion in music with Cirillo's descriptions and criticisms, we can perhaps question whether it was the performance of religious music that was the cause of his complaint, or the substance of the compositions themselves. Modern studies separate represented emotion from induced emotion. Represented emotion is signalled by a range of expressive cues within the music that includes tempo, dynamic range, articulation, vibrato, timbre and so on. Induced emotion is what the listener feels in response to music. One study of induced emotion concluded that listeners responded with five basic emotions – tenderness, happiness, sadness, fear and anger.[23] These are essentially the basic emotions recognised in antiquity and transmitted in sources that would have been familiar to Cirillo.

Cirillo expressed no criticism of dance music, but his point that at the *sound* of these, women started to dance, suggests something about the way in which the music was performed that induced a response. Perhaps he was implying that the performers were more invested in conveying the positive emotions of the dance than Church musicians were, or, that he was aware of the music of pulse in the Galenic sense, and that dance music connected with, and was in correct proportion to, the human pulse, and was therefore more effective. His separation of dance music from Church music raises another question about the effective representation of emotion in instrumental music for dance, as

[23] Patrik N. Juslin, 'Communicating Emotion in Music Performance: A Review and Theoretical Framework', in Patrik N. Juslin and John A. Sloboda, *Music and Emotion: Theory and Research* (Oxford, 2001), pp. 309–337, esp. p. 315.

opposed to the quality of vocal music in church, that for him, failed to induce emotion. If he had been exposed to poorly trained clergy who were unable to sing chant correctly, or to undisciplined and badly trained choirs attempting to sing polyphony, it would hardly be surprising if he was left unmoved by the music. Might we read into his comments that as well as being dissatisfied with the musical substance of Church music, that its performance was also generally poor? In other words, it neither represented nor induced emotion effectively.

The flipside of effective representation of emotion lies with the listener. While human beings have not physiologically changed since Cirillo's day, our social conditioning has, and thus the ways in which we listen to music cannot be assumed to be the same as it was five hundred years ago. We cannot, therefore, equate modern emotional responses to music with what would have been deemed appropriate responses to music in the sixteenth century.[24] Cirillo's position indicates the early modern belief that hearing was a direct channel to the passions of the soul, and suggests a listening habitus shaped by the public or monastic experience of the sacred. The concept of *recte sentire*, the correct listening or understanding that would emerge in the decades following the Catholic Reformation seems to be in play here already, but in a way that harks back to antiquity.

Although citing well-known narratives from classical antiquity, Cirillo would have been reading the ancient accounts through the lens of his own time. His understanding of the concept of affect would have been constructed by sixteenth-century social and linguistic meanings. As a Church man, Cirillo's starting point was no doubt the Church's view on the passions of the soul. Broadly, this was based on Aristotle as elaborated by Augustine and Thomas Aquinas: there was one immortal soul which was divided into three parts – the intellectual or rational, the animal or sensitive (which governed sense perception and appetites) and the vegetative or nutritive (which governed growth and generation). Music appealed to the animal or sensual soul, but intersected with the rational and intellectual. It was on this basis that Augustine appreciated the beauty of Church music as a powerful means of drawing people in, in order for them to then focus on and absorb the meaning of the words conveyed by the music. The emotional trajectory moved from mere sensuous beauty towards the contemplation of the divine. Perhaps the state of mind which Cirillo saw as a desirable outcome for religious music was a parallel to the internalisation and emotional engagement with the experience of saints and martyrs that featured in new devotional exercises, such as those of Ignatius Loyola, that were emerging around the same time.

[24] See Bettina Varwig, *Music in the Flesh: An Early Modern Musical Physiology* (Cambridge, 2023) for discussion of physiological responses to music; and Michael Schwarz, 'Bodies of Transcendence: The Spirit of Affect in Giotto and Piero', in Penelope Gouk and Helen Hills (eds), *Representing Emotions: New Connections in the Histories of Art, Music and Medicine* (Aldershot, 2005), pp. 69–87, for responses to painting.

Cirillo's experience of music as foundation of critique

If the intention of the letter was either to critique polyphony or to try and influence reform of Church music, it raises the question as to what kind of music Cirillo was being exposed to in the churches over which he presided as priest and bishop. He graduated in 1526, thus his formative years coincided with the early years of Lutheran reform. It seems unlikely that he would have avoided debates about reform or have been unaware of the emergence of congregational singing. In contrast to poorly performed polyphony, simple homophonic hymns delivering a text syllabically and conveying a single affect may well have held some attraction. The similarity between Protestant hymns and the laude that had re-emerged as an instrument of reform for the followers of Savonarola in Florence during the 1490s may also have influenced the direction of Cirillo's argument. The Savonarola episode was surely in recent memory during the period in which Cirillo was studying in Rome.

Two of the polyphonic masses named in the letter, *L'homme armé,* and *Hercules Dux Ferrariae* suggest that it was the style of Josquin that Cirillo objected to, although *L'homme armé* was so famous, there were a number of Masses based on it that might be equally likely candidates. The reference to *La Filomena* is probably to the Mass on a motet of that name by Richafort. Taken together, the three titles capture broadly the Franco-Flemish style of polyphony dominant in the first decades of the sixteenth century as the target of his criticism.

Following his studies, Cirillo's appointments at Loreto and at Santa Maria Maggiore in Rome would have exposed him to diverse types of liturgical and devotional music. However, the latter post-dated the indicative date of the letter, thus could not have influenced its contents. His appointment to the position of archpriest of Loreto in 1535 may well have played a part in shaping his views, as he would have been exposed to a different range of musical experiences and practices than those of his student years in Rome.

During the sixteenth century, the shrine of Loreto became an increasingly popular destination for pilgrims of all classes. The devotions of ordinary folk, expressed in music in the form of sung laude and Litanies were no doubt part of the soundscape of this environment. Cirillo's desire to rid the liturgy of complex music may have been reinforced by witnessing the devotion of ordinary people singing simple songs and Litanies. Communal singing, whether modern football anthems or ancient hymns, functions as a uniting force for a social group. The communal singing of simple, repetitive laude, whether sung within confraternities or in the context of specific Marian devotions inspired devotion, piety and penitence.

Laude and Litanies were both expressions of traditions that were deeply oral in origin but that emerged into more fixed, written and, in the sixteenth century, printed, forms. Kendrick has noted that the Litany is a striking example of the interaction between orality and print in early modern devotional practices. There was a profusion of Litany texts in the sixteenth century with over a hundred non-musical prints of texts between 1520–1600. This quantity of source material is not matched by written sources for the chant formula as it was not usually included in antiphoners or graduals. The assumption has to be made that the printers of the texts took for granted that their target audience would have known, and been able to sing, the chant formula.[25]

A parallel to the unwritten chant formula of the Litany can be found in the lauda repertory in the shape of the 'cantasi come' tradition of singing a text to an existing melody, often a secular song. Fitting words to existing music meant that specific poetic structures, often with repeating refrains, were commonly used. The ballata predominated in the thirteenth century but later gave way to the strambotto or barzaletta in the fifteenth century. Like Litanies, the texts of such laude could be transmitted without the need for music. While laude had been the vehicle for Savanarola's public displays of piety in Florence in the late fifteenth century, they were not new then, but found a new outlet in the Dominican friar's attempts at reform. These songs did not disappear with his death. It is not coincidental that new publications of laude appeared in the 1560s triggered by the Tridentine drive for reform.[26]

If Cirillo did not hear laude in the popular devotions at the Santa Casa in Loreto, he would certainly have heard them in Rome as he was a friend of Fillipo Neri. During Cirillo's tenure at the Hospital, Neri was a frequent visitor. He carried out nursing duties in the hospital wards, shaving the beards and washing the feet of patients and making and cleaning beds, overcoming his own fastidiousness about personal hygiene and natural aversions in order to care for the poor and sick. It is also recorded that Cirillo requested Pope Pius V to relieve him of his duties as commendatore and to have Neri take over. Neri refused the honour because for him caring for the sick was just one of the duties of the members of the Oratory (Congregazione dell'Oratorio).[27] Neri's close association with Cirillo raises the question as to whether there was a mutual influence regarding their views on music. Laude were central to the Oratorians' devotions. The easily remembered laude melodies were an ideal medium for the devotional sung prayers of the Oratorians as evidenced by Animuccia's *Primo libro delle laudi spirituali* printed in 1563 for Neri's gather-

25 Robert Kendrick, 'Orality and Sacred Music', in Stefano dall'Aglio, Brian Richardson and Massimo Rosprocher (eds), *Voices and Texts in Early Modern Italian Society* (London and New York, 2017), pp. 229–240, esp. pp. 232–233.

26 There is a considerable literature on the lauda, notably Blake Wilson, *Music and Merchants: The Laudesi Companies of Republican Florence* (Oxford, 1992); Patrick Macey, *Bonfire Songs: Savanarola's Musical Legacy* (Oxford, 1998); Jonathan Glixon, *Honoring God and the City: Music at Venetian Confraternities, 1260–1807* (Oxford, 2003); Giancarlo Rostirolla, Danilo Zardin and Oscar Mischiati, *La lauda spirituale tra cinque e seicento* (Rome, 2001).

27 Alessandro Canezza, *Gli arcispedali di Roma nella vita cittadina nella storia e nell'arte* (Rome, 1933), pp. 103–104.

ings, and which reuses a number of Florentine lauda melodies.[28] The syllabic text-settings, narrow range and stepwise movement of the laude melodies and Animuccia's homophonic reimagining of them result in highly understandable delivery of the texts – texts which in themselves comprise nuggets of doctrine ordered in a repetitive structure.

In contrast, during his tenure at Santa Maria Maggiore in the mid-1550s, Cirillo may well have experienced high-quality polyphonic music on feast days and special celebrations. While his tenure there was brief, post-dating the 1549 letter and therefore irrelevant to its content, Santa Maria Maggiore offers a useful point of comparison with the Hospital of Santo Spirito. Both institutions had close ties to the papacy and enjoyed the benefit of reciprocal borrowing of singers from the papal choirs for the celebration of major feast days. There is also parity in the surviving records as to the date of the first documentation of financial support for the cappella musicale at Santa Maria is 1545, just five years prior to the earliest surviving records for Santo Spirito. The first securely dated documents relating to expenditure for acquiring music date from 1557 and those indicating the presence of instrumentalists from 1581. An inventory of 1624 listing volumes of music in comparison to surviving archival sources allows us a view of what music is likely to have been performed in the basilica in the latter part of the sixteenth century.[29] Perhaps not unexpectedly, the list is dominated by books by Palestrina, Morales, Victoria, Animuccia and composers with close ties to the papal choirs. As will be seen, there are a number of parallels with Santo Spirito.

Cirillo at Santo Spirito: reputation, music, documents

By the time Cirillo arrived at Santo Spirito in 1556, there was at least one long-established tradition that involved music – the processions that formed part of the liturgical celebrations of specific feast days. Although there is nothing in the Rule instructing the members of the Order to celebrate certain feasts with processions or other devotional activities, a general gathering of the Chapter overseeing activities is called for at Pentecost, the feast day of the Order. There is also iconographic evidence of the exposition of young women, referred to as *zitelle,* wishing to take advantage of the offer of a dowry to be married respectably into the community. A fresco in the Corsia Sistina dating to c. 1480 shows an orderly group of young women processing and kneeling in front of the pope to be blessed and to receive gifts.[30] This image, along with another minia-

28 Piéjus, 'Artistic revival', p. 155.

29 Luca Della Libera, 'Repertori ed organici vocali-strumentali nella basilica di Santa Maria Maggiore a Roma, 1557–1624', *Studi Musicali*, XXXIX (2000), 3–58.

30 Howe offers various readings as to the exact date of completion of the hospital building and its decoration. Eunice Howe, *The Hospital of Santo Spirito and Pope Sixtus IV*, PhD, Johns Hopkins University, 1977, *Outstanding Dissertations in the Fine Arts* (New York and London, 1978), pp. 54–56.

ture in an illuminated copy of the Rule dating from the fifteenth century, confirms that it was a long-standing tradition, and it was one that continued until the early eighteenth century when it was supressed after the Apostolic Visitation by Cardinal Leandro Porzia in 1737.[31] The procession of these women took place three times a year on the feast days of St Anthony the Great in January, St Mark in April and most importantly, at Pentecost, seven weeks after Easter.[32]

We know from first-hand accounts that these processions were grand affairs. The Venetian diarist Marin Sanudo recorded his observations of the procession at Pentecost in 1519. He noted the richness of the clothing, the jewels, the canopy of the clerics and the mules carrying the bridal goods, all preceded by 'players of many instruments of music'.[33] Sadly, he did not describe the music, but it is perhaps worth noting that he mentioned instruments but not singers. The group was apparently large enough to make a splendid visual impression.

The English priest Gregory Martin who lived in Rome between 1576–1578, thus coinciding with the end of Cirillo's tenure, described a procession for the feast of St Mark in which the musicians, orphans, young women and clerics of Santo Spirito took part.

> First, they of the great Hospital of S Spirito, which from they infancie are brought up there of almes, as i wil tell hereafter and these of diverse sortes. Of little ones that were carried by men and wemen 100. Boyes that could go alone two and two 61 Girles that did the like (their nurces byside them) 150. Young maydens marriable 70 the whole 381, al in blewe garded by the Popes Swicers byside the quyer which were 20 and the nurces which I number note. Last of this trayne came the principal of the house in blacke, and a great white Crosse upon hys brest, called the grand Prior or commendatore of Santo Spirito.[34]

Martin's account is supported by the financial records that note the payments to the Swiss Guards and to additional priests. It is from the pay records too, that we can build a picture, albeit one lacking in detail, of the men who provided the music on a day-to-day basis for the church and hospital.

31 ASR OSS 3193, f. 49r. http://www.cflr.beniculturali.it/Preziosi/preziosi.php?lar=1600&alt=900.

32 De Angelis in *Musica e musicisti*, p. 17, identifies the January procession as taking place on the Sunday after the Octave of Epiphany. Although in later sources the day is referred to as the feast of St Antony, the procession was originally part of a 'Holy Station' – a privilege given to the Hospital by Innocent III. Pietro De Angelis, *L'Ospedale di S. Spirito dalle origini al 1500*, 2 vols. Collana di Studi Storici sull'Ospedale di Santo Spirito in Saxia e sugli Ospedali Romani (Rome, 1960; 1962), vol. 1, p. 225.

33 '... avanti li muli andavano suonatori di tanti strumenti di musica': *I diarii di Marino Sanuto: (MCCCCXCVI-MDXXXIII) dall' autografo Marciano ital. cl. VII codd* (Padua, 1890), p. 469.

34 Gregory Martin, *Roma Sancta* (1581), ed. George Bruner Parks (Rome, 1969), p. 84.

The musicians

Cirillo was appointed to the position of commendatore of the Hospital in 1556. The financial records of payments to musicians at the time are not systematic, thus groupings of singers need to be reconstructed from individual entries. Allegra and De Angelis note some of the names of these musicians, and Rostirolla has collated their information into a chronological list.[35] However, none of these scholars has evaluated that information in terms of what music these musicians might have provided; if they were employed concurrently, thus suggesting the size of the ensemble; or if they were employed casually and went from church to church as required.

The earliest surviving financial records from the Hospital are volumes of copies of pay slips, known as *mandati,* dating from 1551. The *mandati* for 1555, the year before Cirillo was appointed commendatore, provide a certain amount of information about what kind of music may have been sung. At this time there was no named maestro di cappella, but there was a regular organist, Vincenzo Ferro. Ferro was paid 28 scudi for fourteen months service in a single payment in May of that year, pushing the starting date of his service back to at least the middle of 1554.[36]

Payments to singers were haphazard, but at least two, Costanzo da Perugia and Luca da Gubbio, were paid more or less monthly while others appear in the lists on odd occasions but are paid for several months' service, for example, Paulo Pisano (or Paulo da Pisa) was paid twice for three months' service each time, and Benedetto da Rocca Contrada, a bass, received at least three payments for varying periods of service. Several other singers were paid for two or three months at a time, and thus appear less frequently in the records, though in reality they were probably present alongside the three who were paid more regularly. Antonio Veneziano for example, received nine months' salary in one payment.[37] These scattered records indicate that there was a choir of four or five voices. In the first half of the year, it was staffed by Costanzo da Perugia, Luca da Gubbio, Antonio Veneziano and Paulo Pisano. In the second half of the year, Antonio and Paulo are not recorded but some new names appear instead: Antonio

35 Antonio Allegra, 'La cappella musicale di S. Spirito in Saxia di Roma: appunti storici (1551–1737)', *Note d'archivio,* 17 (1940), 26–38; Pietro De Angelis, *Musica e musicisti nell'arcispedale di Santo Spirito in Saxia dal quattrocento allo'ottocento,* Collana di studi storici sull'Ospedale di Santo Spirito in Saxia e sugli ospedali romani (Rome, 1950); Giancarlo Rostirolla, 'L'Archivio musicale della chiesa annessa all'ospedale di Santo Spirito', *Il Veltro,* XLV:5–6 (2002), 279–343. There are omissions and errors in all three articles.

36 ASR OSS 1894, *Copie di mandati,* 1555, item 1084. Rostirolla notes Ferro's service as 1551 and 1557–1559. With this additional information, it seems highly likely that he was employed for most of the 1550s.

37 ASR OSS 1894, *Copie di mandati,* 1555, item 5026.

da Brescia who was only paid for one month, Benedetto da Rocca Contrada, and Geronimo da Napoli who were both paid for three months.

Alongside the named singers there was also a group of chaplains whose service seems to have been similarly fluid. These clerics would presumably have been able to sing plainchant if nothing else, but the clear separation of singer (*cantore*) from chaplain (*cappellano*) in the financial records perhaps indicates those who were professionals, as distinct from the chaplains who were probably friars in the Order. The singers and chaplains were all paid 75 baiocchi per month – a small salary and considerably less than the 2 scudi paid to the organist each month, perhaps signifying that he was present in lieu of the choir for many of the Masses, or that the singers were working on a very part-time basis. From this scattered information, we can assume that there would have been a group of singers providing sufficient forces to sing four- or five-voice polyphony, not forgetting that the school may have provided boy sopranos. This does not mean that they did sing polyphony at all services, just that the resources were available when it was required.

Similar forces remained in place in the early years of Cirillo's tenure. In the records for 1557, both Luca da Gubbio and Costanzo da Perugia were still the most regularly paid singers, joined by Geronimo da Napoli, Ventura da Fermo and Antonio Bresciano, a bass. The regular organist was Lodovico da Correggio, and the organ was clearly well-maintained as there are payments to 'Agustino organista' for repairing the bellows and for tuning the instrument.[38]

If we compare the list of names from 1555 to those in the pay records for 1557, it is evident that some of the singers that apparently disappeared were instead going for longer periods without payment, and then received a larger lump-sum payment. Costanzo da Perugia, Luca da Gubbio, Antonio Veneziano, Geronimo da Napoli and the bass Antonio da Brescia (or Bresciano) were all still present, along with Ventura da Fermo. Irregular payments are made to them, sometimes only for a single month at 75 baiocchi, sometimes for two or three months with payments of 1.50, or 2.25.[39] The bass Benedetto da Rocca may have been a substitute in 1555, taking the place of Antonio Bresciano who seems to have been the regular bass. Collating and comparing the singers' names supports the conclusion that five voices were the norm at the time that Cirillo was appointed commendatore, and continued to be so.

In 1570, nearly fifteen years into Cirillo's tenure, the financial records seem to suggest that there was less musical activity. As before, there was a regular organist, Robino de Amici, who appears to have taken over from Lodovico da Correggio early in the year. The only other musicians to appear in the payment records are Baldo Antonio da Cesena and Giulio (or Giuliano) da Gubbio, both basses. Baldo seems to have been paid for at least seven months' work, while

38 ASR OSS 1895, *Copie di mandati*, 1557, Items 2160, 3409 and 3536.

39 ASR OSS 1885, *Copie di mandati*, 1557, Items 1045, 1568, 3485 etc.

Giulio was paid for only two. There were various chaplains, but none seems to have been paid regularly alongside any singers.

There could be many reasons for the change, the most likely being financial. The scribe noting the *mandati* at this time provided a monthly tally after the final entry for each month of the year, and then at the end of the year, a calculation for all the expenses for the whole year is written out. This perhaps suggests that there was an economic imperative for change. The expenses for items such as candles are listed in some detail, which is unusual, and there are several more detailed payments relating to the school, for example for books.[40] A telling note is that the prior, not a maestro di cappella, was paid for expenses for Pentecost, amounting to 12 scudi.[41] This is the kind of figure that was listed as payment to various external musicians for Pentecost in the early years of the next century, but we know from scattered references elsewhere that payments were made for a variety of costs associated with the Pentecost celebrations. The sum may therefore have included payment for additional priests, paying the Swiss Guard for their services and expenses relating to the hire or building of temporary structures used for outdoor performance during processions. It would be incorrect to assume that it was only for music.

By 1578, three years after Cirillo's death, the pattern evident in the records of 1555 and 1557 of paying a number of musicians in a scattergun fashion continued. No fewer than ten singers' names appear in the payment records at different times during the year but none seems to have been paid for continuous service. Some appear only once, paid for a single month's service, while others appear three or four times, each time being paid for more than a single month. In January, Dragoni was paid for the music for the previous Christmas, and a month's salary in two separate payments. Paulo Papini, too, also appears only once in the payments, being paid for a full year in January.[42]

The scribe noting the payments also used variants of the names of some of the singers, thus there are payments to an Arcangelo Bergamasco as well as to Arcangelo Crivelli – presumably the same person, and similarly Pietro Borgognone and Pietro Gallo Francese. By working out the length of time for which each man was paid, a regular choir of five voices can be deduced, though the personnel within that choir may have been very mobile.[43] For a period of about six months during the spring and summer, the group can be more precisely

40 ASR OSS 1901, *Copie di mandati*, 1570, Item 146 for candles, Item 2108 for books for the school.

41 ASR OSS 1901, *Copie di mandati*, 1570 Item 894.

42 ASR OSS 1904, *Copie di mandati*, 1578 items 36, 118 and 26.

43 ASR OSS 1904, *Copie di mandati*, 1578. The scribe does not note for which months the singers are paid, so this period is deduced from the date of the payment and the number of months' service listed. As the naming of singers is not consistent either, I have assumed that Arcangelo Bergamasco is the same person as Arcangelo Crivelli and similarly, that Pietro Borgognone is Pietro Gallo Francese.

identified as comprising Cesare Volpi, Pietro Borgognone, Marcello da Bologna, Arcangelo Crivelli and Francesco da Segni. The organist, Giovani Battista Locatelli (or Lucatello) on the other hand was paid for continuous service just as his predecessors had been, and seems to have been a fixture throughout the year.[44] In 1578 then, at least three known composers (Dragoni, Crivelli and Papini), were on the payroll at some point, and it seems a logical conclusion to draw that their music would have been performed during the time they were employed. The survival in the musical archive of only one composition each by Dragoni and Crivelli is perhaps in proportion to their respective length of service compared to that of Papini, whose music survives in larger quantity.

After 1578, there is a complete gap in the financial records until the last quarter of 1595 as neither books of *mandati*, nor the *Libri mastri* or other accounting books have survived. Judging from the way in which the accounting records change after this date, this period was one of considerable change, and one in which music emerged as an activity of major importance to the institution. The chronological span of this gap includes the final years of the tenure of Teseo Aldrovandi as commendatore and of four others including that of Giovanni Battista Ruini, who, as we shall see, was a figure of some importance.[45]

The next surviving financial records are for the last quarter of 1595, by which time there are more stable payments to a maestro di cappella, Paulo Papini, who presumably had been present all through this period; an organist, Camillo Picchi; and singers Ludovico Beltrami, Jacopo Cremonese, Vincenzo Santi, Domenico Aniboni and Antonio Margarita. Each of these singers received a salary of 2 scudi per month, a sum substantially higher than the 75 baiocci paid to singers twenty years earlier.[46] The increase in payment parallels the increases in musicians' salaries at other Roman institutions at this time; for example, at Santa Maria Maggiore, salaries doubled between 1562 and 1602. Rather than indicating a change in status of the musicians, it is evidence of the economic climate in Rome in the last quarter of the century which was characterised by significant inflation.[47]

A further indication of the personnel involved in music-making at the end of the sixteenth century is found in a census document dating from 1595 held in the Biblioteca Nazionale Centrale di Roma that describes the numbers of people resident in each of the hospitals in Rome and their duties.

44 ASR OSS 1904, *Copie di mandati*, 1578.

45 Teseo Aldrovandi, 1575–1582; Giovanni Battista Ruini, 1582–1588; Antonio Migliore, 1588–1591; Michele Mercati, 1591; Agostino Fivizzani, 1591–1594. Sallustio Tarugi was appointed in 1594, holding the position until 1600. For a full listing of all incumbents, see Canezza, *Gli ospedali*, pp. 159–162.

46 ASR OSS 1905, *Copie di mandati*, 1595.

47 Noel O' Regan, 'Sacred Polychoral Music in Rome 1575–1621' (unpublished D.Phil. thesis, University of Oxford, 1988), p. 25.

> There is then the church where there are about sixteen brothers ... of these sixteen there is the Maestro di Cappella, the Prior, the curate, the under-curate [sub-curate] and the sacristan. Other than the said brothers there are four chaplains who sing and say Mass. The rest of the cappella is made up of the same brothers, two of the children mentioned above.[48] Then there is the organist who is secular, there is the sub-sacristan and the innocents who serve at the Mass, there is a preacher sometimes according to the occasion. The confessors are of these brothers who are confessors for the nuns, the children and everyone.[49]

This document counts only those who were living in, not the lay musicians. We can therefore assume that for the major services requiring complex polyphony, other musicians were hired for the job. It also implies that the singing chaplains were not friars but perhaps some of the many singers who took minor orders to sing as chaplains in the churches of Rome. Even so, at least six singers including two boy sopranos plus an organist and maestro di cappella were on hand to carry out musical duties in the church.

The minimum number of four chaplain-singers, organist and a maestro di cappella outlined in Ms.Vitt.Em.721 is mirrored in the payment records dating from the turn of the seventeenth century. The surviving *mandati* for 1599 regularly list four or five singers along with the sacristan, sub-sacristan, curate and organist, although the names of the singers are not consistent, disappearing and reappearing through the year, as they had been in the records of the previous half century.[50] The point that the rest of the cappella is made up of the same brothers suggests that the prior, curate, sub-curate and sacristan were all capable of singing Mass, at least in plainchant, and perhaps supplemented the choir if needed. Further evidence that this was indeed the case is found in the payment records where for example we find 'Vincenzo Spadapani cappellano cantore' but 'Marcantonio Carissimi cantore' which seems to separate those members of the choir who are just singers from those who have other

48 This presumably refers to the orphan children who are described in preceding sections of the document.

49 'Ci è poi la Chiesa ove sono circa 16 frati... fra questi sedici è il Maestro di Cappella, il Priore, il Curato, il sotto curato, et il sacrestano. Oltre a detti frati ci sono 4 Cappellani che cantano et dicono messa. Il resto della Cappella è de medesimi frati, 2 de Innocentini detti di sopra. Vi è l'organista che è seculare, vi è il sottosacristano et gl'innocentini che servano alla messa, vi si predica qualche volta seconda l'occassione. I Confissori sono detti Frati, i quali confessano le Monache, gl'Innocentini, et tutti': *Notizie e Statistiche di Roma sotto il Pontificato di Clemente VIII*, I-Rn Ms Vittorio Emmanuele 721 (henceforth Ms.Vitt.Em.721), fol. 4r (second pagination).

50 ASR OSS 1907, *Copie di mandati*, 1599. The disorganised payments for a single month or for several months in arrears, noted with regard to the early financial records, continue in the early years of the seventeenth century, gradually becoming more orderly.

duties.[51] Again, as before, singers are occasionally identified by voice, such as 'Gio. Jacomo Cremonese basso'.[52]

The implication that the chaplains who sang in the church were a separate category from the chaplains employed in the hospital seems to be supported by a description of the tasks of the chaplains in the hospital. These included taking confessions, giving the holy oil to patients and saying Mass every morning, presumably in the ward chapel. The ambiguity between professional singers and chaplains who sing is one that persists in the financial records, making it difficult to identify those who were non-resident professionals. Taken together, the evidence recorded in Ms.Vitt.Em.721 and the payment records indicate a sufficient number of chaplain-singers took it in turns to sing the Conventual Mass, with enough voices to sing polyphony for the Solemn Mass. This information is broadly supported by Spada's description of the period prior to 1624, to be discussed below. Having an idea of the musical forces available during, and immediately after, Cirillo's tenure goes some way towards evaluating his impact, but there are further documents from which we can deduce to some extent what music was performed.

Inventories

Three sixteenth-century inventories have survived in the Hospital archive. These inventories were identified and transcribed by Melella, without commentary on their potential significance for understanding musical practice during the mid-sixteenth century.[53] Read in parallel with other evidence, they provide a glimpse of the music that was performed at the Hospital during the period roughly contemporary with Cirillo. While none of the inventories date from the period of Cirillo's tenure, the fact that they either pre-date or post-date it offers some indication as to whether any changes in practice might have occurred. The inventories date from 1535, 1546 and 1582.[54]

The 1535 inventory of books kept in the sacristy of the church, as might be expected, lists a number of service books, mostly in manuscript. At this date, printed books would still not have been all that common or cheap. The fact that printed missals, breviaries and a psalter are identified as new might help identify them.

51 ASR OSS 1911, *Copie di mandati*, 1605, item 131.

52 ASR OSS 1907, *Copie di mandati*, 1599 items 369, 503, 708.

53 Patrizia Melella, 'Vita musicale e arte organaria a Santo Spirito in Sassia nel cinquecento: note e documenti', in Bianca Maria Antolini, Arnaldo Morelli and Vera Vita Spagnuolo (eds), *La musica a Roma attraverso le fonti d'archivio: atti del convegno internazionale, Roma, 4–7 giugno 1992* (Lucca, 1994), pp. 507–519.

54 ASR OSS, *Istrumenti* vols. 231, 237 and 29.

An Evangeliary covered in silver on vellum in manuscript with various figures and the arms of S. Spirito[55]

Three large books on vellum viz: a Sanctorale, one of the Resurrection and another of advent finished with brass and one other small one of the Resurrection on vellum[56]

A similar Antiphoner that starts from Advent in plainchant

Another similar Antiphoner on parchment

A large Psalter on parchment newly rebound with brass embellishments

A printed book of Masses in polyphony, used

Two manuscript books of polyphony for Vespers, one old the other somewhat used

Two other books of Masses, one old the other new

A Pontificale on vellum covered in green and illuminated

A printed Pontificale on 'carta bombacina' covered in red and ornamented with brass[57]

A manuscript Missal on vellum illuminated with the arms of Pope Sixtus covered with red and gilded

Three new printed Missals

Nine similar old Missals

Six illuminated manuscript Missals on parchment

A new large printed Breviary

A new printed Psalter including the service for Baptism

Two big old Breviaries

A Martyrology on parchment

A register of dead confrati on parchment

Two old Psalteries on parchment

A manual of Vespers for choir

A large manuscript Psalter on parchment, notated and ornamented with brass

55 The inventory uses the terms 'carta pecora' and 'pergamena' that according to the *Vocabolario della Crusca* (1612) mean the same thing, that is, 'paper' made from the skin of a lamb, calf or other animal. I have used vellum for 'carta pecora' and parchment for 'pergamena'.

56 This description may refer to a Temporale in three parts to go with the Sanctorale.

57 Carta bombacina seems to refer to paper made in the Chinese way.

An Antiphoner of Vespers notated in plainchant on parchment

A book of hymns notated in plainchant on parchment

An old Breviary according to the Use of Santo Spirito on parchment.

A large passion [passionary] of All Saints in parchment covered in red

A large Lectionary for Advent and that which begins 'Visio Ysaie filii annos'

Letters of St Jerome, old, printed

A vellum exposition of Psalms, manuscript and illuminated

Five pieces of books on vellum, old and of little value[58]

If we group these books, we can see that there are three antiphoners, all of which are notated in plainchant; five psalteries plus a commentary on the psalms, none of which indicates the type of music, so presumably plainchant; a book of hymns in plainchant and three books of Masses, one of which is explicitly in polyphony, though the others might be; two books of polyphonic music for Vespers and a 'manual' of Vespers for choir. The latter description is odd, but the identification of it as 'for choir' might suggest its location in the choir of the church or that it was some sort of guide for Vespers. The higher number of psalters in comparison to other books underlines the centrality of psalmody in the life of the Hospital noted in Chapter 3.

Perhaps what is striking about the list is how few of the books are listed as having music in polyphony: two printed books of Masses and two manuscripts books for Vespers are the only items that are securely identified as polyphonic. What this does indicate though, is that even at this stage, Vespers were considered important enough to warrant polyphonic music. Together with the 'printed book of masses in polyphony, used', we have an indication that by 1535, there were sufficient singers to use printed books of polyphonic masses and polyphonic Vespers settings. Or, there were at least sufficient funds and interest in polyphony to hire singers to use such books. In all likelihood, a printed Mass book would contain Franco-Flemish-style polyphony. The earliest prints of Masses produced by Petrucci were of those by Josquin – the first book in 1502, the second in 1505 and a third some years later in 1514, but given the Roman context, the description also fits the Antico print of fifteen Franco-Flemish Masses of 1516 and is a more probable candidate.[59] The 'two other books of masses, one old and one new' I would suggest are likely to be polyphonic settings, as chant settings would have been included in recognisable liturgical books such as graduals.

The item described as a breviary according to the use of Santo Spirito tells us that the Order did indeed have its own particular liturgy – something that presumably was suppressed as the Tridentine reforms took hold and gradually

58 ASR OSS 231, *Instrumenti* fols 38v–39v. For a transcription of the original text see Melella, 'Vita musicale', p. 517.

59 *Liber quindecim missarum*, Rome, Andrea Antico 1516.

standardised practices.[60] The number of separate antiphoners and breviaries compared to the absence of a gradual alongside the missals is possibly of note. It could simply indicate that there was not one in the sacristy at the time of the inventory, but it does raise questions. Fortunately, the listed martyrology has survived in the Hospital archive and, as noted in the previous chapter, should more correctly be identified as a *Liber annualium*.[61] The death of Cirillo on 19 June 1575 is of course noted in its pages.

In 1535, printed copies of liturgical books were still relatively new. Although the first printed liturgical books issued in Italy pre-dated printing music from metal type, for example, a missal containing music was issued by Stephan Planck in 1476, it is reasonable to assume that the printed service books in the inventory date from after the Sack of Rome in 1527, as the church was so badly damaged by fire that it had to be rebuilt.[62]

The 1582 inventory post-dates Cirillo's tenure as commendatore and was compiled in November of that year under Giovanni Francesco Ruini's management. It was far more extensive, including rooms of the friars and the commendatore's offices as well as the sacristy, chapel and choir. A number of the service books listed in the 1535 inventory remained in the sacristy; for example the missal with the red, gilded cover and heraldic arms is listed along with three other similar large missals (possibly the three printed missals from 1535), four smaller ones and seven old and used ones, likely to be among the nine old missals listed in 1535. A number of psalters are also noted in various places, including the pulpit and sacristy, one of which is described as large and on vellum, along with unnamed books of various sizes.[63] A copy of the Rule of Santo Spirito covered in silver is listed together with the silver-bound Evangeliary and Epistolary noted in the 1535 inventory and a similarly bound book with names of the brothers.

The scribe did not list the books in the sacristy in a systematic way as he seems to have been more concerned with the vast quantity of silver, vestments, altar cloths and furnishings, much of which is listed with a description of heraldic embellishments that identify the donor. However, there is enough information to indicate that essentially the same liturgical books evident in 1535 remained in use, bearing in mind that individual items may have moved to one of the chapels, to the hospital or to a different part of the church, in order

60 As noted in Chapter 3, the breviary according to the use of the Order of Santo Spirito was probably similar to other pre-Tridentine breviaries such as that of the Hospital Order of St John of Jerusalem.

61 ASR OSS 72, (pencilled foliation, f51).

62 For information on early printed service books, see Mary Kay Duggan, *Italian Music Incunabula: Printers and Type* (Berkeley and Los Angeles, CA, 1991) p. 83.

63 'Libri vecchi grandi mezzani e piccoli, et ordinata di diverse sorte tra gli un salmista grande in carta pecora'; 'Salmisti piccoli per li preti in sacrestia no 8', ASR OSS 29, f.18r, f20r.

to fulfil their function. Further to the liturgical books in the sacristy, the 1582 inventory of the chapel and choir is more informative about music. Leaving aside the descriptions of the bindings or covers, it lists the following:

Four large books of introits

A book of responsories from Septuagesima to Easter

A psalter

Two large books of antiphons

Two psalters printed in folio

A printed book of antiphons and responses

Two books of antiphons for major feasts of the whole year

An old book of motets by Josquin

Four books of diverse motets

Three books of masses by Giannotto

A book of introits for the mass

A manuscript book of the Magnificat of Morales

A manuscript book of various motets

A printed book of masses by Morales

A book of masses by Jacomo

A printed book of masses of Josquin

A printed book of the Magnificat by Ortiz

A book of masses and Magnificat by Animuccia

A printed book of masses by Costanzo Porta

A big new book of masses and Magnificat by Victoria

A manuscript book of hymns by Costanzo Festa

A manuscript book of Magnificat by Costanzo Festa

A manuscript book of motets by various composers

Two manuscript books of lamentations and other pieces for holy week

A book of responses for holy week

Two manuscript books of Te Deum laudamus by Costanzo Festa

A printed book of Venite exultemus

A collection of printed motets

Various other collections of motets covered in white paper

A book of a mass given to Mons. Ruino

A table [tavola] of the gloria[64]

It is striking that the majority of named composers were employed either in the Cappella Giulia or the Cappella Pontificia for at least part of their careers. This is perhaps testament to the close relationship between the Hospital and St Peter's – a relationship that made mutual borrowing of singers possible for celebrations of specific feast days that required larger musical forces and that can be tracked in payment records in both institutions.

At least some of these items can be identified as printed books that can be precisely dated. In 1966, Feininger published a communication sent to him by the librarian of the Biblioteca Lancisiana, Pietro De Angelis. This document states that apart from the items noted on a list identified as Attachment B, the old archive of the cappella musicale of Santo Spirito no longer existed, because it had been given to Pietro Ravalli who had asked the commendatore Monsignor Cioja to give it to him. Ravalli was a singer in the Cappella Giulia from 1823–1851, and was presenting concerts of sacred music in Rome, so one might surmise that the Santo Spirito music would have been used for that purpose. However, in the De Angelis document, there is only an Attachment A. Feininger assumed that this was a scribal error, and that Attachment A was in fact identical to Attachment B.[65] I will refer to this list as the 'De Angelis' list.[66] It is entitled *Libri di canto ecclesiastico trovati nella Sagrestia di S. Spirito, ed ora riuniti nell'Archivio della cappella di S. Spirito*, and appears to comprise printed books, or at least, manuscript copies of prints. Rostirolla has identified the printers and editions.[67] Several of the books on this list, notably those by Soriano, post-date the inventory by some margin, but most do pre-date the inventory, and there is at least some overlap in the information. There are however, sixteenth-century printed books itemised in the De Angelis list that are not in the 1582 inventory. Given the rather odd circumstances regarding the source of the De Angelis document, it can in no way be taken as indicative of a complete library. While it is the only modern source from which printed items that may have been owned by the Hospital can be identified, there is also evidence that some items were acquired a long time after their first printing. For example, Palestrina's first two

64 For a transcription of the original text in ASR OSS 29, fols 27–28 see Melella, 'Vita musicale', p. 518.

65 Lorenzo Feininger, 'Membra disjecta conjuncta', *Acta Societatis Universalis Sanctae Ceciliae*, 4 (1966), 31–32. Feininger's reading of the document raises some important questions regarding the dissolution of the archive and the more recent research on the surviving music that has not further interrogated the De Angelis document.

66 Note though, that De Angelis did not write the document, he was merely the source for it.

67 Rostirolla, 'L'archivio musicale', pp. 287–288.

books of Masses were printed in 1554 and 1567, and are on the list, but are conspicuous by their absence from the 1582 inventory.

Having said that, in the 1582 inventory, there are also two other entries listing various music books (‘*diversi libri di musica*’) that were in the rooms of the prior and the maestro di cappella at the time the inventory was taken. These are not itemised, but could conceivably be other books on the De Angelis list. Although no financial records from 1582 survive, by 1595, Paulo Papini was acting as both prior and maestro di cappella. Papini had been in post as a singer since at least 1578, so such books may have included his own compositions. Whether the appearance of items from the 1582 inventory in the De Angelis list suggests that they were still in the choir or sacristy of the church, or even still in use in the nineteenth century is an interesting but open question. Items in the inventory that are more difficult to identify are the manuscripts, as the significant majority of the surviving music manuscripts from Santo Spirito archive date from the seventeenth century. There are, however, some notable exceptions – a point to which I shall return.

By comparing known titles and dates of various printed books by the composers named in the inventory, with the listing in the inventory itself, it is possible to identify securely a number of these items. The ‘printed book of masses by Morales’ could only be one of the pair of books he had printed by Dorico in 1544. The first was dedicated to Cosimo I de’ Medici and contains Masses for which those of Josquin are the models. The second, dedicated to Pope Paul III, seems to be the more likely candidate as it makes greater use of abstract contrapuntal techniques including vestiges of isorhythm, and was probably more suitable for use in the papal chapel in which Morales was a singer.[68]

The ‘printed book of the Magnificat by Ortiz’ seems to be a non-musical notary’s way of describing the only printed book of liturgical music by Ortiz – his *Musices liber primus hymnos, Magnificas, Salves, motecta, psalmos*, printed in Venice in 1565.[69] As with Ortiz, there is only one likely candidate for a printed book of Masses by Costanzo Porta, and that is his *Liber primus*, printed in Venice in 1578, which would also have been a new book at the time of the inventory.[70] Animuccia had only one book of Masses printed, the *Liber primus* of 1567. This was followed a year later by a print entitled *Canticum*

68 Information on printed editions in this section is drawn from standard composer entries in *Grove Music Online*, Oxford University Press, and from *Printed Sacred Music Database – Printed Sacred Music in Europe 1500–1800*. Published: 2014 [online] http://www.printed-sacred-music.org DOI: 10.5448/RISM-d-lib-001; Robert Stevenson, revised by Alejandro E. Planchart, ‘Morales, Cristobal de’, *Grove music online* (accessed 22/11/2021).

69 The date is given in the list, thus it is easy to identify this book precisely.

70 Lilian P. Pruett, ‘Porta, Costanzo’, *Grove Music Online* (accessed 22/11/2021).

Beatae Mariae Virginis that also included a *Magnificat quinti toni*.[71] It seems safe to assume that these are the books in the inventory.

The 'big new book of masses and Magnificat by Victoria' suggests his *Liber primus: qui missas, psalmos, Magnificat...* printed in Venice in 1576.[72] Although the De Angelis list notes three volumes by Victoria, two can be ruled out: the *Officium Hebdomodae Sanctae* (1585) post-dates the inventory, and the *Hymni totius anni* (1581) simply does not fit the description of the books in the inventory at all. A third book by Victoria that really would have been new at the time of the inventory is his *Cantica Beatae Virginis vulgo Magnificat quatuor vocibus* printed by Zanetti in 1581. While the Magnificat part of the description is correct, it seems possible that the notary may have misunderstood the rest of the contents. But even the *Liber primus* would have been relatively new at the time of the inventory in 1582, and this is the book that most closely matches the description.

There can be far less certainty concerning the Morales Magnificat, the book of Masses by Josquin and the music by Jacomo and Giannotto. While Morales's *Magnificat cum quatuor vocibus* was printed numerous times in the sixteenth century, and a book of Magnificats by Morales is on the De Angelis list, the inventory is clear that this one is in manuscript. That of course does not rule out a manuscript copy of a print or indeed a copy of another manuscript.[73] There are a number of possibilities for the printed book of Josquin Masses as Petrucci issued three books, all of which went through several reprints. It does seem feasible though that this item may also be the only printed book of Masses listed in the 1535 inventory.

The 'three books of masses' by Giannotto suggests that whoever Giannotto was, he was well enough known for a quantity of material to be in the collection. It seems likely that this refers to Palestrina whose nickname was 'Giannetto'.[74] He is a good fit chronologically as his first three books of Masses had all been printed by 1570, and for the quantity of material in the inventory. The scribal reference to him by a misspelt nickname is odd, but his absence from such an inventory would perhaps be even more so. 'Jacomo' on the other hand,

71 Lewis Lockwood, revised by Noel O'Regan, 'Animuccia, Giovanni', *Grove Music Online* (accessed 16/12/2021).

72 Robert Stevenson, 'Victoria, Tomas Luis', *Grove Music Online* (accessed 16/12/2021).

73 Morales, *Magnificat cum quatuor vocibus* (Venice: Gardano, 1545 with reprints in 1559, 1563, 1568 etc.). A number of manuscript copies of Magnificat settings have survived, for example, in the Vatican library, British Library, Bibliothèque nationale de France and the Bibliothèque Royale de Belgique.

74 Lewis Lockwood, Noel O'Regan and Jessie-Ann Owens, 'Palestrina [Prenestino] Giovanni Pierluigi da ['Giannetto']', *Grove Music Online* (accessed 01/02/2023). Palestrina is referred to as Giannetto in the inventories of S. Rocco of 1581. Noel O'Regan, 'Music at the Roman Archconfraternity of San Rocco in the Late Sixteenth Century', in Bianca Maria Antolini, Arnaldo Morelli and Vera Vita Spagnuolo (eds), *La Musica a Roma attraverso le fonte d'archivio* (Lucca, 1994), pp. 521–552.

suggests three possible candidates – Jacobus de Kerle, Jachet of Mantua and Jachet de Berchem. The latter is least likely (though not impossible) as he wrote very little sacred music.[75] Items by de Kerle and Jachet of Mantua are on the De Angelis list. The inventory item is a book of Masses, which rules out the Jachet *Magnificat* on the list, though not necessarily other works by him. The inventory description does not indicate whether the book is printed or manuscript. Printed books of Masses survive for both composers. Jachet's first book was issued by Scotto in 1554 and a second book in 1555. A volume entitled *Messe del fiore* followed in 1561.[76] All of these publications fit the time frame, as does Jacobus de Kerle's *Sex missae suavissimis modulationibus referte* which was printed in Venice by Gardano in 1562.

The manuscript books of Masses and hymns by Festa are of interest as much of his music was written during his tenure in the Capella Pontificia to which he was appointed in 1517. Only a handful of his Masses have survived in manuscript. The presence of Festa's music at Santo Spirito would at least indicate that his music was sung beyond the papal chapel.[77] However, no manuscript music attributed to Festa has been identified by Rostirolla or by earlier scholars attempting to trace the contents of the musical archive of Santo Spirito. Table 4.1 lists the items from the 1582 inventory that can be identified with some certainty.

Table 4.1 Securely identified books in the 1582 inventory.

Composer	Title	Date
Morales	*Missarum Liber primus, Liber secundus*	1544
Giannotto [Palestrina]	*Missarum Liber primus, Liber secundus, Liber tertius*	1554, 1567, 1570
Animuccia	*Missarum Liber primus*	1567
Animuccia	*Canticum Beatae Mariae Virginis... Magnificat quinti toni*	1568
Ortiz	*Musices liber primus hymnos, Magnificas, Salves, motecta, psalmo*	1565
Porta	*Missarum Liber primus*	1578
Victoria	*Liber primus: qui missas, psalmos, Magnificat...*	1576

75 The motet 'Ave virgo gloriosum' in D-Rp BH6003 is one of only nine securely identifiable sacred pieces by him.

76 These are listed in both RISM, https://opac.rism.info/metaopac/refineSearch.do?id=subject_facet&methodToCall=filterSearch&subval=Masses, and the Kurtzman and Schnoebelen catalogue. Jeffery Kurtzman and Anne Schnoebelen, *A Catalogue of Motets, Mass, Office, and Holy Week Music Printed in Italy, 1516–1770*, https://sscm-jscm.org/instrumenta/instrumenta-volumes/instrumenta-volume-2/ (accessed 17/12/2021).

77 James Haar, 'Festa, Costanzo', *Grove Music Online* (accessed 22/11/2021).

Manuscript sources

This leaves unidentified quite a number of books listed in the inventory in vague terms, such as 'a manuscript book of various motets', or 'a manuscript of motets by various composers'. It seems probable that a large manuscript choirbook in the Bischöfliche Zentralbibliothek, Regensburg is one of these. D-Rp BH 6003 is a compilation of items, comprising two Masses, a Requiem by Richafort and a number of motets, all anonymous except for one by Francesco Roselli. A number of the anonymous items have been identified as pieces by Franco-Flemish composers such as Gombert, Jachet de Berchem, Willaert, Verdelot and Lheritier, all of whom were dead by 1570, thus making a date compatible with the inventory possible. The paper and watermarks too are consistent with a date of 1560–1600. The book has signs of having been rebound, or perhaps various separate sections of slightly different sizes being bound together, as the pages of the first section containing the two Masses have been cut down. There are at least eight scribes, which might also suggest the possibility that there were originally several smaller books or sections that were bound together.[78] The financial records for 1557 note a large payment of 80 scudi recorded to a 'librario' for binding a book of canto figurato.[79] At that price, it must have been a large choirbook format and a good quality binding, such as of leather. This could conceivably be a book such as BH 6003.

It seems possible that one or more of four other undated manuscript choirbooks now in Regensburg may also have been included in the inventory. If they were compiled over a period of time, and the presence of a number of different scribes and different papers suggests that they were, then sections of several of them might easily be described as 'a manuscript book of various motets'. These choirbooks, BH 6004, BH 6005, BH 6006 and BH 6008, include music by Papini and Palestrina, alongside single items by Morales and Matelart and a considerable number of anonymous pieces in similar style. The choirbooks are difficult to date precisely but they may well contain sections roughly contemporary with the inventory. As a group, they were unquestionably compiled in the last quarter of the sixteenth century. As such, they are indicative of the style used at Santo Spirito in the years after Cirillo's death.[80]

78 Dieter Haberl has described the scribes, watermarks and paper, and provides a thematic list of the pieces contained in the manuscript identifying the composer where possible. Dieter Haberl, *Bischöfliche Zentralbibliothek Regensburg, Thematischer Katalog der Musikhandscriften, 7 Bibliothek Franz Xaver Haberl Manuskripte BH6001 bis BH 6949*, Kataloge Bayerischer Musiksammlungen, Herausgegeben von der Bayerischen Staatsbibliothek, Band 14/7–8, (Munich, 2000).

79 ASR OSS 1895, *Copie di mandati*, 1557, item 3609.

80 The choirbooks were mentioned in passing by Canezza, (*Gli archispedali*, p. 62) and by Allegra who referred only to Canezza ('La cappella musicale', p. 27) They were bought by Haberl in 1884, but since 1940, there appears to have been no scholarly investigation of them.

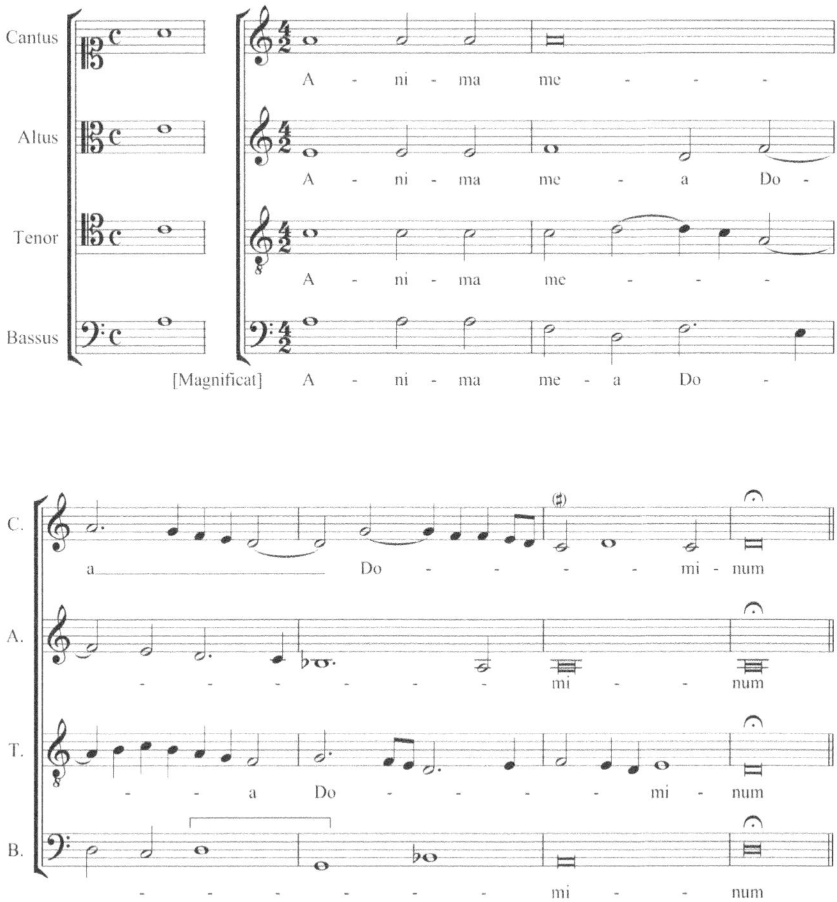

Example 4.1 Papini, *Magnificat primi toni*, D-Rp BH 6006, fol. 106v–107r, opening section.

The books are dominated by the music of Palestrina. Second to him is the work of a man who was employed at the Hospital from at least 1578 until his death in 1603, and that is Paulo Papini.[81] Papini was a friar of the Order of Santo Spirito, and at some point, he became both prior of the Order, and maestro di cappella. His presence in the financial records is more difficult to trace for that reason, as references to those who held office tend to be made to the title and not the person occupying that position. His status is evident in the various manuscripts, as he is referred to as 'Frater' in the choirbooks and as 'nostro' in the financial documents. Several of Papini's laude were included in printed

[81] The earliest payment to Papini that has come to light is ASR OSS 1902, *Copie di mandati*, 1571, item 130.

anthologies, with one, 'Vergin ben posso dire', appearing in two different collections.[82] These are typical of the genre with simple melodies in strophic form, and largely homophonic textures. His inclusion in these collections suggests that his music aligned with the principles of collective singing of devotional songs as expressed by the Oratorians.

Papini's music in the Regensburg choirbooks perhaps gives a sense of the way musical style may have developed within the Hospital in the years following the death of Cirillo. The four-part *Magnifcat primi toni* in BH 6006 f106v–109r, for example, is strictly modal and consonant except at cadences where some controlled dissonance appears. Papini avoids repeating words or phrases of the text, but does use some melismas as seen in Example 4.1.[83]

In another of the volumes, BH 6005, there are several motets ('Salve Regina', 'Miserere mei Deus', 'Benedictus dominus') composed in a style that is essentially a written-out falsobordone. The texts are set syllabically and homorhythmically using repeated chords that only change at cadence points. In this choirbook, several of the items are designated for eight voices, but the pages are laid out for a choir of four, suggesting that a companion volume may have been lost. There are further settings that seem to combine falsobordone with simple counterpoint, resulting in a declamatory, largely homorhythmic style punctuated by cadences that are more active rhythmically.

Although a full evaluation of Papini's music is yet to be made, it seems to adhere closely to the ideals of Tridentine reform as much of the music in these choirbooks appears to be in a stripped-down polyphony. If we add the Regensburg manuscript items to the list of music securely identified in the inventory, we arrive at a repertory of music that would have been used at Santo Spirito in the last quarter of the sixteenth century, that is, the period immediately after Cirillo's death. It is perhaps worth noting that music by the one composer who has been identified as closely connected to Cirillo, namely Annibale Zoilo, is conspicuous by its absence.

Table 4.2 Probable repertory of Santo Spirito c. 1570–1600.

Composer	**Title**	**Date**
Morales	*Missarum liber primus, Liber secundus*	1544
Giannotto [Palestrina]	*Missarum liber primus, Liber secundus, Liber tertius*	1554, 1567, 1570

82 *Tempio armonico della Beatissma Vergine* (Rome, 1599); *Nuove laude ariose della Beatissima Vergine scelte da diversi autori a quattro voci per il rever. D. Giovanni Arascione piemontese da Cairo prete secolare* (Rome, 1600).

83 Haberl, *Bischöfliche Zentralbibliothek Regensburg, Thematischer Katalog*, 14, suggests that this Magnificat was for eight voices, but there is no indication to that effect in the source. It is however laid out with two verses on a single opening, each of which has a calligraphic initial letter, making it look like the incipits of eight separate parts.

Animuccia	*Missarum Liber primus*	1567
Animuccia	*Canticum Beatae Mariae Virginis... Magnificat quinti toni*	1568
Ortiz	*Musices liber primus hymnos, Magnificas, Salves, motecta, psalmo*	1565
Porta	*Missarum Liber primus*	1578
Victoria	*Liber primus: qui missas, psalmos, Magnificat...*	1576
Gombert, Richafort, Verdelot etc.	Masses and motets D-Rp BH 6003	c. 1570?
Papini, Palestrina, anon	Masses, motets, magnificats D-Rp BH 6004, BH 6005, BH 6006, BH 6008, BH 6009	c. 1578–1603

Cirillo's impact on music

Taken together, the two inventories that chronologically frame Cirillo's tenure as governor of the Hospital do seem to indicate a change in the musical repertory. The surviving manuscript choirbooks support that shift. It might be inferred that the changes in the last quarter of the sixteenth century were a direct result of Cirillo's influence, but it would be imprudent to assert that his influence was the only factor.

The financial records are incomplete, and the 'blip' in 1570 that suggests a reduction in financial support for music is hardly indicative of a shift away from complex polyphony back to chant and alternatim performance with the organ. Cirillo's own account of the institution written in 1571 notes how he had had to deal with the poor condition of the buildings and expenditure to deal with significant problems.[84] One of Cirillo's accomplishments as commendatore was restoring the financial stability of the Hospital and overseeing the repair of the buildings, thus a dip in spending on music cannot, in the wider view of his tenure, be interpreted as an aesthetic choice.

Rather, the similarity of forces and payment patterns in 1557 and 1578 compared to those of 1570 is strong evidence for continuity of practice. The brief change in 1570 is far more likely to be indicative of a change in scribal or accounting practice, or that normal staffing was interrupted by other circumstances, such as changes in the economic climate.[85] Further argument

84 V-CVbav Ottob Lat. 2473, fols.179–204, Cirillo, *Relatione della fabrica e casa di S. Spirito di Roma* (1571).

85 Sella notes the rising farm prices and land values, land acquisition by the wealthy at the expense of rural communities, the decline in shipping and ship building followed by a series of poor harvests that triggered high food prices and famine in the 1590s.

for continuity of practice is found in the observations of those external to the organisation who testify to the quality and beauty of musical embellishment of the liturgy. Such comments were included in guidebooks to ensure such visitors witnessed the best of Rome, or written by those who did actually visit, such as Gregory Martin. Panciroli's description of the institution targeted at visitors suggests that the Offices were celebrated with music as a matter of course.[86]

If evidence of Cirillo's influence on music at the Hospital is inconclusive, there are nonetheless conclusions that can be drawn regarding music at Santo Spirito under his tenure. First, the practice of hiring of professional musicians for the major celebrations, especially Pentecost, was uninterrupted in spite of the economic conditions, while the salaried singers and chaplains of the Order supported by an organist provided the basic services. Second, the salaries of musicians at the Hospital mirror those paid to singers in other Roman institutions. The lower salaries of the singers compared to that of the organist in this period is likely to indicate duties that were not particularly onerous – perhaps one daily Mass and Vespers on feast days.[87] The continuous presence of an organist, and the comparatively higher salary for this post, suggests that this role carried greater responsibilities. If this was the case, chanting in alternatim with the organ seems likely as a norm for everyday Offices and Masses, and that the organist was perhaps the glue that held the small ensemble of singers together when more complex music was required. Third, putting the information about musicians together with the evidence of the inventories and the surviving choirbooks, we can conclude that for feast days at least, polyphonic music was sung.

There are more polyphonic settings than plainchant in the later, 1582, inventory, but music by composers with connections to the papal choirs, and the style favoured by Tridentine reformers, seem to emerge as a trend. The music in the Regensburg choirbooks is further evidence of that trend. However, while it might be inferred that Cirillo was the driving force for the shift in style, it cannot be proved conclusively, as the music at Santo Spirito echoes the fashion in other churches, and indeed, other charitable institutions across Rome at the same time. A comparison with the repertory at Santa Maria Maggiore over a similar time frame indicates a leaning towards the same composers, all of

---

Domenico Sella, *Italy in the Seventeenth Century* (Abingdon, [1997] 2014), pp. 21–23.

86 'Per non essere lungo, tacerò la divotione, con che si celebrino qui con canti e musici i divini officii e la richezza de i loro paramenti.' 'So as not to be longwinded, I will be silent on the devotions which they celebrate here with songs and music of the divine Offices and their rich embellishments': Ottavio Panciroli, *I tesori nascosti nell'alma città di Roma* (Rome, 1600), pp. 770–775; Gregory Martin, *Roma Sancta*, p. 84.

87 The source documents for information concerning the duties of chaplains and singers post-date this period, but sung Mass and Vespers, especially on feast days, were probably already established. See Chapter 5.

whose music focused on the clarity of the text within polyphonic textures and avoided paraphrase and parody Masses on secular melodies.

Whether Cirillo's impassioned rhetoric about music influenced the upper echelons of Church hierarchy is impossible to ascertain. His own institution does not particularly stand out as leading by example, but rather as one of several including Santa Maria Maggiore, the Oratorians at Santa Maria in Vallicella, S.S. Trinità dei Pellegrini, all moving in the same direction. Although the utilitarian polyphony and written-out falsobordone style of Papini, an 'insider' of the Order of Santo Spirito, suggests that at the very least, there was a close adherence to the principles of reform, it cannot be assumed that Cirillo's governorship instigated the change. However, if one were to look for an individual whose work might reflect a direct influence, Papini is the most likely candidate.

The direction of travel in these institutions may of course betray intersecting circles of patronage or other allegiances. As noted above, Cirillo was briefly employed at Santa Maria Maggiore and also enjoyed a close friendship with Filipo Neri. The Zoilo family connections with the Hospital of Santo Spirito during the later years of Cirillo's tenure may also have been a channel for influencing practices, as Annibale, who also provided music to SS. Trinità dei Pellegrini, was entrusted by Pope Gregory XIII to work with Palestrina on reforming chant.[88] Within these interlocking relationships of like-minded individuals leading particular institutions, it is unwise to identify a single individual as a causal point of influence. It would perhaps be fair only to say that the Hospital of Santo Spirito and its collegiate church was an early adopter of music that conformed to Tridentine ideals. The extent to which Santo Spirito was a laboratory for promoting Tridentine reform only becomes evident as other evidence is taken into consideration.

88 Noel O'Regan, *Institutional Patronage in Post-Tridentine Rome: Music at Santissima Trinita dei Pellegrini 1550–1650* (London, 1995), p. 31.

5

Music in the Church of Santo Spirito in the Seventeenth Century

The last three decades of the sixteenth century, including the final years of Cirillo's tenure as commendatore, encompassed a period of considerable change for Rome, and specifically for the Hospital of Santo Spirito. Between Cirillo's death in 1575, and 1600, the leadership of the Hospital passed to six new commendatori in relatively quick succession. The buildings bear witness to the fact that several of them were keen to make their mark physically. Further, the consolidation of the ideals of the Council of Trent was starting to take effect.

Much important information about this period in the history of Santo Spirito is found in the retrospective report written by Virgilio Spada in 1660 entitled *Stato della Casa dell'Archiospedale di Santo Spirito di Roma*.[1] Spada's tenure as commendatore of the Hospital in 1660–1662 was brief, but provides a neat bookend to that of Cirillo a century earlier. Thanks to his character and education, his observations are of considerable value.[2] Like Cirillo's *Relatione della fabrica e casa di S. Spirito di Roma* written nearly a century earlier, and the more generic report on all the institutions of Rome written in 1624 for Urban VIII, Spada's *Stato della Casa* was probably required by the papal authorities as a report in response to an Apostolic Visitation to present a justification of expenditure.[3] This four-inch-thick manuscript book held in the Archivio di Stato in Rome considers the ways in which all aspects of the institution were run, including their costs. The account on the one hand looks backward, giving an overview of the institution's history, and on the other, describes how the institution was operating at the time at which it was written. It thus offers scope for comparison with earlier periods; a point of reference

1 Virgilio Spada, *Stato della Casa dell'Archiospedale di Santo Spirito di Roma, 1661*, ASR OSS 47.

2 Spada was a polymath with many connections in scientific and artistic communities, including the Academia dei Lincei, and Borromini and his circle. See Giuseppe Finocchiaro, *Il museo di curiosità di Virgilio Spada: Una raccolta romana del seicento* (Rome, 1999); Anna di Falco, *Francesco Borromini, Virgilio Spada e la costruzione della Casa dei Filippini. Contributi per la storia costruttiva dell'Oratorio a seguito dei lavori di restauro e di alcune fonti inedite* (Rome, 2015).

3 V-CVbav Ottob Lat. 2473, ff.179–204, Cirillo, *Relatione della fabrica e casa di S. Spirito di Roma* (1571); V-CVaav Misc.Arm VII / 77 *Stato temporale delle chiese di Roma fatto nel pontificato di Urbano VIII l'anno 1625.*

for activities in the decades that followed it; and an overview of the running of both the church and the hospital in the mid-seventeenth century. Though neither Spada nor Stefano Vai, the other commendatore of major importance in the mid-seventeenth century, mention the Tridentine reforms specifically, it is evident from what they do say that it was a fundamental consideration in their respective periods of governorship.

Musicological discussions of post-Tridentine music were, until fairly recently, one-dimensional, focusing on the necessity for clarity of text. The myth of Palestrina as the saviour of Church music, though having been categorically debunked, still hovers in the background. As noted by Bertoglio, Monson and others, it was the reinstatement and reinforcement of doctrine in parallel with the reform of liturgical texts that underpinned musical changes.[4] The desire of the Council to create a uniform liturgy across the Catholic world led to the publication of the new breviary and missal in 1568 and 1570 respectively.[5] The work was instigated by Pius IV but completed under Pius V, who issued a Bull that presented the new missal as returning the liturgy to a purer state by collating ancient sources and codices.[6] The invocation of ancient authority for the reformed missal perhaps reflects the interest in paleo-Christianity that had engulfed Rome at the time, and was pursued in particular by one of the new organisations set up to improve the education of the clergy, that is, the Oratorians – an organisation with which both Bernardino da Cirillo and Spada were closely connected.

A crucial change in the reformed breviary was the suppression of dozens of feast days and their Octaves that had accumulated in the medieval calendar. The aim of this alteration was to restore the weekly recitation of the psalter through the Offices for ferial, that is ordinary, days. The value of daily psalm singing as a means of prayer, teaching, and overcoming the negative passions of the soul had been emphasised in Patristic writings. Reaching back to the authority of antiquity by the Church hierarchy aligned with the secular revival of interest in classical philosophy. These trends, that were already evident in Cirillo's views in the mid-sixteenth century, become obvious in the liturgical music performed at Santo Spirito after 1600.

4 For a detailed consideration of reforming trends following the Council of Trent, see Craig Monson, 'The Council of Trent Revisited', *Journal of the American Musicological Society*, 55:1 (2002), 1–37; J. W. O'Malley, 'Early Modern Catholicism: The State of Research', in Daniele V. Fillipi and Michael Noone (eds), *Listening to Early Modern Catholicism* (Leiden, 2017); Chiara Bertoglio, *Reforming Music: Music and the Religious Reformations of the Sixteenth Century* (Berlin and Boston, 2018), Chapter 9.

5 *Breviarum Romanum ex decreto Sacrosancti Concilii Tridentini restitutum* (Venice, 1568); *Missale Romanum ex decreto Sacrosancti Concilii Tridentini restitutum* (Rome, 1570).

6 The Bull 'Quo primum' also essentially made the use of the 1570 missal a 'law' for all Catholic churches. Anthony Chadwick, *Missa Tridentina: The Reform of the Roman Liturgy in the Sixteenth Century*, http://civitas-dei.eu/Mass_of_St_Pius_V.pdf.

Parallel to the renewed observation of the Offices, actions were taken to reinforce doctrine, the most important elements of which were spread to clergy, and thence to the laity, in a new Catechism completed in 1566.[7] The *Catechism of the Council of Trent for Parish Priests* emphasised the correct understanding of the sacraments and was presented in four parts – the Creed, the Sacraments, the Ten Commandments and the Lord's Prayer.[8] Those teaching doctrine often harnessed music to do so. Filippi has accumulated a significant amount of evidence to suggest that sung Catechism was not only popular, but also that the teaching of doctrine through singing had a missionary dimension, especially for the Jesuits, and was as likely to happen in public spaces as in schools and churches.[9] The potential for music to reinforce doctrine, especially the sacraments, was not missed in more local contexts.[10] As will be seen in Chapter 6, the organ played an important role in underlining the sacrament of the Eucharist, but music could also play a role in the missionary aspect of teaching doctrine.

Evidence of musical activity at Santo Spirito can be gleaned from the musical archive, from documentary records and from the building itself. I will use all of these sources to argue that the church of Santo Spirito conformed closely to Tridentine reforms. The non-linear nature of the evidence shapes the structure of this chapter, which will start with an account of *musica straordinaria* for the patronal feast of Pentecost, before considering the more everyday music in the church and the professional singers who provided it, and finishing with Spada's defence of music which offers a backward look at music before 1660. This jigsaw of data presents a picture of shifting fortunes for the singers, chaplains and instrumentalists who worked at the institution under successive commendatori, each of whom imposed their own views of reform.

Although there remain significant gaps in our knowledge of printed materials, liturgical books and music from the sixteenth century and earlier that may have been owned by the institution, the seventeenth-century manuscript collection has, to a large extent, been traced, notably by Feininger, and, more recently, organised into a systematic list by Rostirolla.[11] Using the list created

7 *Catechismus ex decreto SS. Concilii Tridentini ad parochos PII V. Pont. Max. jussu editus* (Catechism of the Council of Trent for Parish Priests Issued by Order of Pius V, the Supreme Pontiff).

8 Robert Fastiggi, 'The Contributions of the Council of Trent to the Catholic Reformation', *Perichoresis*, 18:6 (2020), 3–20.

9 Daniele V. Filippi, 'Catechismum modulans docebat: Teaching the Doctrine through Singing', in *Listening to Early Modern Catholicism* (Leiden, 2017), pp. 129–148.

10 For example, Carlo Borromeo's reforms in his Milan diocese.

11 A number of scholars have attempted to locate the lost musical archive of Santo Spirito, including Guido Mattei-Gentili, *'Membra disjecta' dell'archivio musicale di Santo Spirito in Saxia* (Rome, 1937); Raffaele Casimiri, 'Il disperso archivio musicale di Santo Spirito in Saxia', *Note d'archivio*, XV (1938), 140–144; Antonio Allegra, 'La cappella musicale di S. Spirito in Saxia di Roma: Appunti storici (1551–1737)', *Note d'archivio,*

by Rostirolla as a basis for data analysis, various patterns emerge concerning the type of music and the forces required for its performance. However, the list does not include music from the Regensburg choirbooks, nor any printed material. It also contains some music that may not originally have been in the Santo Spirito library, but was sold off with it, and for which the evidence for its inclusion in the collection is somewhat inconclusive. The results of the analyses below are therefore indicative rather than definitive.

Pentecost and the propaganda of reform

Following the death of Pius V in 1572, Gregory XIII Boncompagni was elected pope. Gregory had an enthusiastic if not zealous desire to reunite the Eastern and Western Churches and to regain Christians lost to Protestantism. His leadership promoted a missionary attitude to both conversion of non-Christians and re-conversion of Protestants. A key moment in the early history of Christianity was the day of Pentecost, as it was from this moment that the followers of Jesus were empowered to build the Christian Church through preaching, baptism and healing. The book of the Acts of the Apostles that recounts this event became the model for this new mission. Gregory XIII's enthusiasm was founded on his study of the Eastern Church Fathers – John Chrysostom, Basil and especially Gregory of Nazianzus – and their exegeses of the Pentecostal narratives, and of the nature of the Holy Spirit within the Holy Trinity. These ancient authorities were all points of reference for the Tridentine reaffirmation of Catholic Trinitarian doctrine.

The reformed missal of 1570 had already established a new liturgy for Pentecost, formally recognising and including the sequence 'Veni sancte spiritus', one of only seven such medieval accretions to be retained.[12] As the text of this hymn is attributed to Innocent III, its use at the Hospital would have been even more meaningful.[13] The new missal also established the response 'Emitte tuum' and Communion antiphon 'Et repleti sunt omnes spiritu sanctu loquentes magnalia Dei'.[14]

XVII (1940), 26–38; Lorenzo Feininger, 'Membra disjecta riperta', *Acta Societatis Universalis Sanctae Ceciliae*, 3 (1964); Lorenzo Feininger, 'Membra disjecta conjuncta', *Acta Societatis Universalis Sanctae Ceciliae*, 4 (1966); Giancarlo Rostirolla, 'L'archivio musicale della chiesa annessa all'ospedale di Santo Spirito', *Il Veltro*, XLV:5–6 (2002), 279–343.

12 *Missale Romanum* (Rome, 1575) p. 361.

13 For the complete Latin text and translation see https://www.preces-latinae.org/preces.html.

14 Louise Smith Bross, 'The Church of Santo Spirito in Sassia: A Study in the Development of Art, Architecture and Patronage in Counter-reformation Rome' (unpublished PhD thesis, University of Chicago, 1994), p. 405.

In response to the reforms of Pius V and Gregory XIII, depictions of the descent of the Holy Spirit on the day of Pentecost in paintings changed in the last quarter of the sixteenth century. In particular, they started to include representations of the Trinity of God the Father, the risen Jesus and the Holy Spirit in the form of a dove, as part of the scene, as well as larger groups of people including women other than the Madonna all receiving the gifts of the spirit. These changes are evident in the frescoes commissioned for the decoration of the church of Santo Spirito in Sassia – a church for which Pentecost was the 'patronal' feast day.[15]

Gregory XIII took a great deal of interest in the Hospital of Santo Spirito as he realised that it could promote his campaign of conversion, and on Cirillo's death appointed Teseo Aldrovandi, a fellow Bolognese, as commendatore. Aldrovandi's tenure was relatively short, but he lost no time in commissioning the decoration of the palazzo housing the administrative centre for the commendatore that had been built under Cirillo. Gregory seems to have intervened, appointing Ignazio Danti as his agent to oversee the decoration of the church. The contract between Aldrovandi and the artist Jacopo Zucchi was signed only days before Aldrovandi's death. Thus it was another of Gregory XIII's appointees, the apparently devout but cultured art lover Giovanni Battista Ruini who oversaw the completion of the frescoes in the tribune, apse and half-dome of the church. While the financial records for this period have been lost, the contract has survived and suggests that the costs were substantial.[16] Bross, Valone and Pillsbury provide detailed analyses of the stylistic aspects of these paintings and their importance in the output of the artist Jacopo Zucchi, who was apparently borrowed from Cardinal Medici to do the work in a very short time period.

For the purposes of this study, the frescoes provide a different perspective of activity within the Hospital, as they were completed in 1583 and were therefore contemporary with the inventory discussed in the previous chapter. Unlike the more modest memorials to various commendatori in the church, the name of Giovanni Battista Ruini is placed conspicuously where all can see it in the frescoed arch above the altar steps.[17] The narratives of Zucchi's frescoes are perhaps evidence of renewed dedication to the founding purpose of the Order, but are also indicative of the importance of music within that purpose.

The frescoes behind, above and around the altar of the church present a coherent programme of images based on the biblical narrative of the descent

15 Carolyn Valone, 'Pentecost: Image and Experience in Late Sixteenth-century Rome', *Sixteenth Century Journal*, XXIV (1993), 801–828.

16 The contract is published in full in Edmund Pillsbury, 'Jacopo Zucchi in S. Spirito in Sassia', *The Burlington Magazine*, 116:857 (1974), 434–444.

17 Although Ruini did not commission the fresco, the assumption is that they were complete by 1583 when this panel was painted. The terms of the contract are outlined by Pillsbury.

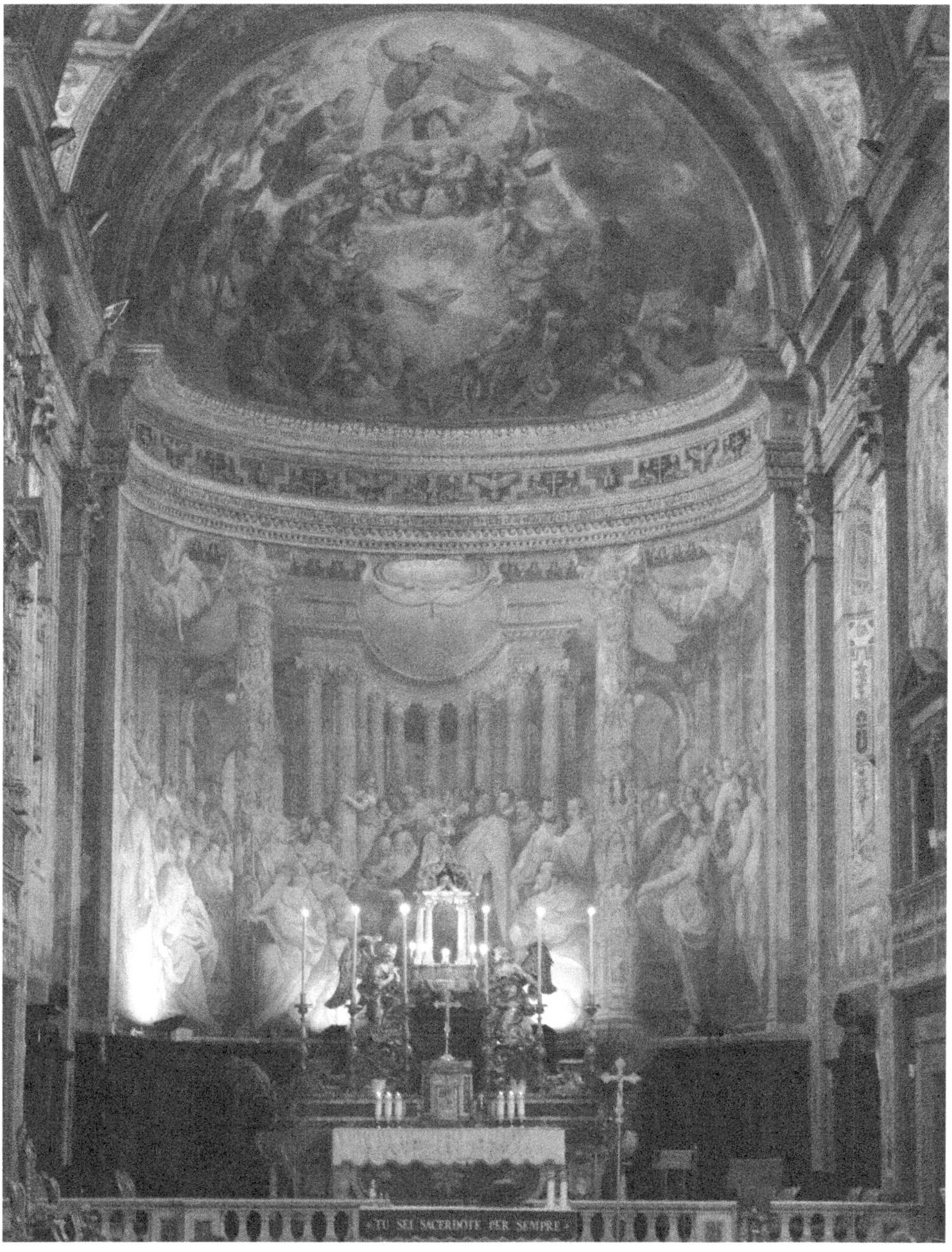

Plate 5.1 Church of Santo Spirito in Sassia, High Altar with Pentecost frescoes by Jacopo Zucchi. Photo © Chris Churnside and the author, used with permission of ASL Roma.

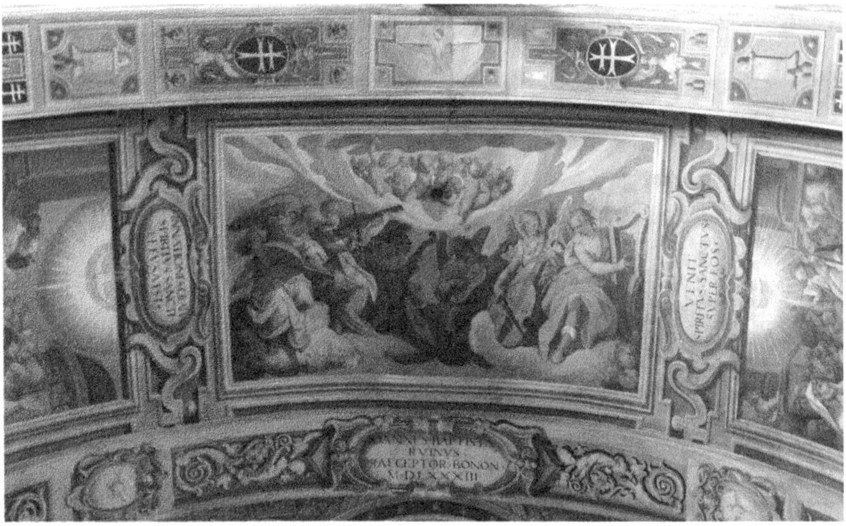

Plate 5.2 Church of Santo Spirito in Sassia: Jacopo Zucchi, fresco of angel musicians in barrel vault above the altar. Photo © Chris Churnside and the author, used with permission of ASL Roma.

of the Holy Spirit onto the followers of Jesus following his crucifixion and resurrection. According to the account in the second chapter of Acts, Jesus's disciples were gathered together in an upper room, when an influx of the Holy Spirit in the form of flames of fire and light caused them to speak in multiple languages. In the biblical narrative, the disciple Peter then explained the phenomenon as the fulfilment of an Old Testament prophecy. In so doing, he quoted Psalms 16 and 110 to reinforce his point, making an explicit connection between their assumed author King David, and Jesus, his direct descendent whose resurrection he foresaw.[18] As a result of this event, many onlookers were immediately baptised and became followers of Jesus, giving up their own possessions to live together as Christians. They then went on to heal the sick as Jesus had done. Pentecost thus marked the beginning of the Church as a community, and its growth through preaching and baptism. A point often overlooked is that Pentecost also marked the conferral on the disciples of Jesus of the power to heal the sick. The remainder of the book of Acts is a narrative of the early history of the Christian Church and the healing activities of the disciples. As they were able to cure the sick, they drew to the new Christian movement more and more followers, thus establishing the Church.

Although the image of God the Father is placed in a tondo at the highest point of the barrel vault above the altar, the vault of the semi-circular apse is

[18] Acts 2:25–28, 34–36. Psalm 110 is 'Dixit Dominus', many settings of which survive in the musical archive.

dominated by the figure of the resurrected Jesus. Beneath his feet, a circle of angels and saints surround the descending Holy Spirit, depicted as a white dove in a mandorla of golden light, with rays going out from it in all directions. The curved wall behind the altar continues the narrative in the earthly realm. The rays of light descending from the apse fall across a cartouche bearing the words 'Veni sancte spiritus' into a room filled with a crowd of people, both men and women. Some fall on their knees, others look startled. The painted architectural features of classical columns and steps serve to link the picture space with the physical space around the altar and to the onlooker in the nave. The fictive space and the real space merge, giving the effect of the light of the Holy Spirit falling on those in the actual building, in particular the space that would have been occupied by the members of the Order seated in the choir. Although they are later replacements for a large ciborium that originally partially obscured the image, the monstrance and cross on the altar appear to become part of the image. From a viewpoint in the nave, the consecrated host, illuminated by candles, effectively becomes the endpoint of the falling rays of light.

If one were in any doubt about what the images were about, angels float in swags above the columns bearing plaques with the Latin texts 'et repleti sunt omnes spiritu sanctu' and 'Et loquebantur verbum Dei cum fiducia'. Together they present the verse 'and they were all filled with the Holy Spirit and spoke the word of God boldly'.[19] These texts reinforce the liturgy as they are extracts from the Lessons for Pentecost in the revised missal. The barrel vault above the altar is decorated with two bands of illusionistic images. The one nearest the altar includes the tondo of God the Father, while that towards the nave contains three rectangular paintings, executed in the illusionistic style known as *quadri riportati*. The decorative borders separating the three images bear texts further expounding the story of the descent of the Holy Spirit empowering the new Christian movement and explaining the images adjacent to them. On the left, 'in nationes gratia Spiritus Sancti effusa est' is taken from the account of Peter preaching and converting the gentiles, and on the right 'venit spiritus sanctus super eos' from a similar account of Paul converting the Greeks in Ephesus.[20] The first of these texts, again, is included in the reformed missal as a reading for the second day of Pentecost.

In the central panel above the altar step, a group of angel musicians accompanies the influx of light falling on Peter and Paul and the newly converted believers depicted in the panels on either side. The implication that angelic music accompanied the descent of the Holy Spirit seems significant in the light

19 Acts 4:31.

20 Acts 10:44–46: 'While Peter was still speaking these words, the Holy Spirit came on all who heard the message. The circumcised believers who had come with Peter were astonished that the gift of the Holy Spirit had been poured out even on the Gentiles.' Acts 19:6: 'When Paul placed his hands on them, the Holy Spirit came on them, and they spoke in tongues and prophesied.'

of other evidence about the celebration of Pentecost, to be discussed below. These angel musicians play a variety of string instruments – violin, viola da gamba, harp, lute and guitar. The predominance of stringed instruments is striking, and perhaps also has a classical reference to the music of Apollo, the ancient god of healing. Apollo, like King David, is often depicted with a lyre or harp, and in mythology was supposed to have despised the wind instruments of Dionysian rituals that were played by Pan and Marsyas, who had challenged his authority.

The left pendentive above the altar facing the nave continues the musical association as it depicts King David with his harp accompanied by the text 'Emitte tuum', an abbreviation of Psalm 103:30, 'emitte spiritum tuum et creabuntur et renovabis faciem terrae'.[21] King David was associated with healing as he played his harp to sooth King Saul. The pairing of David the harp-playing prophet-healer with musical angels accompanying the descent of the Holy Spirit invokes music as a fundamental part of the Pentecostal experience, and by extension, music as having the capacity to heal.

On the opposite pendentive, a prophet looks towards the text 'effundam spiritum meum super semen tuum', a quote from Isaiah.[22] This is slightly odd as the book of Acts refers to the words of Joel that prophesy the coming of the Holy Spirit and the speaking in tongues framed in words that are remarkably similar: 'effundam spiritum meum super omnem carnem'.[23] Whether the intention was to depict Isaiah or Joel, the pairing of this prophet with David frames the narrative of the day of Pentecost both visually and textually. The surviving music from the library of the church indicates that the texts would have been repeated in the music that was sung, thus reinforcing the message.

The Regensburg choirbooks, compiled in the late sixteenth century, contain no less than three settings of 'Veni sancte spiritus', perhaps prompted by the sanction of this text in the revised missal. A further setting, not of the hymn sequence, but of the brief prayer that starts with the same words, is shown in Example 5.1. It is included at the end of two collections of thirty-two and thirty-six motets for processions in manuscript partbooks, I-Rsc G.MSS. 796–805 that date from the late sixteenth century. In the Cantus partbook, the invocation is followed by the versetto 'Emitte tuum' in plainchant. Stylistically this setting of 'Veni sancte spiritus' is essentially a written out falsobordone, and is prefaced by the instruction, 'This is sung in the Pentecost procession kneeling in front of the altar in the middle of the hospital'.[24] This tiny piece of evidence confirms

21 'When you send your spirit, they are created, you renew the face of the earth': Psalm 104:30; (Psalm 103 Vulgate).

22 'I will put my spirit upon him and he will bring justice to the nations': Isaiah 42:1.

23 'I will pour out my spirit upon all people, your sons and daughters will prophesy, your old men will dream dreams, your young men will see visions': Joel 2:28. Zucchi's paintings in another part of the church, the Tolfi chapel, the first chapel on the right, specifically depict Joel.

24 'Questo si canta nella processione della Pentecoste inginocchioni avanti l'altare in mezzo all'ospedale.'

that the celebration of Pentecost, perhaps as part of the new missionary element, embraced not only the local streets through the processions, but also the sick in the hospital. It is perhaps not insignificant that although the setting is simple, the initial invocation in imperfect time is followed quickly by a longer section in triple metre. The symbolism of triple metre as an aural assertion of the Trinity in this context is surely not a coincidence.

These four settings are among the earliest of a number of settings of key Pentecostal texts in the musical archive that include the texts that appear in the frescoes, bringing together the visual and the aural in an effort to move the populace to devotion.

Financing Pentecost celebrations

The cost of providing music for Pentecost is further evidence of the importance of the celebrations, and, from 1570 onwards, the records are increasingly regular, enabling comparisons to be made over time and with other churches. As noted in Chapter 4, in 1570 a payment of 12 scudi was made to the prior to cover the costs associated with Pentecost. Although music is not listed, it seems a safe assumption that at least part of that figure was paid to extra singers. From around 1600 when there were better records, and more of the financial documents have survived, the cost of music for Pentecost can be contextualised using other costs and salaries as comparators. Further, there is eye-witness evidence in the form of a chronicle of the visit to Rome in 1608 by the Irish Earl of Tyrone and his entourage. The chronicle notes the splendour of the music on Pentecost Sunday that included a fine choir, two or three organs and instruments. O'Regan has concluded that the 12 scudi paid to the maestro di cappella, Giovanni Francesco Anerio, would have funded additional singers to make up three groups of singers supported by the three organs, and four instrumentalists. These forces would have been used for at least one of the items.[25]

During the period in which Cesare Zoilo was maestro di cappella in the early decades of the seventeenth century, the same amount of 12 scudi was paid annually from 1610–1618 to cover costs of musicians for Pentecost.[26] Zoilo's normal salary was 6 scudi 66 baiocchi. The regular salary of a singer at that time was 3 scudi, and the organist 2.50.[27] As the musicians for a single celebration of Pentecost cost four times the monthly salary of a singer, we can deduce

25 Noel O'Regan, '"Blessed with the Holy Father's Entertainment": Roman Ceremonial Music as Experienced by the Irish Earls in Rome, 1608', *Irish Musical Studies*, 2 (1993), 41–57. O'Regan has also suggested possible musical items that might have been performed on this occasion, one of which is a Magnificat by Anerio now in the Biblioteca Casanatense, Ms 5406.

26 ASR OSS 1914, *Copie di mandati*, 1612, item 908; ASR OSS 1915, *Copie di mandati*, 1614, item 619; ASR OSS 1919, *Copie di mandati*, 1618, item 772.

27 ASR OSS 1913, *Copie di mandati*, 1610, item 827.

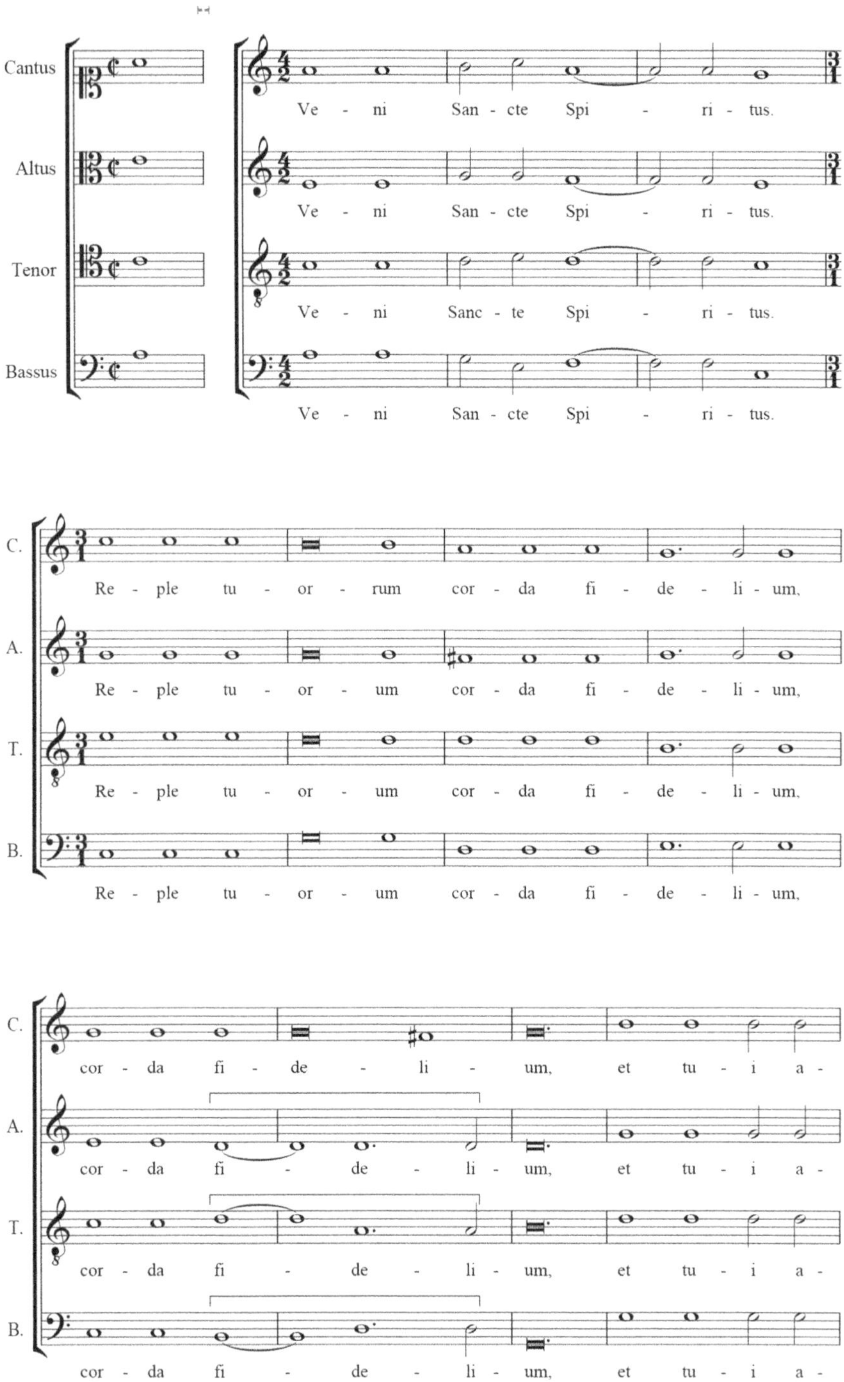
Cantus
Altus
Tenor
Bassus
Ve - ni San - cte Spi - ri - tus.
Ve - ni San - cte Spi - ri - tus.
Ve - ni Sanc - te Spi - ri - tus.
Ve - ni San - cte Spi - ri - tus.
C.
A.
T.
B.
Re - ple tu - or - rum cor - da fi - de - li - um,
Re - ple tu - or - um cor - da fi - de - li - um,
Re - ple tu - or - um cor - da fi - de - li - um,
Re - ple tu - or - um cor - da fi - de - li - um,
C.
A.
T.
B.
cor - da fi - de - li - um, et tu - i a -
cor - da fi - de - li - um, et tu - i a -
cor - da fi - de - li - um, et tu - i a -
cor - da fi - de - li - um, et tu - i a -

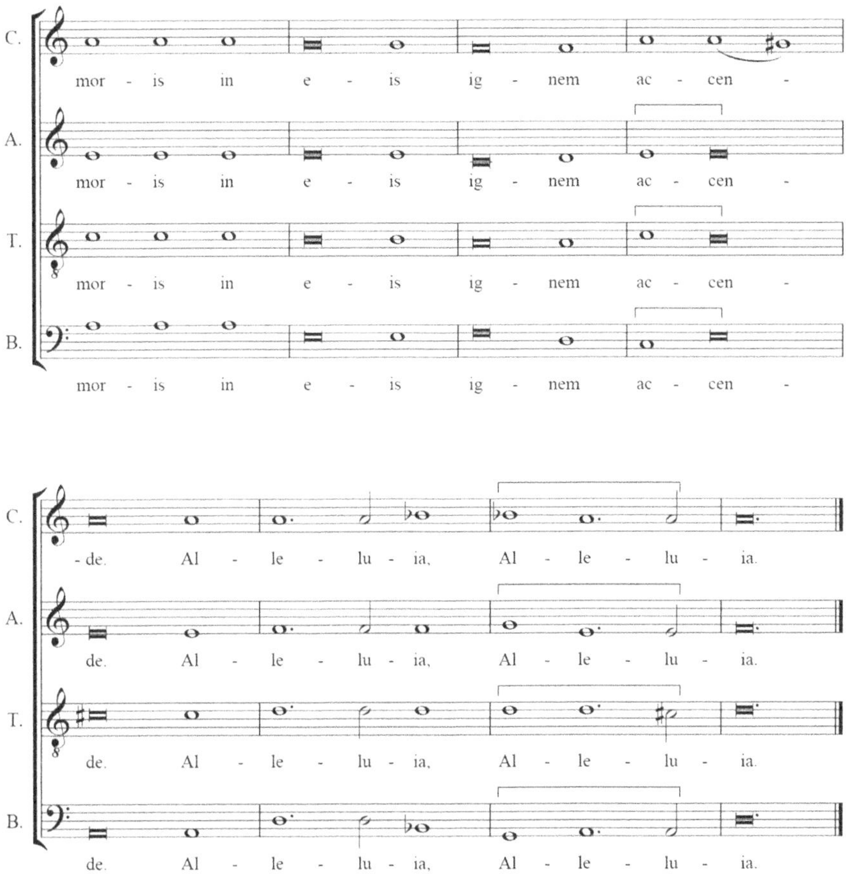

Example 5.1 'Veni sancte spiritus,' I-RsC G.MSS. 796–805.

that a fair number of musicians were hired for the occasion. It would probably also cover the cost of hiring additional organs and for building the *palchi* or wooden platforms that singers and instrumentalists might use in spaces not normally used for music.

A sixteen-voice choir could feasibly have been funded by the amount paid to Zoilo, especially if all the singing chaplains of the Order were called on to supplement the professional singers. That sixteen voices were used for important occasions is supported by the number of surviving musical items from the Santo Spirito music library that are scored for such forces. The choir of twenty that Gregory Martin claims to have witnessed in the 1570s is probably not too much of an exaggeration if viewed in relation to the financial records and the Irish chronicle.

Payments made for Pentecost celebrations were reduced to 5 scudi in the early 1620s and rose again in 1625, when Paolo Troiano was briefly in charge, acting as maestro di cappella.[28] This cutback coincides with Anselmi's reduction of professional singers noted by Spada (discussed below) and perhaps indicates that his economies included expenditure on the patronal feast. Fortunately, we have evidence of a more exact breakdown of costs for one year, 1628, that can provide a point of comparison for calculations of costs relative to the number of musicians. In 1628 there was no salaried maestro di cappella, and a Don Matteo, presumably one of the friars, was paid for his expenses in hiring the musicians. In this case we have names for the musicians, all of whom were identified as from St Peter's. There were nine singers: sopranos Ciero and Francesco; Matteo and Santi (contralto); Annibale, Gabrielo and Jacomo, all tenors; Angelo and Pierluigi basses; and an anonymous 'maestro di cappella di S. Pietro'. The full names of the singers who can be identified are Francesco Bardi (soprano), Matteo Carlucci and Santi Moschetti (contralto), Annibale Fazi and Giacomo Bontempi (tenor) and Angelo Santa Croce (bass). Santi Moschetti had been a singer at Santo Spirito and moved on to St Peter's in 1623, as did Angelo Santa Croce.[29] These singers were accompanied by a violinist, Lionardo, a cornetist, Giorgio and Frescobaldi, identified as organist of St Peter's, though he was previously an employee of Santo Spirito.

This is the only record that has come to light in which the additional musicians are named. The records generally only note payments made to the maestro di cappella for 'external musicians', or even more vaguely, for payments made to 'more singers' for Pentecost.[30] What this unique entry tells us in addition to

[28] ASR OSS 1922, *Copie di mandati*, 1621, item 926; ASR OSS 1923, *Copie di mandati*, 1623, item 904 (Zoilo paid 5 scudi) ASR OSS 1924, *Copie di mandati*, 1625, item 691 (Troiano paid 12 scudi). Paolo Troiano may have been a relative of Giovanni Troiano, a composer active in Rome in the first decades of the seventeenth century.

[29] These singers were all listed in the Cappella Giulia in June 1627. Giancarlo Rostirolla, *Musica e musicisti nella basilica di San Pietro: cinque secoli di storia della Cappella Giulia*, 2 vols (Rome, 2014), vol. 1, p. 381.

[30] 'per tanti ne ha pagati a più musici forestieri per la festa di Pentacosta...': ASR OSS

names is the amount each individual was paid. Six of them, including the maestro di cappella and Frescobaldi, were paid 2 scudi, the rest of the singers and instrumentalists were paid 1.50, making the total bill 22.50 – a not insubstantial sum. Even taking into account the fact that the Pentecost celebrations were not confined to a single day and that the vigil, Sunday, and both the Monday and Tuesday following were marked by services and of course the procession to St Peter's and celebratory Masses, the payments to the individuals were half to two-thirds of a month's salary at the normal rate of pay within the institution.

By the third decade of the seventeenth century the size of the regular choir had expanded to six adult singers, and they, along with the organist, were all still paid the same salary as the employees of the 1620s. While salary levels remained stable, the cost of the Pentecost celebrations, in contrast, rose. In 1644, 17 scudi was paid; by 1651 it had gone up to 36 scudi.[31]

The *mandati* for 1651 offer another nugget of valuable information, in that the recorded payment for Pentecost notes that the amount paid was for music in four choirs with instruments for first Vespers, Mass and second Vespers.[32] This is the only time note is made of the specific services for which singers were hired. At this time there doesn't appear to have been a maestro di cappella listed in the usual group of singers and chaplains, but Pietro Fabrizi is named as maestro di cappella for Pentecost. Fabrizi was clearly a singing priest and a member of the Order of Santo Spirito. He had other duties for which he received a salary, the most significant of which was as the 'commissario di balie', in charge of overseeing the welfare of the wetnurses in the orphanage.

There is a similar entry for the Pentecost of 1655, noting that the payment was for music in four choirs with instruments, but it lacks the detail of specific services. The musicians named in the pay records in 1655 include Ercole Bernabei as organist, and Florido de Silvestris as one of the singers. The others are Giovanni Antonio Schiave, Girolamo Barluzzi, Don Nicolo, Bartolomeo Canesti, Filippo Sota, while the soprano is listed simply as 'Giuseppe soprano'. As there were already six voices, and the music for Pentecost was for sixteen, plus instruments, there would presumably have been ten additional singers, potentially supporting instrumentalists and up to three additional organists, though of course the personnel for Mass and for the procession are likely to have been different.[33]

1919, *Copie di mandati*, 1618, item 772; 'per pagamenti a più cantori per la festa della pentecoste': ASR OSS 1920, *Copie di mandati*, 1619, item 734.

31 ASR OSS 1942, *Copie di mandati*, 1644, item 715; ASR OSS 1948, *Copie di mandati*, 1651, item 716.

32 'A Pietro Fabritii nostro Maestro di Cappella, trentasei scudi fanno pagare ad effetto che cioe … per faceva la musica fatto per diversi instrumenti a quattro cori nella nostra chiesa alle quale date ne debito per la festa di Pentacosta per la prima vesperi del lunedì, messe cantate di detto giorno e per la seconda vesperi come poi di veda nel sottoscritto con pigliare ricevuta': ASR OSS 1948. *Copie di mandati*, 1651, item 716.

33 ASR OSS 1952, *Copie di mandati*, 1655, item 584.

The surviving repertory of music for Pentecost

Only a small number of settings of texts for Pentecost from the reformed missal have survived in the musical archive, but they do perhaps hint at the kind of music that was performed for this key feast day. The quantity of surviving settings of these texts is shown in Figure 5.1.

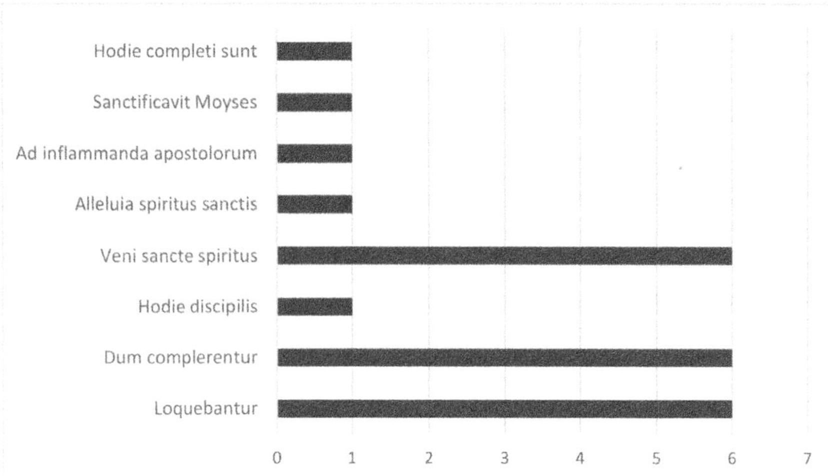

Figure 5.1 Musical settings of texts for Pentecost (including those in the Regensburg choirbooks).

While there are a number of Mass Ordinaries for twelve or sixteen voices, the forces for these settings are more varied. For example, a setting of 'Dum complerentur' attributed to G. B. Anselmi, although for four choirs, is actually for four pairs of voices, soprano and bass, with organ, rather than four SATB choirs.[34] The reduced polychoral texture would have retained the effect of surrounding the participants with sound, but perhaps have been more economical. In contrast, an anonymous eight-part setting of the hymn sequence 'Veni sancte spiritus' in the Feininger collection uses a somewhat monolithic block-like alternation of choirs (see Example 5.3, pp. 106–109 below).[35] Another, a setting of 'Ad inflammanda apostolorum', is almost a mini-cantata, with successive sections of solo voices with continuo, finishing with the full ensemble of three voices – two sopranos and a bass – with organ.[36] Several of these settings take advantage of the opportunities for word painting. In the anonymous 'Ad

[34] I-TrFeininger FP 122/1–15 attributed to G. B. Anselmi, 'Dum complerentur'.

[35] I-TrFeininger FP 121/1–10 Anon, 'Veni sancti spiritus'.

[36] I-TrFeininger FP 130/1–4 Anon, 'Ad inflammanda apostolorum'.

inflammanda apostolorum', the opening section includes melismas that imitate in sound the descent of the Holy Spirit through sequences of descending running semiquavers, while the tongues of fire described in the text are mirrored in ascending and descending semiquavers that almost create the rising and falling shape of flames on the page (see Example 5.2). In somewhat similar fashion, Bernabei's setting of 'Loquebantur variis linguis' uses the 'speaking' of 'loquebantur' to develop melismatic passages that pass between the choirs, the effect no doubt intended to mimic the babble of many voices.[37]

If the items scored for three or four choirs were sung from the galleries and choir stalls, the effect of sound surrounding the onlooker would have provided an aural parallel to the painted depictions of heavenly light falling from the fictive spaces of the walls and vaults into the real space of the tribune of the church. The descent of the Holy Spirit perceived as real and fictive light, sound and, in addition, smell in the form of incense, would have been a powerful statement of doctrine and probably quite an emotional one for the congregation, or at least for those close enough to the tribune to experience it.

Valone has noted that as the religious climate of the early seventeenth century changed from optimism about the reunification of Christendom to realistic confrontation with the Protestant revolt, the iconography of Pentecost reverted to an earlier type depicting a much reduced group of disciples and apostles receiving the gifts of the spirit.[38] In contrast, at Santo Spirito the musical celebration of Pentecost not only continued, but over the course of the next century must have become increasingly sophisticated as the recorded costs of the music alone spiralled. By 1700, the music for Pentecost cost more than 97 scudi, while the monthly salary of the singers remained static at 3 scudi.[39]

An overview of liturgical music from the Santo Spirito library

While music for Pentecost was evidently large-scale and a display of splendour, the surviving musical archive indicates that it wasn't the only feast celebrated with elaborate music. Although around half of the surviving music is anonymous, by using music that does carry an attribution and/or a date, some indication of the level of activity across time can be extracted. A purely numerical count of items that can be securely attributed and therefore placed within a likely chronological timespan relating to the active life of the composer demonstrates the patterns of musical activity at the Hospital. The data here needs some context. Rostirolla lists over 500 items that once belonged to the music library of Santo Spirito, all in partbook format. He does not include the Regensburg choirbooks, which contain a further 185 items. Aside from

37 I-Rc Ms 5404.

38 Valone, 'Pentecost: image and experience', p. 828.

39 ASR-OSS 1995, *Copie di mandati*, 1700, item 495.

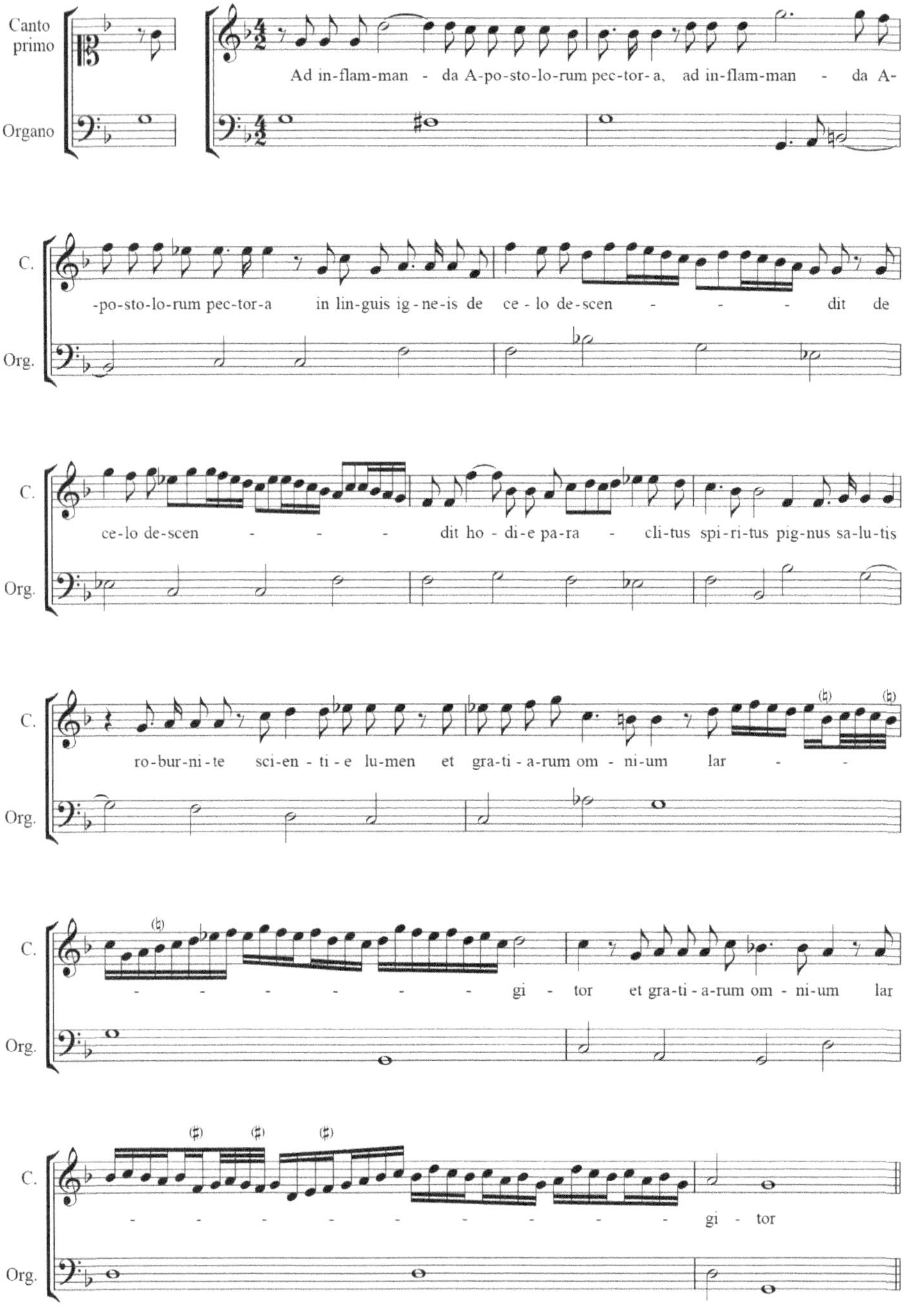
Canto primo
Organo
Ad in-flam-man - da A-po-sto-lo-rum pec-tor-a, ad in-flam-man - da A-
C.
Org.
-po-sto-lo-rum pec-tor-a in lin-guis ig-ne-is de ce-lo de-scen - - - dit de
ce-lo de-scen - - - dit ho - di-e pa-ra - cli-tus spi-ri-tus pig-nus sa-lu-tis
ro-bur-ni-te sci-en - ti - e lu-men et gra-ti - a-rum om - ni-um lar - -
- - - - - - gi - tor et gra-ti - a-rum om - ni-um lar
- - - - - - - - - gi - tor

Example 5.2 Anon, 'Ad inflammanda apostolorum,' I-TrFeininger, FP 130/1–4, opening section.

four Cifra Masses, all the music contained within the Regensburg choirbooks, including the anonymous material, dates from before 1603, although some of the material was copied between 1625 and 1637. The music without composer attributions listed by Rostirolla cannot be given blanket dates and would need careful stylistic study in order to establish even approximate dates.

Over 60% of the surviving music listed by Rostirolla that carries a composer attribution can be dated to the period 1600–1660. The marginally fewer compositions in the timespan 1630–1660 represented in Figure 5.2 (30.5% as opposed to 31.5%) is somewhat misleading as some composers such as Carissimi were active mid-century and the dates of specific outputs impossible to ascertain. After 1660, the number drops quite sharply, and drops again after 1700. These late manuscripts may have entered the library around or after the suppression of the professional choir, and for the purposes of this study are not included.

Using the 62% of the surviving material that falls within the date range 1600–1660 and collating this data with information about the vocal forces required, the activity becomes more sharply defined. Before 1600, music for more than five voices was the exception rather than the rule. After the turn of the seventeenth century, music for six or more voices was common, if not the norm. This further nuancing of the data is presented in Figure 5.3, where the proportion of music for five voices is shown in comparison to music for more than five voices.

If music from the Regensburg choirbooks is included in the data, the shift in vocal forces over this period of time becomes even more marked, as can be seen in Figure 5.4.

By including all the anonymous and undated pieces in the data, the vocal forces that were favoured becomes even clearer, as shown in Figure 5.5. There is a sizeable group of pieces for a small number of voices with organ, along with the expected four- and five-voice settings typical of late-sixteenth-century sacred polyphony, a significant proportion of which is contained in the Regensburg choirbooks. However, 74% of the material not in the choirbooks is for six or more voices, with items scored for only six voices making up a tiny fraction of that percentage. A significant quantity of surviving music is scored for double choir with and without additional instruments stipulated as 'ripieni' or 'concertato'.

Although eight-voice settings dominate the large-scale compositions, there are a number of items for double choir in nine voices and for twelve or sixteen voices, distributed in three or four choirs, sometimes 'concertato' rather than just with organ bass. Only around 8% of the 501 items in the manuscript listings are for twelve to sixteen voices in three or four choirs. This figure rises to 14% if music for nine or more voices is included.[40] Dixon suggests that this kind of music was circulated largely in manuscript rather than in printed for-

40 There are no settings for more than eight voices in the Regensburg choirbooks.

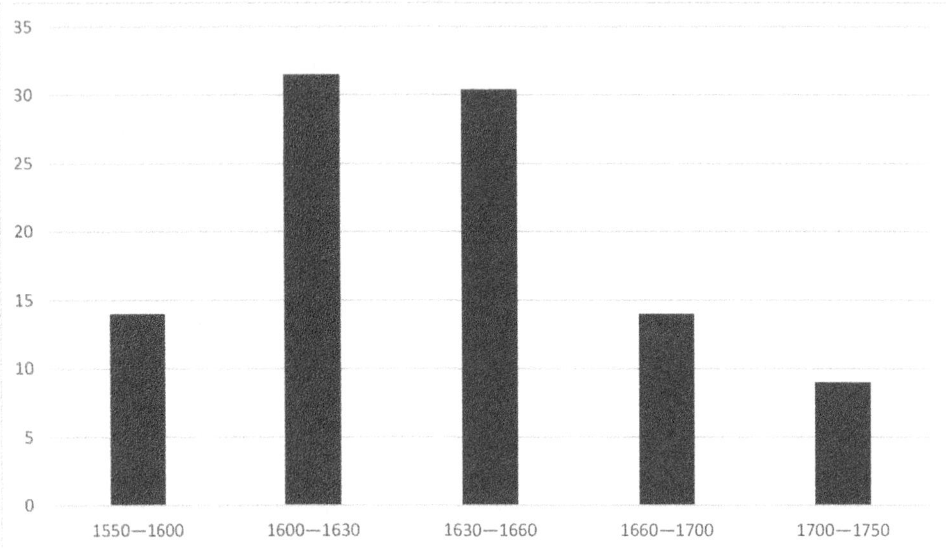

Figure 5.2 Distribution of music manuscripts dated by composer attribution expressed as percentages but excluding the items in the Regensburg choirbooks which pre-date 1600.

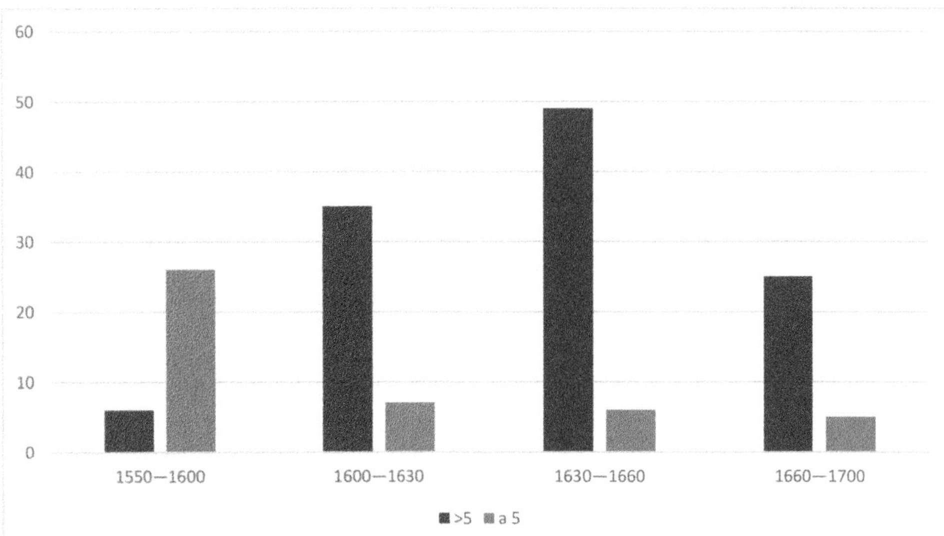

Figure 5.3 Numerical count of music manuscripts for five voices and more than five voices dated by composer attribution, excluding material from the Regensburg choirbooks.

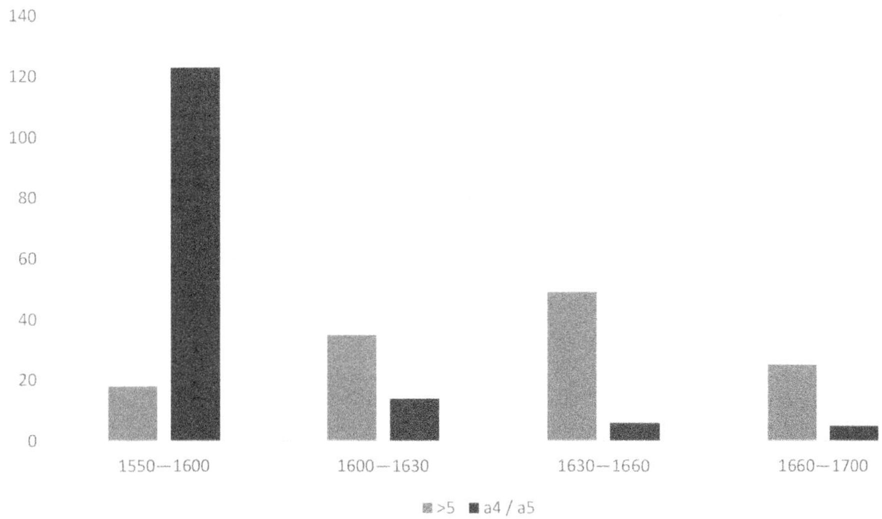

Figure 5.4 Numerical count of manuscript items for four to five voices compared to larger forces, including material from Regensburg choirbooks.

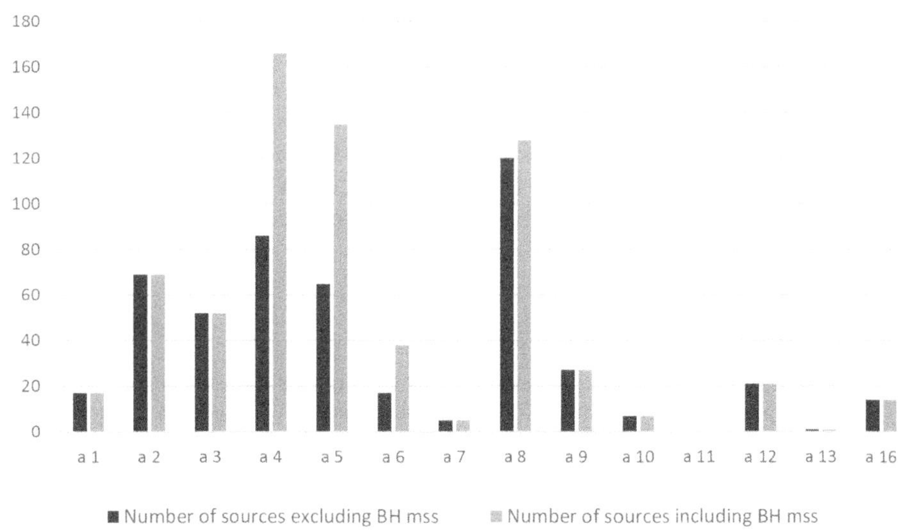

Figure 5.5 Vocal forces required in surviving music manuscripts.

mats because few institutions could afford music of this scale. The small market meant that printed books were not financially viable.[41]

This data is indicative that the church of Santo Spirito adopted the Roman polychoral style that had first appeared in the 1570s, such as in Palestrina's second and third motet collections, and that flourished in the final decades of the sixteenth century.[42] However, it seems to have taken up the style somewhat later than some other Roman churches such as S. Luigi dei Francesi. Nevertheless, there are indications that at Santo Spirito the style was retained for a long period of time. The so-called 'colossal baroque' style using multiple choirs had become popular for celebrating important feast days at various churches in Rome by the 1620s, but at Santo Spirito, payment records for the celebration of Pentecost suggest that they continued to employ very large numbers of musicians for their patronal feast day, even as late as 1700.

Additional evidence for the use of polychoral music

Architectural spaces too, were adapted to accommodate new styles of music. Morelli notes the positioning of pulpits or galleries for singers in fifteenth- and sixteenth-century buildings, and how new churches such as Santa Maria in Vallicella (the Chiesa Nuova, consecrated in 1599) and Sant'Ivo alla Sapienza (1642–1660) were built with multiple singing galleries (*cantorie*) specifically to accommodate polychoral music. In older churches, platforms (*palchi*) for groups of singers or instrumentalists were built and placed in different positions in the nave, side chapels and galleries, using existing architectural spaces to maximise the effect of the new musical style. In addition, organs were moved to different positions to facilitate polychoral singing. [43]

Santo Spirito followed the trends of the time and can be added to the major Roman basilicas discussed by Morelli. Various payments to a 'festarolo' or the major-domo for building platforms or other apparatus are scattered throughout the financial records. In 1604, Luca and Stefano Blasi were paid for moving the bellows of the large nave organ to create more space for singers.[44] Both the

41 Graham Dixon, 'The Origins of the Roman "Colossal Baroque"', *Proceedings of the Royal Musical Association*, 106 (1979–1980), 115–128.

42 The organisation and use of Palestrina's motet collections is discussed in detail in Noel O'Regan, 'Palestrina's Mid-life Compositional Summary', in E. Rodriguez-Garcia and D. Filippi (eds), *Mapping the Motet in the Post-Tridentine Era* (Abingdon, 2019), pp. 102–122.

43 Arnaldo Morelli, *Teatro della vista e dell'udito: La musica e i suoi luoghi nell'età moderna* (Lucca, 2017), pp. 71–98.

44 Morelli, '*Teatro della vista*', p. 23; Furio Luccichenti, 'Luca Blasi (c. 1545–1608): Profilo di un organaro', *L'Organo*, XIX (1981), 113–131; Melella summarises the notarial records in Patrizia Melella, 'Vita musicale e arte organaria a Santo Spirito in Sassia

organs were tuned regularly, and in 1636 Ennio Bonifatio was paid for replacing the bellows on the small organ.[45] Two years later, in 1638, he was paid 50 scudi for work done, and to be done, on a new organ. It was probably at this latter time that the small organ was replaced and repositioned in an enlarged balcony or pulpit on the left (east) side of the tribune – the position in which it is depicted in an engraving in Saulnier's book of 1649, and in which it has remained.[46] The potential for dramatic musical interchanges between the organ and singers in the nave and a similar group above and to the left of the altar may well have been exploited in the music for eight or more voices found in the Santo Spirito musical archive. One could easily imagine the anonymous 'Veni sancti spiritus' (Example 5.3) for double choir creating a majestic effect if performed in this way, but a close analysis of the body of music from Santo Spirito is needed to evaluate more accurately how it might have been performed in this space.

There was a salaried choir of eight recorded in the payment books for most of the second half of the seventeenth century (see below). The continued use of polychoral music at the Hospital indicates that Santo Spirito followed the practices in other Roman institutions such as S. Luigi dei Francesi and Santa Maria dell'Anima.[47] Double, triple and quadruple choirs, often with supporting concertato groups would have been costly, even if only for three or four major feasts, and speaks to the priority of these celebrations in the liturgical year.

An analysis of the eight-voice settings by genre suggests that music for Vespers was the most common use for eight-voice compositions. The disposition of these compositions by genre is illustrated in Figure 5.6. There are 109 eight-voice pieces, of which just over half have an identifiable composer. Eight-voice mass settings account for only 8% of the total, while motets account for 30% and psalms for 45%. The remainder is made up of Magnificats (13%) and miscellaneous liturgical pieces (one hymn, one setting of the improperia etc.) (4%).[48] The prominence of eight-voice music aligns with the eight-man choir listed in financial records from the middle of the seventeenth century. The bal-

---

nel cinquecento: note e documenti', in Bianca Maria Antolini, Arnaldo Morelli and Vera Vita Spagnuolo, *La musica a Roma attraverso le fonti d'archivio* (Lucca, 1994), pp. 507–519. For more on the nave organ, see pp. 136–138.

45 '... per haver fatto due mantici novi per l'organo piccolo della nostra chiesa': ASR OSS 1934, *Copie di mandati*, 1636, item 646.

46 '... di diversi lavori d'organista fatti, e da farsi intorno all'organo novo della nostra chiesa': ASR OSS 1936, *Copie di mandati*, 1638 item 1486.

47 For material on S. Luigi dei Francesi, see Jean Lionnet, 'La musique a Saint-Louis des Français de Rome au XVII° siècle', *Note d'Archivio*, III (1985), supplement. Celebrations of the patronal feast of S. Luigi dei Francesi continued to use very large forces into the 1660s. See Florian Bassani Grampp, 'On a Roman Polychoral Performance in August 1665', *Early Music*, 36:3 (2008), 415–433.

48 I have followed Rostirolla's genre assignations to generate these figures.

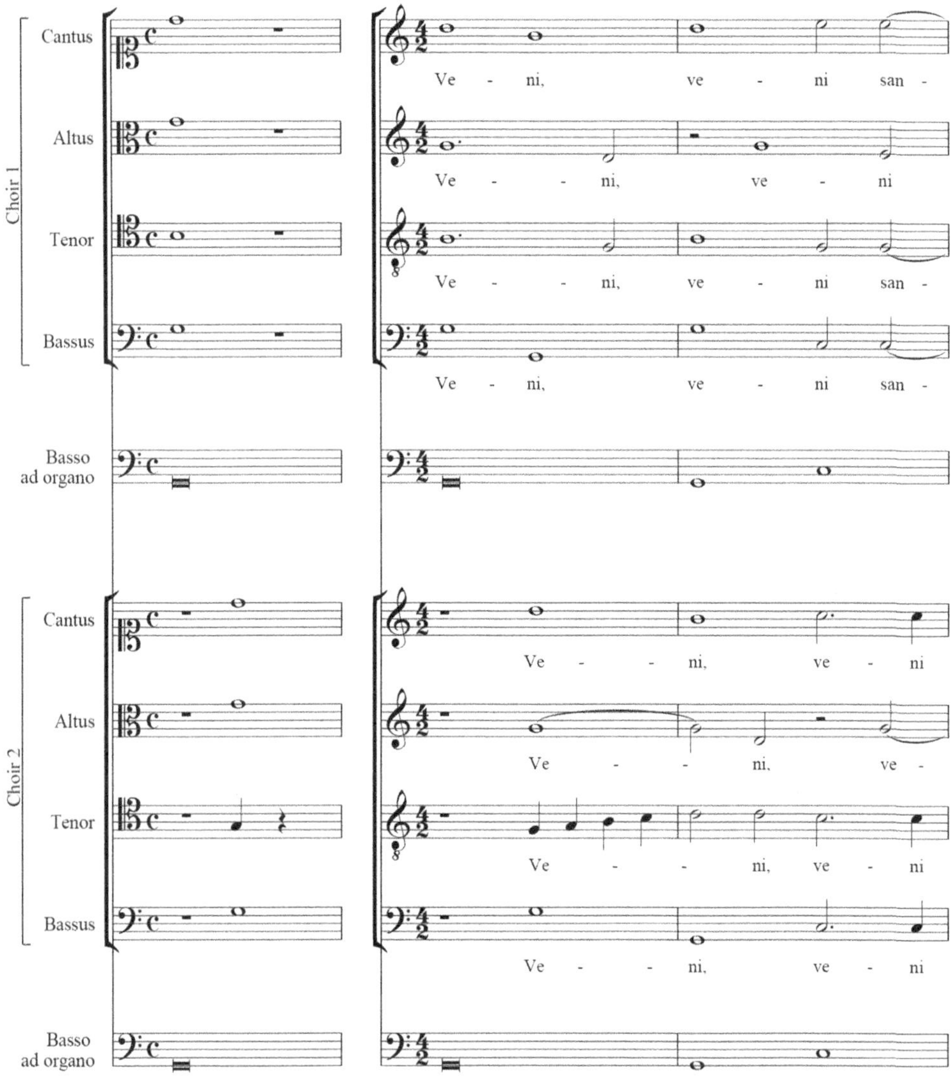
Choir 1
Cantus
Ve - ni, ve - ni san -
Altus
Ve - - ni, ve - ni
Tenor
Ve - - ni, ve - ni san -
Bassus
Ve - ni, ve - ni san -
Basso ad organo
Choir 2
Cantus
Ve - - ni, ve - ni
Altus
Ve - - ni, ve -
Tenor
Ve - - ni, ve - ni
Bassus
Ve - - ni, ve - ni
Basso ad organo

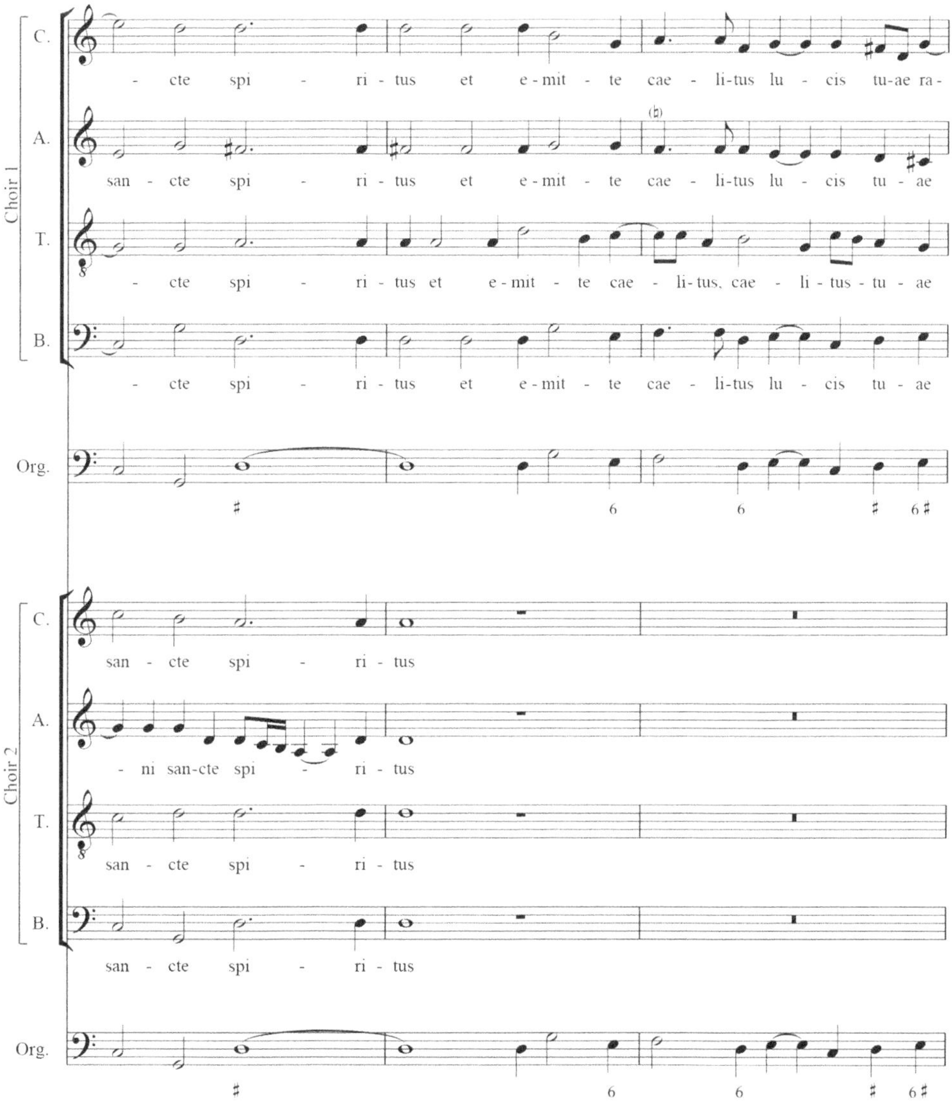

Example 5.3 Anon, 'Veni sancti spiritus,' I-TrFeininger FP 121/1–10, bars 1–11.

(Example 5.3 continued)

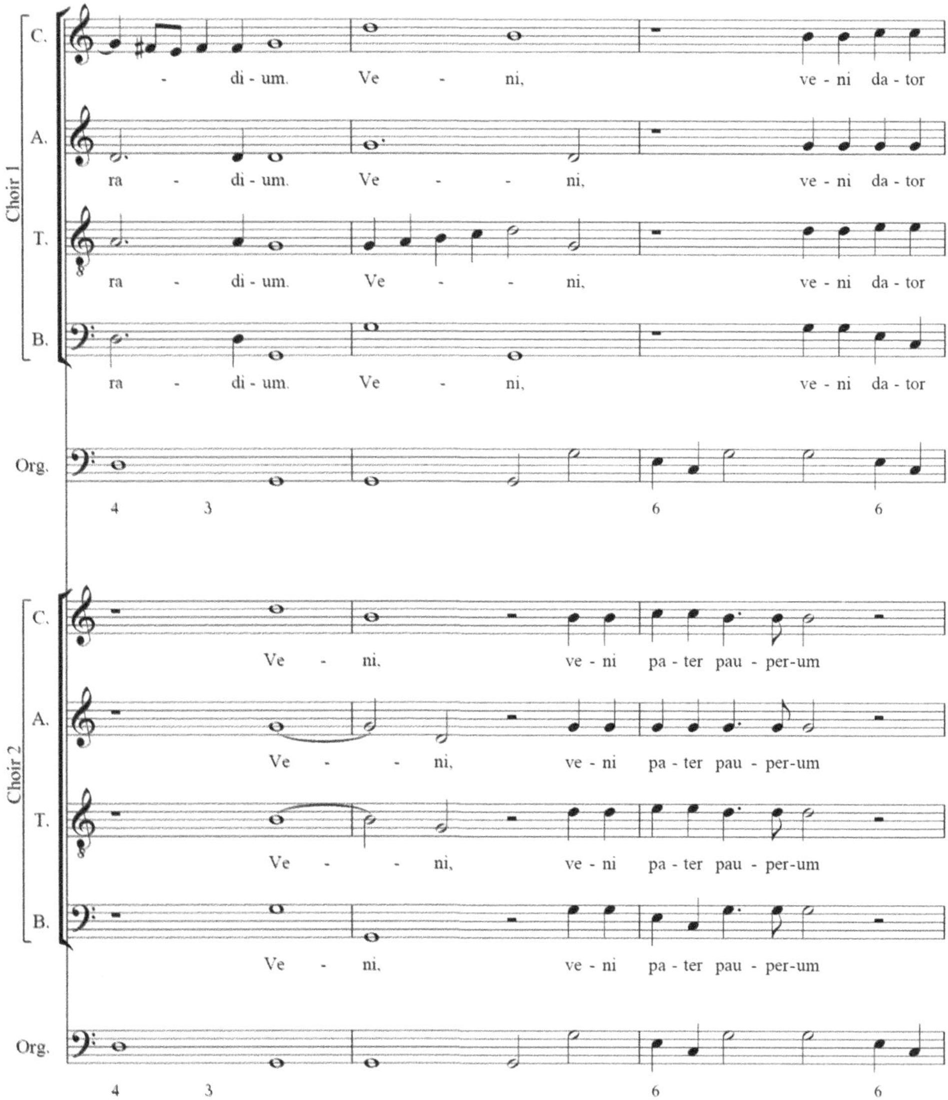

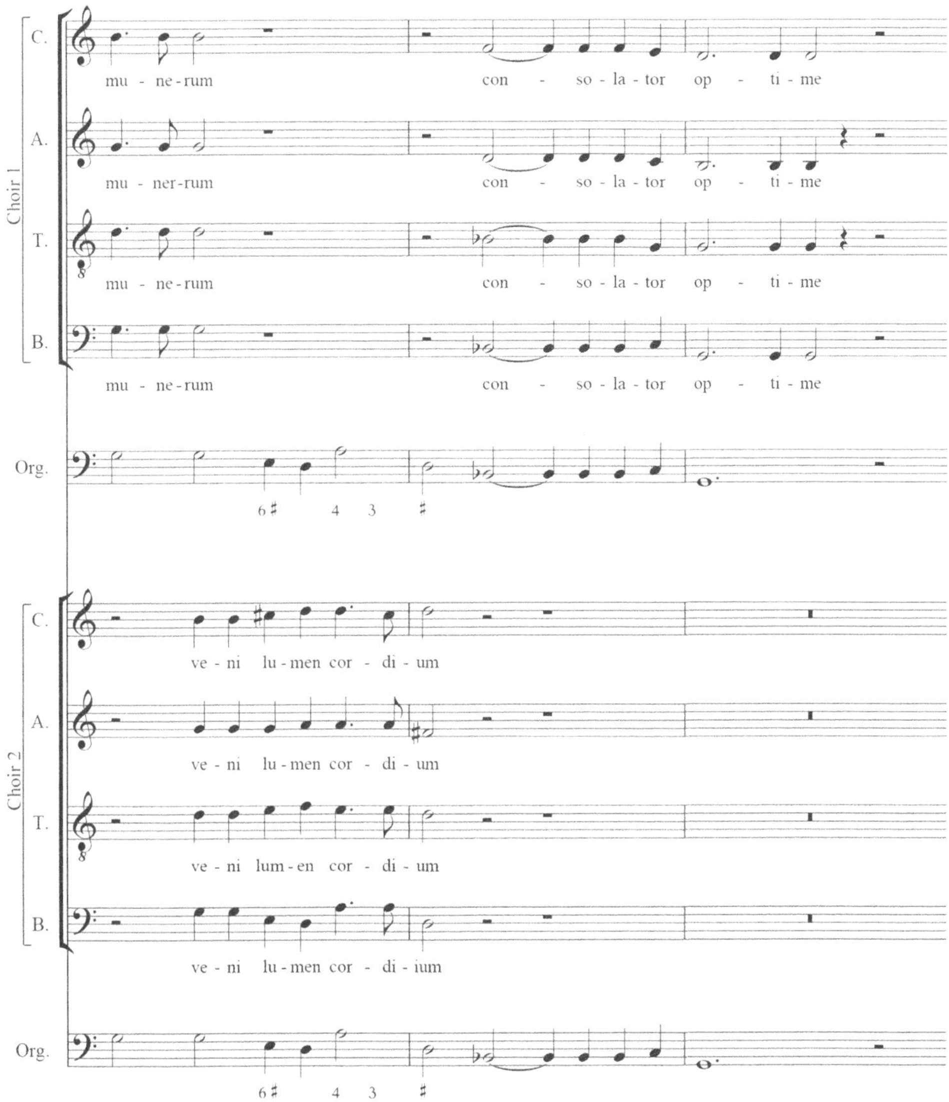
Choir 1
C.
mu - ne-rum con - so - la - tor op - ti - me
A.
mu - ner-rum con - so - la - tor op - ti - me
T.
mu - ne-rum con - so - la - tor op - ti - me
B.
mu - ne-rum con - so - la - tor op - ti - me
Org.
6♯ 4 3 ♯
Choir 2
C.
ve - ni lu - men cor - di - um
A.
ve - ni lu - men cor - di - um
T.
ve - ni lum - en cor - di - um
B.
ve - ni lu - men cor - di - ium
Org.
6♯ 4 3 ♯

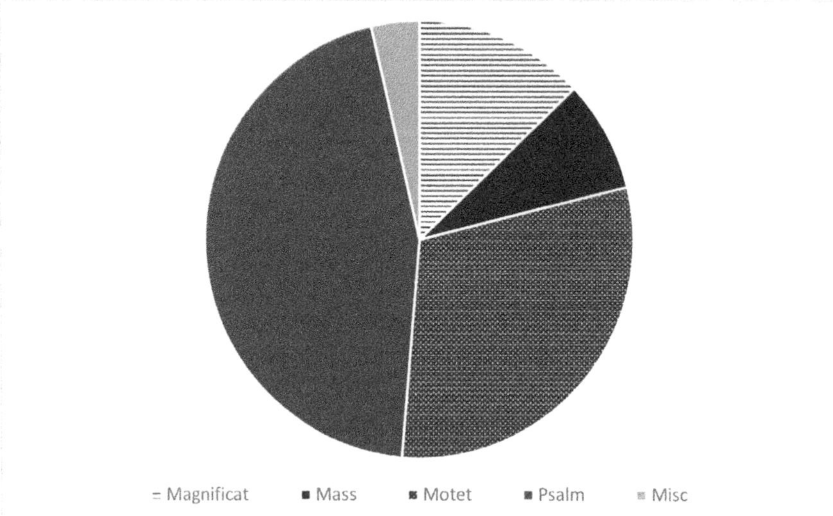

Figure 5.6 Distribution of eight-voice settings by genre.

ance of genres suggests that those that offer the possibility of affective expression, that is the various psalm settings and motets, were most likely to be sung with larger forces on special occasions. This leaning towards expressive potential might also suggest that it was music for Vespers rather than Mass that was accorded the most elaborate setting.

In the years following the publication of the revised breviary in 1568, numerous composers produced collections of music to fulfil the need for music for Vespers that included hymns, psalms and Magnificats. New motet collections too were organised according to the liturgical year and reflected the suppression of certain feast days. Motets were not strictly necessary to the liturgy, but the texts they used could comment on or provide exegesis of the scriptural texts that were proper to the day, though of course such exegeses would only have been accessible to those with a knowledge of Latin.[49] They were most commonly sung during the Offertory, Elevation, Communion and at the end of Mass and the end of Vespers, but, as O' Regan has pointed out, motets could have a variety of uses, not just liturgical. Motets were, for example, sung in the institution-specific context of the *Possesso* (a special service for the installation of a new commendatore). The term 'motet' itself is problematic in this period, thus the term 'sacrae cantiones' may be viewed as an equivalent.[50]

Further, the motet was seized upon as a vehicle for creating music that would move the emotions whether to sorrow and penitence, to joy and praise,

[49] David Crook, 'Proper to the Day: Calendrical Ordering in Post-Tridentine Motet Books', in Rodríguez-Garcìa and Filippi, *Mapping the Motet*, pp. 16–35.

[50] O'Regan, 'Palestrina's Mid-life Compositional Summary', pp. 102–122, esp. p. 114.

or to inspire pious devotion. An understanding of the text was not necessary if the right emotions were elicited in the listener.[51] With this emotional function in mind, motets may well have been used in the hospital wards, as will be discussed in the next chapter. It is not surprising, therefore, that motets form the largest group of items in the surviving music manuscripts. In itself, the collection of motets from the Santo Spirito music library deserves close study in terms of text choice, organisation with regard to liturgical use, and style.[52]

Music for Vespers

After the revision of the breviary, public musical celebrations of the Offices tended to become restricted to Sunday Vespers, and it was for these services that professional singers were required.[53] In addition to Sunday Vespers, Vespers for feasts of the Blessed Virgin Mary, of the apostles, evangelists and martyrs; for Corpus Domini and a church's patronal or dedication feast would have required more lavish musical accompaniment. However, some psalms were common to celebratory Vespers for many days of the year; thus fourteen psalms and the Magnificat were constantly recurring items and mostly likely to have been sung in polyphony. Eleven of these psalms served for Sundays or for categories of feasts as noted in Table 5.1. A further three were used for Corpus Domini and Christmas.

The importance of Vespers at Santo Spirito is supported by documents outlining the duties of the organist who was required to play daily for Mass and for Vespers on Sundays and feast days and for the Saturday Litanies. Further, the contents of the surviving music library provide proof of the quantity of music created or collected for use in this Office. There are 140 settings of Vespers psalms and thirty-five Magnificats among the surviving music manuscripts from Santo Spirito listed by Rostirolla.[54] In sharp contrast, of the approximately 180 items included in the late-sixteenth-century Regensburg choirbooks, only six are psalm settings.[55]

51 Bertoglio, *Reforming Music*, p. 468.

52 It is beyond the scope of this book to examine these motets, but as a body of music from a single institution they are a rich resource.

53 John Harper, *The Forms and Orders of Western Liturgy from the Tenth Century to the Eighteenth Century* (Oxford, 1991) p. 158.

54 These figures take Rostirolla's information at face value and include sources that may not have been in the Santo Spirito library in the seventeenth century. They also do not include the Regensburg choirbooks.

55 There is also a single verse of *In exitu Israel* (*Mare videt*) by Papini in BH 6005 and BH 6006. These two sources are identical apart from the addition of a 'sicut erat' in BH 6005. This incomplete setting of the text has not been included in this statistic.

Table 5.1 Core Psalms for Vespers.*

Psalm	Sunday Vespers	BVM	apostles, evangelists & martyrs	Dedication	2nd Vespers apostles, evangelists & martyrs
Ps 109 Dixit dominus	✓	✓	✓	✓	✓
Ps 110 Confitebor	✓		✓	✓	
Ps 111 Beatus vir	✓		✓	✓	
Ps 112 Laudate Pueri	✓	✓	✓	✓	✓
Ps 113 In exitu Israel	✓				
Ps 121 Laetatus sum		✓			
Ps 126 Nisi Dominus		✓			
Ps 147 Lauda Jerusalem		✓		✓	
Ps 116 Laudate Dominum			✓		
Ps 115 Credidi propter quod					✓
Ps 125 In convertendo					✓
Ps 139 Domine probasti					✓

*Information redacted from Harper, *The Forms and Orders of Western Liturgy*, pp. 157–161.

A relatively high number of the first four psalms for Sunday Vespers are also used for First Vespers for feasts of apostles, evangelists and martyrs. The remaining psalms, 'In exitu Israel' for Sundays and 'Laudate Dominum' for feasts of apostles, evangelists and martyrs respectively, exist in far fewer settings. In contrast, the psalms for Second Vespers for apostles, evangelists and martyrs are all present, albeit in smaller numbers. The numerical breakdown of the psalm settings is shown in Figure 5.7.

We might conclude from this information that Santo Spirito followed the practice of the papal choir, and that not all the psalms were sung polyphonically for every Vespers even on feast days.[56] A further conclusion is perhaps that psalms that served more than one liturgical purpose were more likely to attract polyphonic settings.

One complete collection of psalms composed by Francesco Beretta who served as maestro di cappella is perhaps indicative of this practice as it might have been performed in the second half of the seventeenth century. As Beretta also served as maestro di cappella at St Peter's we might infer that Santo Spirito followed the same practices. The collection is dated 1688 and contains eight-voice settings of the first four psalms for Sunday Vespers, plus a setting of 'Laudate Dominum'. The opening 'Dixit Dominus' in the collection exemplifies this functional music in the Roman polychoral tradition. The two choirs alternate in short, homorhythmic phrases with very little contrapuntal activity, delivering the text efficiently. See Example 5.4.

Collating the information regarding the function of the psalm settings, 110 items, that is 78.5%, are of the five psalms used for Sunday Vespers, four of which are also used for feasts of the apostles, evangelists and martyrs, and dedication. These would thus have been multi-purpose items. The additional psalms required for other feasts make up a much smaller proportion of the whole.

The proportion of psalms used only for Vespers of the Blessed Virgin is small compared to the multi-purpose Sunday psalms, at only 13.5%. The amount of music for these feasts that has survived in relation to that for Sundays and other feasts implies that there was less music for them to start with, and perhaps that the music might have been recycled and reused over a period of time as only a few Marian feasts were celebrated. Again, on any single feast day, probably not all the psalms were sung in polyphony. As a group, the psalm collection mirrors the frequency of their use in the revised breviary. This information is represented graphically in Figure 5.8.

These statistics offer a window into the way in which an institution that was tied by patronal relationship to the papacy responded to the Tridentine reforms. As already noted in Chapter 3, the instructions issued by successive governors to sing the psalms with devotion, and to be often in the choir,

[56] The practices and statistics for Vespers music in the papal choir are given in Noel O' Regan, 'Sacred polychoral music in Rome 1575–1621' (unpublished D.Phil. thesis, University of Oxford, 1988), p. 85.

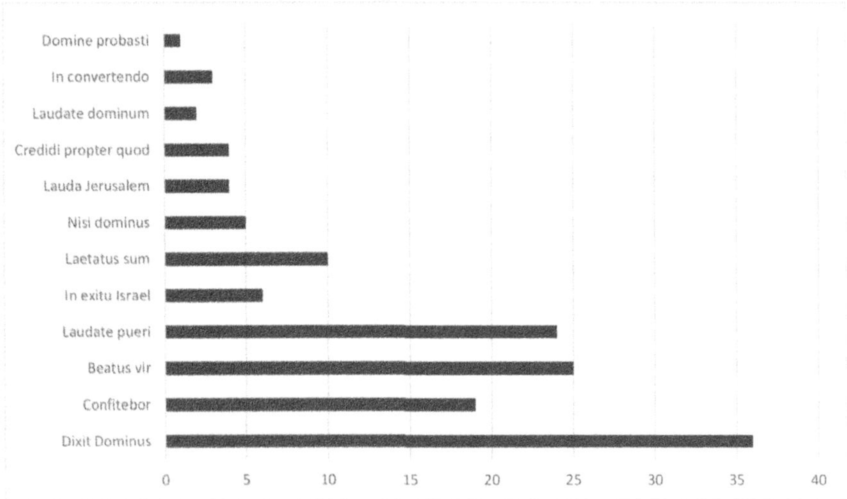

Figure 5.7 Numerical breakdown of manuscript psalm settings.

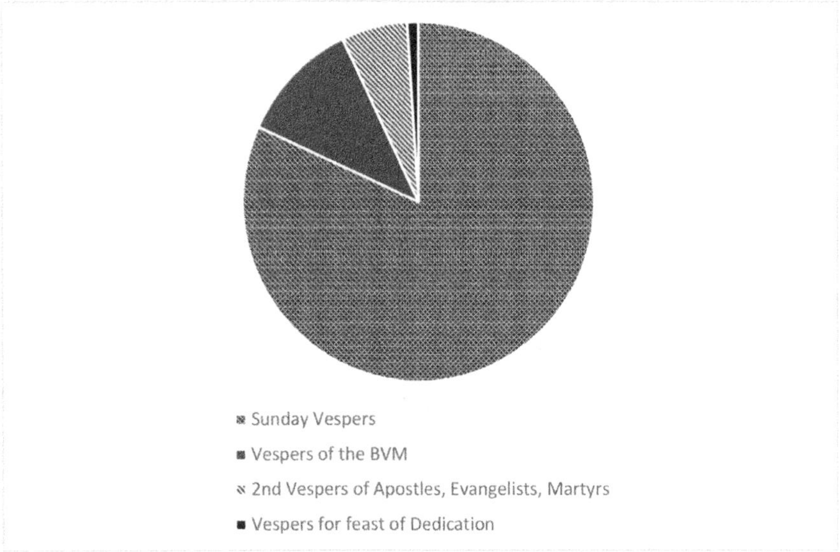

Figure 5.8 Uses of Vespers psalm settings.

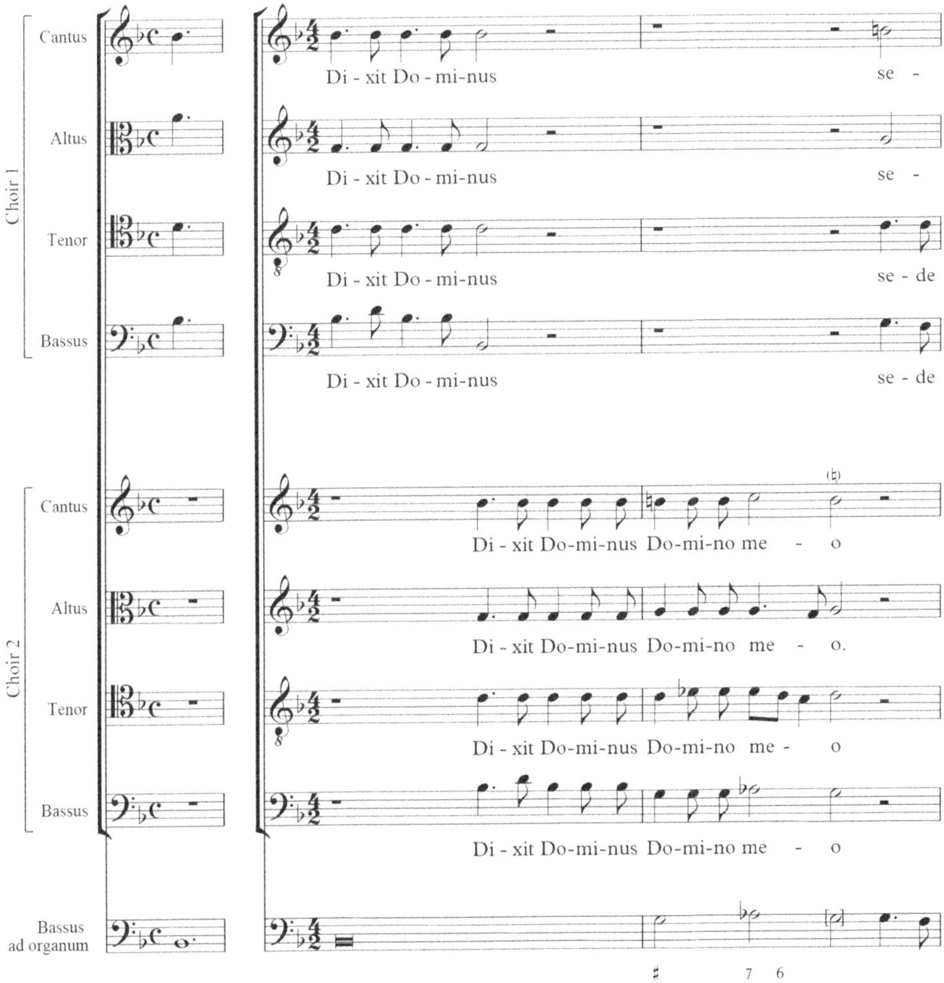

Example 5.4 Beretta, 'Dixit Dominus,' I-Rsc G. MS. 082, bars 1–4.

(Example 5.4 continued)

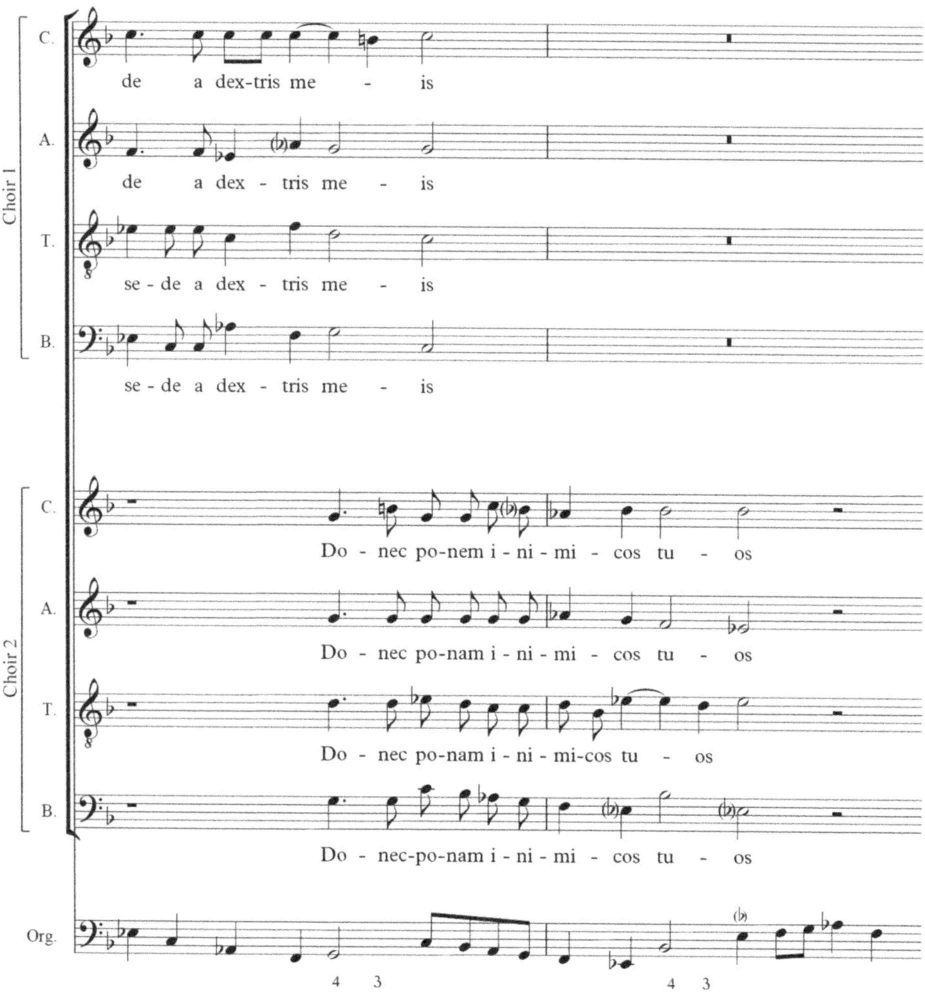
Choir 1
C.
de a dex-tris me - is
A.
de a dex - tris me - is
T.
se - de a dex - tris me - is
B.
se - de a dex - tris me - is
Choir 2
C.
Do - nec po-nem i - ni - mi - cos tu - os
A.
Do - nec po-nam i - ni - mi - cos tu - os
T.
Do - nec po-nam i - ni - mi-cos tu - os
B.
Do - nec-po-nam i - ni - mi - cos tu - os
Org.
4 3
4 3

reinforce a desire to conform to the Tridentine reforms. The centrality of the psalms to the religious life of the Order is further underlined by the fresco, noted above, in which the biblical King David, author of the psalms, musician, harpist and healer, is visually connected to the narrative of Pentecost. The financial records and musical data are supported by other documents in the Santo Spirito archive, especially Vai's decree (to be discussed in Chapter 7), and Spada's *Stato della Casa*.

Historical evidence for the Cappella Musicale: Spada's *Stato della Casa* and the archival record

The most important section of Spada's *Stato della Casa* from the point of view of tracking musical activities is Chapter 5, which reports on the church of Santo Spirito, its history, its personnel and the costs involved in running it.[57] At the end of the chapter, Spada adds an appendix entitled 'Discorso sopra la musica nella chiesa' that is fundamentally a defence of music, justifying its continuity in spite of the expenses involved. This account can be cross-referenced to the surviving financial records and mapped onto the statistics extracted from musical sources. A transcription and translation of the 'Discorso' is given in full in Appendix A below.

Spada's chapter proceeds in a series of numbered paragraphs, the first two of which give a brief historical outline of the foundation of the church drawn from Saulnier's book. He then neatly jumps to the period a mere twenty years or so before his tenure, noting that over time the church had been embellished by many past commendatori, mentioning especially Stefano Vai who had commissioned the walnut furnishings for the sacristy as well as beautiful paintings. Mentioning Vai's contribution to the beauty of the church is Spada's way into a discussion of Vai's decree concerning the correct procedures to be observed in the celebration of the liturgy, and from thence to an analysis of how the church was running at the time of his writing. It is clear that the purpose of the document is to demonstrate obedience to regulations, and to evaluate costs and opportunities for saving money.

Although Spada asserts that the church can be praised for the accuracy with which Vai's decrees have been observed and the devotion given to recitation of canonical praise, he goes on to make some observations about the number of singers and what they are paid. He notes the small number of friars present at the Offices due to other duties they have to fulfil in the hospital and elsewhere. To perform the Offices he states that 'the present need is met by eight singers who are not only paid, but also at least six of them are priests who eat in the

[57] Chapter 4 on the role of the commendatore includes an appendix on the ritual of the *Possesso* which includes reference to the music used. ASR OSS 47, Spada, *Stato della Casa*, pp. 101–102.

refectory of the priests.' He goes on, 'Nowadays, the maestro di cappella is one of the friars, and, consequently, there are nine of them. Indeed, including the organist, who is paid, they are ten.'[58] In addition, he notes that 'those singers we have in the house, as well as their board are given 3.40 scudi each, but they are obliged to perform the church service every day, with just one day off in a week. The two non-resident singers are given 2 scudi a month, a sum which can vary according to their skills.'[59]

In the 'Discorso sopra la musica della chiesa' a few pages later, Spada offers a slightly different view of the number of musicians. Here he lists seven ordinary chaplain musicians who get board and lodging in the house, a non-priest soprano, paid monthly without board, and an organist paid monthly without board, all of whom serve alongside the sacristan, curate and minor church officials. Spada's instructions as to who should carry out which services are recorded in the equivalent of a minute book, noting decisions and instructions made by the Chapter.[60]

Further to these paid singers, Spada notes in item ten of his chapter on the church that there were '12 putti, sons of the House,' who served in the church from the first bell of the morning until Mass. Of those, four helped as singers. He then bizarrely adds, that 'it would be good for a couple of them to learn how to sing, but so far there is none.'[61] If they were singing with the choir, one would assume that they already could sing, so perhaps he means that it would be good for a couple of them to learn to sing as professionals and therefore to earn a living from singing, given that the orphan boys were all taught a trade of some sort.

By putting this information together, we can build the picture of six or seven resident friar singers and a friar maestro di cappella, plus one or two additional singers, of whom at least one is a soprano, and an organist. Both of the latter are 'secular,' that is, not living in. We can add to these the 'putti.' Perhaps one or two worked the bellows for the organist, others acted as acolytes, and

58 '... viene nondimeno supplito al necessario bisogno da otto Cantori, non solo stipendiati, ma anche almeno Sei che sono Sacerdoti alimentati nel Tinello de Preti. Il Mastro di Cappella hoggi è uno de Frati, di maniera che con esso sono 9, anzi con l'organista parimenti stipendiato giungono al numero di 10' : ASR OSS 47, p. 120.

59 'A quelli Cantori, che habiamo in casa, oltre il Tinello si danno scudi 3 et 40 per ciascheduno, ma sono obbligati a celebrare ogni giorno per servizio della Chiesa con vacanza d'un solo giorno la settimana. Alli 2 non residenti, si danno scudi 2 il mese più o meno secondo si trovano megliori o manco buoni': ASR OSS 47, pp. 120–121.

60 ASR-OSS 137, *Spedizioni e decreti, Rubricella atti*, 1657–1660, fols 133r–144v.

61 'Per servigio della Chiesa sono destinati 12 putti, figli di Casa, quali dal segno del mattino sino al segno della Messa risiedono in Chiesa, servendo Messe, e facendo cio che gli è comandato, quattro de quali aiutano al Choro in grado di Cantori, e complirebbe che almeno un paro sempre imparassero di cantare, ma hoggi non ven'è alcuno': ASR OSS 47, p. 123.

some sang. They would of course not be paid. The payment records support the description given by Spada.

The salary lists for the date at which Spada was writing in 1660 confirm his report that there were six or seven musicians plus a soprano, and an organist. The scribe noting the payments refers to them in this instance not as chaplains and singers (*cappellani e cantori*) but as *musico*. In April of 1660, the singers who were paid were Girolamo Amatore, Bartolomeo Antonietti, Nicola Corradi, Camillo Nebbia and Carlo Fei, along with Matteo who is simply identified as 'musico', while a further singer, Alessandro, was paid by a third party as he was leaving (or had left). The second soprano is specifically identified as one Ludovico. Giovanni Battista Fede was the organist at this time. The singers were indeed paid 3 scudi 40 baiocchi each, the soprano 2 scudi and the organist 2.50. In June of the same year and the months thereafter, there were eight singers. The maestro di cappella is not named, nor listed among the singers, which corroborates Spada's note that the role was carried out by one of the friars. The quantity of music for eight voices in the period up to 1660 thus aligns with the available choir of eight noted in the financial records. However, if the testimony of Francesco Massonetti, a singer, assistant surgeon and chronicler who worked at Santo Spirito as a teenager ten years later in the 1670s is to be taken as a norm, these singers would only have been on duty every other week, and all eight would only be required for more important celebrations.[62]

The total cost of salaries for the singers and the men required for services (curate, sacristan, sub-sacristan, etc.) varied between 42 and 57 scudi. Although the salaries for the individual posts remained stable, not all the singers were paid in full at the same time, and occasionally one of them might be paid for two months or a month and half, which of course alters the total. Given the total cost of running the entire institution, the figure for staffing the church is quite small, amounting in total to about one third of the hospital employees' salary bill.

Spada's financial justification of the expenditure of the present is contrasted with practices of the past. He notes that the friars were supposed to sing at least one Conventual Mass per week each, but were too busy with their other duties, so this job was left to other chaplains. He sketches out past practices making references to particular people. From these, a rough chronology can be deduced and the information aligned with evidence from other sources dating from the same time frame.

> As it had been done before, to keep the choir they had brought in guest Priests under the title of ordinary chaplains, and since Vespers, and sung Masses were sung with polyphony, and also the Lauds on solemn feasts, not only chaplains, but also lay musicians were paid a salary.

62 Giancarlo Rostirolla, Livia Martinoli Santini and Candida Santoro (eds), *Musica, medicina, cronache di corte al tempo di Arcangelo Corelli: Il diario di G. A. Francesco Massonetti, 1659–1729* (Rome, 2021) p. 60.

> But at the time of Urban VIII of sacred memory under Commendatore Monsignor Anselmo it was considered more useful for the House that the same chaplains were musicians, and so after removing the lay musicians they have always employed chaplain choristers, although of very poor quality.[63]

Commendatore Giuseppe Anselmi was indeed in post under Pope Urban VIII, having been appointed in 1624, remaining there until his death in 1630. The inference of what had been done before, that is, that they had guest priests and lay musicians in order to fulfil the duties of singing polyphonic masses and Vespers, thus appears to refer to a period prior to 1624.

Evidence of the period prior to the 1620s that should be less biased than internal documents is found in the manuscript census document for 1595 noted in the previous chapter (I-Rn Ms.Vitt.Em.721). Although the descriptions in the census are far from detailed, the document does give an indication of the separate functions of chaplains in the different parts of the organisation and that the chaplains were friars, that is, members of the Order.[64] In summary, the organist was a lay person and hired to work alongside a minimum of four singers who were also chaplains. A further point to note from the 1595 description is that children served at Mass and sang.[65] These were presumably the 'putti' referred to by Spada, probably orphan children from the school who had shown musical talent and were used to support the singing of Mass. The census document makes it clear that music was taught to the orphans, some of whom remained in the institution.[66] Although sopranos are noted from time to time in the *mandati*, they are not a continual presence in the payrolls. During the tenure of Cesare Zoilo as maestro di cappella, which post-dates the census by fifteen years, but pre-dates Anselmi, there were often two sopranos recorded in pay documents. Presumably if children from inside the institution were used, they would not necessarily appear on salary rolls, which must imply that at times adult sopranos or boys from outside the institution were used.[67]

Spada's account continues with a description of the period under Anselmi, who considered it would be more useful to only have chaplains who were also musicians. Anselmi's tenure coincided with the period in which Soldi was operating his print shop at the Hospital, and when Frescobaldi was working

63 Spada, *Stato della Casa*, ASR OSS 47, pp. 231– 231, Appendix A p. 203.

64 The function of the hospital chaplains is described on fol. 3v.

65 See p. 68.

66 '... et come sono alla detta età si mettono con altri à varii essercitii, ma se ne allieva sempre tanti per la musica, che sono sempre dieci, ò dodici, che rimangano in casa.' '... and when they are of that age, they are put with others of various trades, but they always teach music to many, of which there are always ten or twelve who remain in the house': I-Rn Ms.Vitt.Em.721, fol 2 (second pagination).

67 Francesco Massonetti was not an orphan in the hospital but served as a soprano in 1675, getting paid 2 scudi for the job. Rostirolla, Santini and Santoro, *Musica, medicina, cronache di corte al tempo di Arcangelo Corelli*, p. 60.

as the organist at both the Cappella Giulia and the Hospital. Frescobaldi's sporadic presence, apparently juggling the two positions until 1628, perhaps says something about Anselmi's employment practices.[68] According to Spada, after removing the lay musicians, Anselmi employed chaplain choristers of poor quality. The dismissal of salaried musicians in the 1620s maps onto the payment records. From around 1605 to 1618 there is a pattern of singers remaining on the payroll for long periods of service, many of them more than ten years. From 1620, when a number of long-serving singers disappear from the payroll, and up to 1625, periods of service are short, often only a year or even a few months. A number of singers, including Bartolomeo Nicolini in 1620, and Angelo Santa Croce and Santi Moschetti in 1623, disappear from the Santo Spirito records and appear in the account books for the Cappella Giulia, while Girolamo Navarro in 1624 and Curtio Tanicoli in 1629 are noted in the records of an Apostolic Visitation to the Cappella Pontificia in 1630 that gives the date on which they started their service there.[69]

From 1625 the payment records use the formula 'cappellano cantore' for all the singers listed, and the report on the churches of Rome made for Urban VIII in that year notes that Santo Spirito employed six chaplains who also served as singers, supporting the evidence of the financial documents.[70] There follows a period of relative stability in the workforce at least until 1630, but there was no maestro di cappella serving for any length of time between 1623 and 1630, and those that do appear in the financial records were not paid regularly.

Spada does not seem to take into account what happened in the period following Anselmi's reductions, even though he is at pains to underline how well the church has carried out the decrees of Stefano Vai (see Chapter 7 and Appendix B). Vai was appointed commendatore of the Hospital of Santo Spirito in 1632 by Urban VIII Barberini, remaining in post until his death in 1650. The period of his tenure in the 1630s and 1640s was more stable in terms of the musical leadership of the community than the previous decade. In 1630 Orazio Benevoli was appointed maestro di cappella and remained in post for eight years. For at least some of that time he was also the organist, and enjoyed a slightly larger salary of 7.50 scudi per month. He was succeeded by Antonio Carpani (Carpano) who likewise served for at least eight years, but at a

[68] For an analysis of Frescobaldi's career at this time, see Naomi J. Barker, 'Frescobaldi at the Ospedale di Santo Spirito: Evidence of a Portfolio Career in Seventeenth-century Rome', *Early Music*, 49:3 (2021), 395–412.

[69] ASR-OSS 1913–1928, *Copie di Mandati*, 1610–1630; V-CVbav ACSP – CG 73 (1620) and CG 77 (1624); V-CVaav Misc.Arm VII/ 113, *Acti Sacrae Visitationis Apostolicae S.d. N Urbani VIII*, 1630.

[70] '... Tiene sei cappellani quali anco servono per cantori...': *Stato temporale delle chiese di Roma fatto nel pontificato di Urbano VIII l'anno 1625*, V-CVaav Misc.Arm VII /77, f.643.

reduced salary of 5 scudi.[71] Indeed, the maestro di cappella's salary from 1638 and throughout the 1640s was lower than it was when Cesare Zoilo was in post in the first decades of the century.[72]

The continued presence of a single maestro di cappella after 1630 contrasts quite markedly with the 1620s. The payments for Pentecost were also lower, with Benevoli being paid just 5 scudi in 1636–1638; however, there were larger payments of 12 scudi for the celebration of the feast of Santa Tecla, the patronal celebration of the chapel of the nuns and women.[73] The list of personnel for 1645 remained broadly similar to that of 1640. By 1651 after Vai's death, the choir had increased to eight voices, and by 1655 the cost of music for Pentecost had more than doubled to 39 scudi 50 baiocchi – an amount that paid for music in four choirs plus instruments.[74] All of this information suggests that there were different priorities, rather than a general financial squeeze. The salaries of other employees, notably the physicians and medical staff, remained exactly the same.

The appearance of figures such as Orazio Benevoli, Antonio Carpani and Florido de Silvestris on the payrolls from the 1630s onwards rather undermines Spada's assertion that the chaplain singers were of poor quality. Perhaps he wanted to ignore the fact that costs had risen again at that point in time. What he does say is that more recently, perhaps meaning in the decade between Vai's death and his own appointment, up to six additional chaplains were employed, but as they were not mentioned in the most recent Apostolic Visitation, Spada notes he has given orders to dismiss them to save 384 scudi a year. At this point he gives the list of personnel noted above – that is seven chaplain singers, a non-priest soprano and an organist.

Something that emerges in the payment records that is not mentioned by Spada is that from the late 1620s, the salary listings stipulate the specific duty of singing the Litanies, either against individual names or as part of the description of the person, for example, 'chaplain and singer and for the Litanies'.[75] Prior to 1628 there is no mention of specific duties for the singers in the salary records and each singer-chaplain is paid the same flat rate. From 1628 there are two regular monthly payments to the musicians in the copies of the *mandati* rather than the single payment recorded previously. One is for the salaries and lists the

71 The change in salary is particularly evident in 1638 as there are payments to Benevoli in the first half of the year, and to Carpani in the second half of the year. While Benevoli also acted as organist, Carpani had 'Leonardo' as his organist. This was probably Leonardo Castellani. ASR OSS 1936, *Copie di mandati* 1638, items 217, 405, 732, 1107, 1342 etc.

72 ASR OSS 1947, *Copie di mandati,* 1649, items 9, 156, 299 etc.

73 ASR OSS 1936, *Copie di mandati* 1638, items 789, 1209.

74 ASR OSS 1952, *Copie di mandati,* 1655, item 584.

75 'cappelano e cantore e per le letanie': ASR OSS 1942, *Copie di mandati,* 1644, item 148; ASR OSS 1948, *Copie di mandati,* 1651, item 484.

chaplains and singers alongside the maestro di cappella and organist in the same way as for the previous three decades, but a second payment is made to 'singers who sing the Saturday Litanies in our church'.[76] Thus the same singers who appear in the salary listing are paid a second time for a specific service. The two payments made to the singers add up to the same sum as that listed in the single payments in the earlier records, and the amounts paid to the maestro di cappella and organist also do not change with this shift in the accounting practice. Even in the 1640s, the lists of chaplain-singers to be paid includes the phrase 'and for the Litanies' against the names of particular singers, usually four of them.

Spada's defence of church music

Spada's account of the church personnel is broadly corroborated by the financial records of monthly payments, and there are plenty of contemporary musical sources that are suitable for the size of the choir recorded. However, regarding the musical traditions such as the celebration of Pentecost, the weekly sung Litanies and sung Vespers, Spada says nothing. His awareness of specific music used in the *Possesso,* a service performed only sporadically, contrasts starkly with the complete lack of information about the celebration of Pentecost which happened annually, or the Litanies that happened weekly. Given that the *Stato della Casa* was above all a report aimed at providing financial information about the running of the Hospital, these omissions, all of which were costly, are something of an anomaly in his report. Further, all of these traditions seem to have been consolidated in the second half of the sixteenth century, prompted by the Church reforms that reshaped religious thought and practices with impacts across society as a whole. They were, in other words, well-established during and before the period of Anselmi, thus within the scope of the period covered by Spada's account. Were they left out of the calculations because they were fundamental to post-Tridentine Church politics and were to be continued regardless of cost?

The final section of Spada's 'Discorso' is essentially a defence of the music in church and a justification for continued expenditure on it. It reads as though the music was under attack, particularly because of its expense, and that he must of necessity defend it. Providing appropriate music for the Offices and Masses was obviously becoming something of a burden on the institution, or at least had triggered concern with the authorities.

It is perhaps in this final section that we glimpse a little of the man himself. In order to take up the position of commendatore, Spada had been forced to leave the Oratorians, the Order to which he was deeply committed, and which was well-known for the way in which it used music to encourage worship. To

[76] 'cantore che cantano letanie per il sabato in nostra chiesa': ASR OSS 1926, *Copie di mandati*, 1628, items 230, 389, 532.

defend the music in church, Spada sets out the arguments for and against it in an almost forensic way, displaying some rhetorical skill. He starts by recounting the costs of music and that although music was introduced to draw people to divine worship, apparent lack of attendance means that music is a waste of money. He gives the impression of being on the side of those who are critical of maintaining music in the church.

> Against music you can say that 'every agent acts for its end'[77] but that the music of this church has no purpose whatsoever, since it was introduced to draw people to divine worship; but this church being (you can say) outside the city, and in an uninhabited part today and crowded with poor people, many of them cannot go to Mass even on feasts for lack of clothes, let alone at weekdays, music is completely no use, and in fact very few people attend it at weekdays; above all since there is [Santa Maria in] Traspontina, which is in a more frequented street, and the church of Saint Peter, the only one which draws people in these suburbs.[78]

His rebuttal is laid out in three points:

> On the contrary it could be considered that
>
> i) To efface an old and deep-rooted tradition can cause great complaints and grumbles, and that to have to face the burden of so many masses means to keep chaplains, and keeping them, spending a bit more money you can find priests, who are able to sing, as it is done at present.
>
> ii) Even if at weekdays there are just a few people in the church, nevertheless on feasts and in the morning, and on the days with Vespers there is a great number, so money is not wasted.
>
> iii) That dismissing musicians and using friars who can only sing Gregorian chant would spoil the singing of the Divine Office, and they would make themselves ridiculous, that anyway a compromise could be found that is to say that instead of seven or eight chaplain musicians, only four should be kept, who were musicians, and with Prior, Sacristan and four novices there would be the full chorus, of at least ten priests, and on feasts four more choristers could be employed with two scudi a month each.[79]

The first point is a neat rhetorical twist, arguing that keeping the music would avoid complaints about the loss of a tradition. At no point previously had he mentioned musical traditions within the Hospital, but it is evident from the way he uses this angle in his argument, that there was an awareness of it, perhaps

77 *omne gens agit propter finem* is a philosophical axiom about moral and intellectual agency, acting for the sake of an end, discussed at length by Thomas Aquinas but Aristotelian in origin.

78 Spada, *Stato della Casa*, ASR OSS 47, pp. 236–237, Appendix A, p. 204.

79 Spada, *Stato della Casa*, ASR OSS 47, pp. 238–239, Appendix A, p. 205.

even a sense of the value of music within the community. The tension here is between the requirement of quantity versus quality.

The second point is about attendance, which amounts to confronting the argument that there is no point in singing if there is no audience. The idea that music would draw people to worship underpins Spada's response. His argument is that at Vespers and on feast days there is a great number of people, so the money is not wasted. This is another useful indicator that there was indeed an audience for the music performed during the Sunday Mass and Offices at this period, likely to be for eight voices for at least some parts of both Mass and Vespers.

His final point, if musicians are dismissed in favour of friars who only sing Gregorian chant, they would spoil the singing of the Divine Office and make themselves ridiculous is indicative of Spada's desire for quality music in church. He then skilfully buttresses his argument for keeping the music by offering a money-saving solution, that is to reduce the number of paid singers, so instead of seven or eight only four should be kept, and on feast days four more choristers could be employed. In sealing his suggestion, he describes what happens at San Girolamo della Carità, the location of the Spada family chapel which he and his brother Bernadino renovated in 1654–1657, and in so doing provides an insight into both institutions.

A key piece of information required to unpick this defence is that increasing numbers of Masses of obligation were required of the chaplains. These Masses were stipulated in bequests, by charitable donors and pious parishioners. It is extremely likely that several Masses may have taken place simultaneously in the various side chapels of the church in order to fulfil these obligations. Spada even gives a list of the Masses of obligation required which runs to several pages. These Masses would not have required any great musical skill, therefore could be handed over to ordinary priests. If this were done, then the main Conventual Mass of the day and the main Mass in the hospital and women's chapel could be covered by the 'normal' cohort of chaplain-singers. The financial records support this information as various chaplains are paid for singing Masses in specified chapels.

If financial concerns drove Spada's defence of music, it is not entirely surprising. The patterns in the payment records shift fairly dramatically over a century. In the mid-sixteenth century the books of *mandati* are dominated by regular payments to large numbers of women who nursed and raised infants and young children as well as needy women. By the 1660s, there are payments to hundreds of employees on farms and vineyards, in the stables, the gardens and so on as well as to suppliers of all manner of food and clothing, maintenance for the building, supplies to the dispensary and any other expense one might imagine for a modern business. While the *mandati* of the 1550s list as many as fifty or sixty wetnurses ('balie') in any one month, each identified by name and the name of the child in their care, by 1660 those payments are largely absent or included in a single payment to a 'commissario di balie' or maestro da casa for 'balie'. At this date, the hospital and church in some respects seem to have become only a small part of a very large organisation.

Although Spada's *Stato della Casa* is quite clear regarding concerns about the cost of the music in the church, there is no evidence that things changed in the years following his death. In 1670 there was still a choir of eight paid on a regular basis each month. There is no regular maestro di cappella listed, so this role must have continued to be taken by one of the friars in the way that Spada noted. The salary records are detailed enough to identify who sang which voice parts, as first and second contraltos, tenors and basses are listed as well as the two sopranos. The latter, being paid somewhat less, were probably boys or teenagers. Francesco Beretta, identified as of our Order ('di nostra religione'), was paid as maestro di cappella for the Pentecost celebrations of that year, including money to be paid to the musicians he hired for that feast.[80] At 44 scudi 10 baiocchi this was no small amount, more than the monthly salary bill for the regular choir and organist which amounted to a figure just short of 30 scudi. If we assume one-off payments of just 1 scudo per musician, it would imply at least doubling the size of the choir and having a similar number of instrumentalists to accompany them, probably with enough money left to hire extra organs or organetti for processions, or to copy or buy new music. Beretta, as a composer himself, may of course have used his own music, some of which has survived in manuscripts now in the Conservatorio di Santa Cecilia and the Biblioteca Casanatense.[81]

Ten years later in 1680, the pattern of payments is virtually identical.[82] Instead of identifying voices of the singers, the scribe simply numbered them, referring to 'primo cappellano' through to 'sesto cappellano' with the two sopranos listed together afterwards. Perhaps Spada's idea of identifying musicians as chaplains had finally taken effect. For Pentecost, Beretta is still the named maestro di cappella, although his name never appears in the lists of regular singers. The monthly payments indicate that a choir of eight was the norm.

Even in 1700 the payments to the choir remain almost the same as those of twenty years earlier. Alongside the maestro di cappella, Pompeo Cannicciari, there were six adult singers, two sopranos and the organist, still receiving the same salary.[83] This financial outlay did not of course take into consideration the extraordinary costs of feast days and, as noted above, in 1700 the cost of Pentecost celebrations was astronomical. Whatever the financial concerns were that triggered Spada's defence, nothing happened to curtail costs for at least four decades after it was written.

80 ASR OSS 1966, *Copie di mandati*, 1670, items 163, 255, 511, etc. The payment for Pentecost is item 354.

81 For example, Berretta, *Psalmodia*, 1688, I-Rsc G. MS 082 see pp. 115–116; Berretta, *In exitu Israel*, I-Bc Ms 5434.

82 ASR OSS 1976, *Copie di mandati*, 1680, items 264, 462, 809, etc.

83 ASR OSS 1995, *Copie di mandati*, 1700, items 144, 242, 777, etc.

What does emerge from Spada's discourse is a tension between what he saw as the essential function of music as an integral part of worshipping the divine; the demands of the Offices and Masses that the chaplains were obliged to provide alongside their other duties; and the costs involved. His calculations of the costs of music are less than the reality, as the extraordinary payments for extra musicians for feast days are ignored, perhaps deliberately, so as not to draw attention to the expense. At the same time, he emphasises how much is done regarding the singing of all the many Masses of obligation. Spada, the manager, is presenting the good news of how well they are doing for so little money, offering a solution that might save some more on things that are perhaps less important to him, and by virtue of omission, the great feast days continue to be celebrated at some cost.

There are also hidden inferences and assumptions in his points regarding Vespers. The surviving daily schedules of activity in the Hospital indicate that this Office was observed unusually early, no doubt because of the major operation of serving the evening meal to patients, children, women and of course the friars themselves. Regular Vespers would therefore not be well-attended, but on Sundays and feast days, the working public would have been more able to attend, and no doubt leave financial offerings at the same time. The expense of a lavish musical Vespers no doubt generated more charitable giving by drawing larger crowds of better-off people. The splendour of music for Vespers was perhaps part of the public face of the business of charity. The message Spada seems to be giving in defence of musical Vespers is a somewhat managerial, even cynical, 'spend to earn'.

The managerial expertise with which Spada makes his case is evident, but his aesthetic sense also emerges in his defence of music. His dismissal of the idea of having only friars to sing plainchant as it would spoil the divine worship, and his pointed comment that Anselmi only appointed poor quality chaplain-singers, is indicative that the quality of musical performance mattered to him. Was the music still intended to move the listener to piety and devotion? Spada's view that the novice should attend frequently in the choir suggests that conceptually at least, he still maintained a view that music had a place in the spiritual life of the institution, as noted above (p. 49). There is plenty of evidence of badly behaved church choirs and poorly sung liturgy reaching back to the fifteenth century. Perhaps the music at Santo Spirito had reached a standard of which Spada approved, either as a result of the reforms of his predecessors which he praised so highly, or through judicious hiring of good quality musicians, and he did not want to let standards slip. Or perhaps the reality was different, and his defence foreshadows the more robust scrutiny that was to come in the 1730s.

His comments about the quality of singing raise the question as to who the singers were singing for. Bonnie Blackburn asked this question regarding first-person texts in fifteenth-century psalteries and prayer books.[84] Here, the question is in one sense literal and, at that level, can be answered by the many locations in which Masses were held – for the sick in the hospital, for the girls and women in the women's chapel (of Santa Tecla), in the oratorio for the members of the Confraternity and so on. On another level, it addresses the fundamental reasons for singing in these spaces, and that is that music needed to reach these audiences in a visceral way, to move the passions of the soul, to act on the humours in order to relieve mental and physical pain, to change or improve behaviours, and to induce piety and devotion in charitable labour. Would a choir made up predominantly of brothers committed to the Order and its charitable purpose have performed their music in such a way as to enhance its emotional content better than lay professionals who may have been singing simply for the money? We will never know.

The implication of Spada's defence is that even if there were no other people present, the quality of the worship was what mattered to him, and that the beauty of the worship and its music was important in and of itself. Documentation of Spada's lengthy engagement with the architect Borromini during the rebuilding of the Casa dei Filippini for the Oratorians situated next to the church of Santa Maria in Vallicella (the Chiesa Nuova) provides ample evidence of a man to whom beauty mattered. Indeed, the notion attributed to Borromini that just as the beauty of music depends on the proportions that it embodies, so too architecture must embody musical proportions, is likely to have initially come from Spada and not the architect himself.[85]

As an Oratorian, Spada would have been fully aware and committed to their use of music as a force for the renewal of the Church, for fostering devotion, for teaching spiritual lessons and so on. Just as the passions of the soul were the primary target for the musical mission of the Oratorians, and in Cirillo's argument for better quality church music written more than a century before, so too the power of good quality music to move the emotions is implicit in Spada's defence of music. The spiritual health, and therefore the physical health of the community depended on it.

84 Bonnie J. Blackburn 'For Whom do the Singers Sing?', *Early Music* 25:4 (1997), 593–609.

85 di Falco, *Francesco Borromini*, pp. 35–36.

6

Music for Body and Soul

The requirement for music that moved the emotions that was articulated by both Cirillo and Spada resonates across the medical and religious remit of the Hospital. Affecting the passions was more critical than simple entertainment, it was the means of regaining wellbeing, both bodily and in spirit. A healthy soul was the gateway to a healthy body, and both could be reached by music. While the desire to move public emotions towards a renewal of devotion and piety is especially evident in the celebration of Pentecost, it also surfaces in other music written in response to Tridentine liturgy and doctrine.

Pius V not only revised the breviary and missal in order to clarify and unify the liturgy, which as noted in Chapter 5 transformed the celebration of Pentecost, he also issued a Bull that would have an impact in hospitals. This Bull, dated 1566, and titled *Super gregem dominicum*, forbade doctors to treat patients who refused confession for more than three days. Several sessions of the Council of Trent had discussed the sacramental process as 'medicamentum'. The underlying assumption was held that disease was caused by sin, and that confession and taking Communion were in themselves a medicine.

From earliest times the Eucharist – the re-enactment of the Last Supper in which Jesus shared bread and wine with his disciples before his crucifixion, instructing them to take and eat it as it was his body and blood – was deemed a 'mystery', but it was, and is, central to Catholic belief.[1] The consecrated bread and wine was regarded as holy food as it contained the truth of the Word of God. Any fraudulent use of it was a crime that resulted in a gruesome death.[2] The doctrine of transubstantiation, first conceived by theologians in the twelfth century, was formalised into an official statement by the Council of Trent. This doctrine insisted that at the moment of consecration, the bread and wine became the actual body and blood of Christ and were not just sacred symbols or representations as declared by Protestants. Further, that if anyone

1 All four canonic Gospels give an account of the last supper: Matthew 26, Mark 14, Luke 22, John 13–14. The account in John lacks the detail of bread and wine, but includes other details.

2 For substantial literary references and contemporary accounts of the mystical nature of the consecrated Host and its centrality in Catholic dogma see Piero Camporesi, *The Fear of Hell: Images of Damnation and Salvation in Early Modern Europe*, trans. Lucinda Byatt, ([Milan, 1987] Cambridge, 1990).

denied this, he should be 'anathema'.[3] The doctrine of transubstantiation was challenged not only by Protestants, but by the third decade of the seventeenth century, by new scientific thinking and discoveries that threatened to undermine it. Aristotelian scholasticism, in particular, the atomic conception that understood all things to have a dual nature comprising 'substance' – that is the essential properties of what make an object what it is – and 'accident', meaning the object's observably physical characteristics, underpinned the notion of transubstantiation. The Aristotelian notion that substance and accident could be separated was overturned by Galileo's atomic model. By 1624, an anonymous criticism of Galileo's *Il Saggiatore* (*The Assayer*) made it clear that Galileo should be condemned because the book went against this teaching.[4]

While the doctrine of transubstantiation and of the sacramental process as 'medicamentum' was formalised at Trent, it was not new, as the concept of *Christus medicus* reaches back to the early Church Fathers. St Ambrose described the body of Christ present in the consecrated bread as 'the sure protection and health of soul and body, the remedy for all spiritual and physical ills'.[5] In medieval hospitals it was a given that physicians worked alongside priests to treat the whole person, body and soul. The patient who had confessed his or her sins and taken Communion was not only prepared to receive the last rites should it be necessary, but was also relieved of the fear of dying, and thus psychologically more likely to respond to treatment. Hospital wards were designed so that patients could see and hear Mass and especially be able to gaze at the consecrated Host. The Aristotelian concept of *katharsis*, the purging or therapeutic cleansing of bad emotions, was taken up by early Christian writers, and connected to confession and Communion, as well as to the experience of music and song.[6]

Roman hospitals had always been spaces of exchanging of ideas between people of different nationalities coming to the city for all manner of reasons, but in the face of the threat of Protestantism, Pius V noted that they additionally presented an opportunity for conversion or re-conversion. By the middle of the seventeenth century, the requirement of confession before admittance to hospital became a route for forcing conversion or re-conversion of sick people.

3 The decrees and canons regarding the Eucharist were established at the thirteenth session of the Council of Trent in 1551. Eternal Word Television Network, https://www.ewtn.com/catholicism/library/thirteenth-session-of-the-council-of-trent-1479.

4 White and Redondi argue that it was this, and not heliocentrism, that was the reason for Galileo's trial and subsequent condemnation for heresy. Michael White, *Galileo Antichrist* (London, 2007 (rep, 2009)); Pietro Redondi, *Galileo Heretic* (Princeton, NJ, 1987).

5 Cited in Carol Rawclife, 'Christ the Physician Walks the Wards', in Matthew Davies and Andrew Prescott (eds), *London and the Kingdom: Essays in Honour of Caroline M. Barron* (Donington, 2008), pp. 91–92.

6 Philip E. Stolzfus, *Theology as Performance: Music, Aesthetics, and God in Modern Theology* (New York and London, 2006), pp. 37–39.

Protestant travellers were even warned about the practice when embarking on a journey to Rome.[7]

The celebration of Mass and the distribution of the sacrament in the Hospital of Santo Spirito would have been accepted as a treatment for the patients alongside whatever other remedies were administered by the doctors. The architectural design of the Sistine wards with an imposing altar positioned in its central octagonal space ensured there was no boundary between the sacred chapel space and the wards on either side of it. Indeed, the sacred space was also the focal point for anyone entering from the street. It was also here that an organ was built, cementing the place of music at a nexus between the sacred and secular worlds.

Although the use of music in hospitals, and in medicine more generally, was well documented in the Islamic world in the medieval period, the knowledge of music as part of a holistic treatment of patients was not transmitted to the West. The Hospital of Santo Spirito was unique in this respect in the Latin early modern world.[8] The organ in the hospital ward is first mentioned in documents dating from after 1600 that tell of its therapeutic uses, which will be discussed below.

The organ

We cannot establish exactly what the organ in the ward would have sounded like as the instrument no longer exists, neither have any documents concerning its construction come to light. Camiz, the only scholar to have attempted any investigation of proto-music therapy in the Hospital, has assumed that it was built at around the same time as the large organ in the church and by the same builder.[9] As the hospital and the church were both badly damaged in the Sack of Rome in 1527, and the necessary repairs and renovations of the buildings only completed by the middle of the century, the organ is unlikely to have been installed much before 1550. It is probably a fair assumption that providing an organ for the newly reconstructed church would have been prioritised over that

7 Irene Fosi, 'The Hospital as a Space of Conversion: Roman Examples from the Seventeenth Century', in Giuseppe Marcocci, Aliocha Maldavsky and Wietse de Boer (eds), *Space and Conversion in Global Perspective* (Leiden, 2015), pp. 154–74, esp. p. 170.

8 Peregrine Horden, 'Religion as Medicine: Music in Medieval Hospitals', in Peter Biller and Joseph Ziegler (eds), *Religion and Medicine in the Middle Ages* (York, 2001), pp. 135–154.

9 Franca Trinchieri Camiz, 'Music Performance and Healing in Renaissance Rome Revealed by Text and Images', in Katherine A. McIver (ed.), *Art and Music in the Early Modern Period: Essays in Honor of Franca Trinchieri Camiz* (London & New York, 2016 (1st edn 2003)), pp. 353–366.

of the hospital, so a date of 1548 is probably a reasonable *termine post quem*, but it may well have been built in the decade after 1550.

We do know from documented observations that the organ was a large instrument and in a prominent position. This is supported by illustrations that give an impression of an imposing instrument that would have been visible from almost any point in the wards. Today there is a shadow on the wall above the main door that outlines where the organ was before it was removed in the nineteenth century. The shadow covers the frescoes which were completed sometime in the 1480s, indicating that the over-door position of the organ was later than the decoration as it is unlikely that it would originally have been positioned to cover newly decorated walls. The organ is shown in this position over the main doorway from the street and between the two halls of the ward in a lithograph illustration in a nineteenth-century volume describing the institutions of Rome to the potential 'Grand Tourist' (Plate 6.1).[10] A high position is consistent with the seventeenth-century eyewitness accounts discussed below.

The description of the organ in Saulnier's history of the Order and its hospital is somewhat ambiguous but seems to suggest that the organ was located behind the altar.[11] Although the organ is no longer extant, the altar remains in place. The construction of an extension to the ward, connected to it by a doorway behind the altar, perhaps necessitated moving the organ from an earlier location.[12] Saulnier's illustrations offer a visual documentation of the buildings in the early to mid-seventeenth century, including a plan of the site (See Plate 1.1) and a number of images of the interiors, one of which is of the hospital ward (Plate 6.2). His image of the chapel looking towards the ward does not give a clear view of an organ, but there is a structure at the head of the ward that is more clearly visible in the nineteenth-century lithograph in the foreground to the right. De Angelis describes this as the old cantoria and it could well have been a structure akin to a gallery for singers. If so, it would suggest, for practical reasons, that the organ was in close proximity, perhaps the pipework above it, with the keyboard located in the middle of the cantoria.[13] If, on the other hand, the organ was in the over-door position, and singers in a gallery on the opposite wall, it would suggest performing practices that might have

10 F. Benoist el al, *Rome dans sa grandeur: Vues, monuments anciens et modernes*, vol. 2 (Paris, 1870).

11 Pierre Saulnier, *De capite sacri ordinis Sancti Spiritus dissertatio* (Lyon, 1649).

12 The dates of completion of the frescoes on the walls behind and opposite the altar, and of the extension to the ward, are not clear, but are discussed by Eunice Howe, *The Hospital of Santo Spirito and Pope Sixtus IV* (New York and London, 1978), pp. 98–101. Howe also dates the installation of the organ to 1546–1552, when Alessandro Guidiccioni was commendatore. Howe, *The Hospital of Santo Spirito*, p. 129.

13 Pietro De Angelis, *L'architetto e gli affreschi di Santo Spirito in Saxia*, Collana di Studi Storici sull'Ospedale di Santo Spirito in Saxia e sugli Ospedali Romani (Rome, 1961), p. 61.

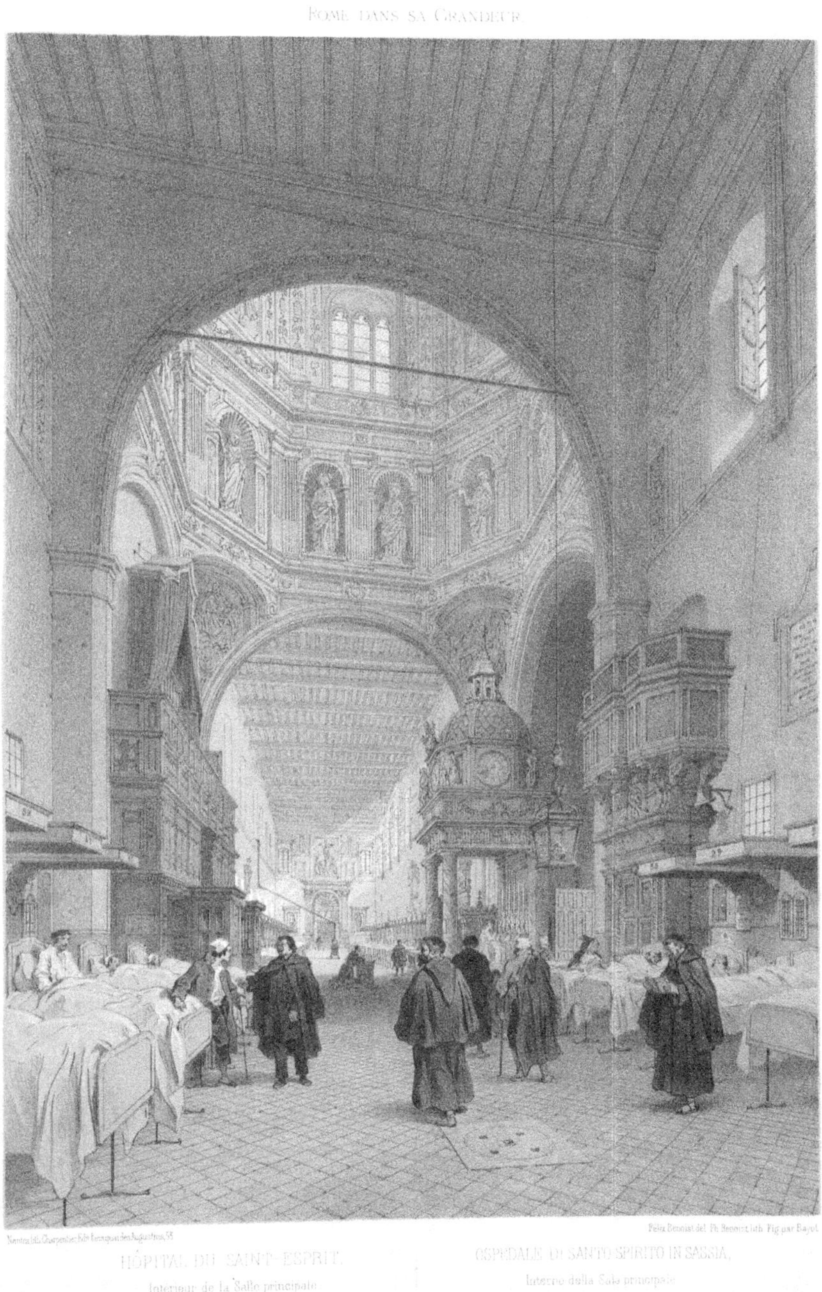

Plate 6.1 Hospital of Santo Spirito in Sassia: view of the Corsia Sistina looking from the ward to the central octagon, showing the organ on the left, opposite the altar. F. Benoist et al, *Rome dans sa grandeur: Vues, monuments anciens et mondernes* (Paris, 1870), vol. ii, p. 6. London, British Library © The British Library Board, Cup.652.a.1.

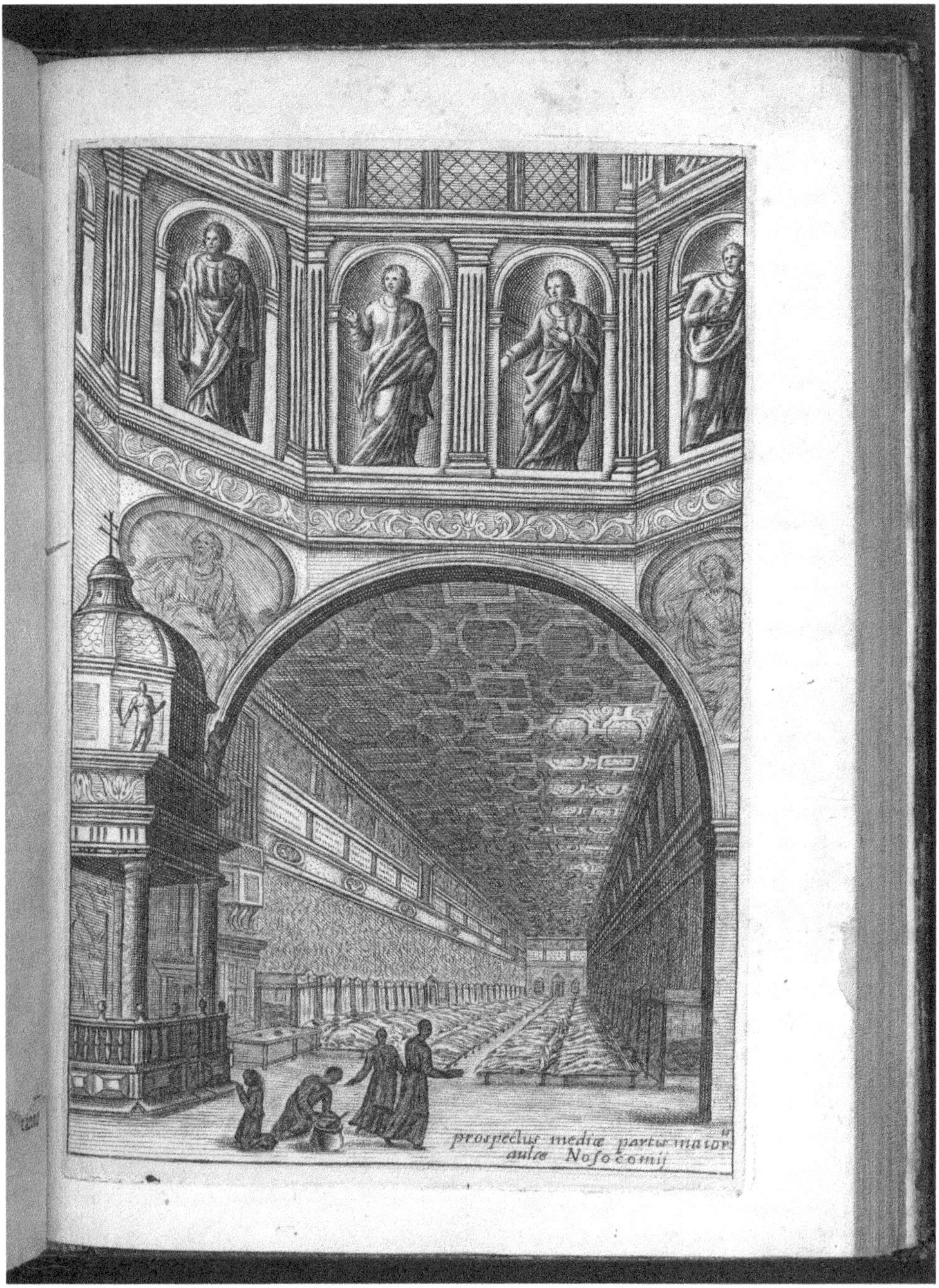

Plate 6.2 Hospital of Santo Spirito in Sassia: view of the Corsia Sistina from the central octagon showing the altar and 'old cantoria' on the left. Saulnier, *De capite sacri ordinis S. Spiritus dissertatio* (Lyon, 1649), plate 15. London, British Library © The British Library Board c.183.c.13.

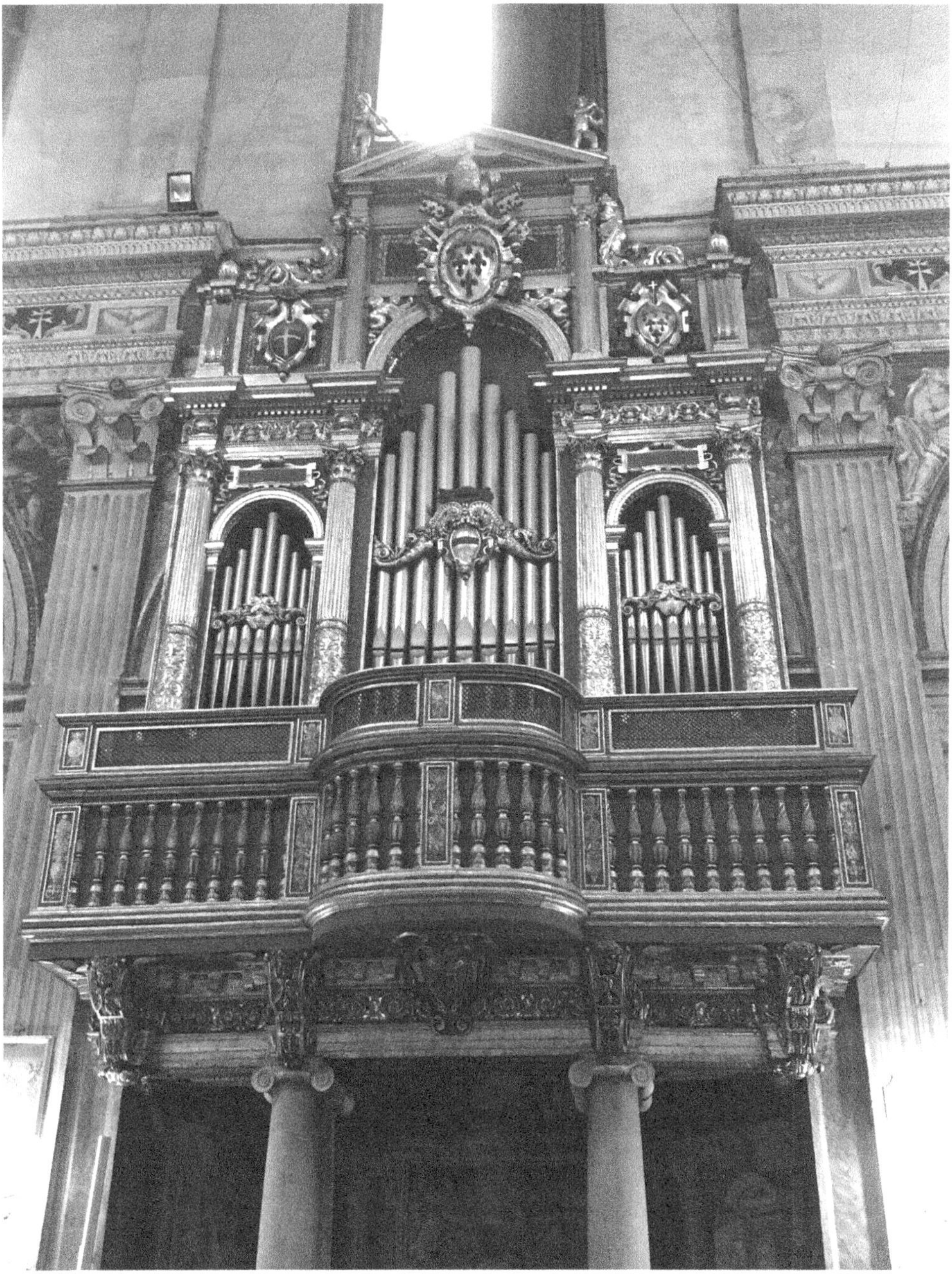

Plate 6.3 Church of Santo Spirito in Sassia: Organ case attributed to Antonio da Sangallo the younger. Photo © Chris Churnside and the author, with permission of ASL Roma.

made use of spatially distant groups of musicians, a practice already noted as a feature of music for the church especially in the seventeenth century.

While we have no documents concerning the organ in the hospital ward, the situation with regard to the organs in the church of Santo Spirito is somewhat different. Notarial records of contracts with Nicolò Tezzani of Cremona survive in the archive, as does the case of the instrument itself (Plate 6.3). The description given in the contract indicates that it was a typical instrument of its time and type. The organ case, which has been the focus of art historical research, has now been attributed to Antonio da Sangallo the younger, who also designed the church when it was rebuilt in the first half of the sixteenth century.[14]

A contract for the sale of an old organ, also built by Tezzani, to Santa Maria dell'Anima in June 1546, and one for the construction of a new one, to be paid for by September 1546, were both signed by Pietro Santi, the commendatore of the time.[15] By 1547 a new contract was drawn up between Tezzani and the commendatore Alessandro Guidiccioni for an organ for the then still new church, to be built to particular specifications within six months. The contract twice specifies that the instrument should be an excellent one, first noting that it should be 'a good and perfect organ and of high quality'. Following the precise stipulation of registers and size, the necessity for a quality instrument that is 'good and beautiful according to the judgement of skilled men and expert in the art such as players and singers' is emphasised.[16]

The cost of building the instrument was 400 scudi, with an initial payment of 100 scudi, followed by 300 scudi for the case and decoration. A separate contract for the decoration of the instrument was drawn up in July 1547 between Guidiccioni and Francesco Credenza of Naples. This includes gilding and an explicit instruction for 'azzuro fino', that is, fine blue, rather than the cheaper smalt blue ('smalto'); and for engraved designs in red.[17] Although final payments were only made in April 1548, the organ was almost certainly finished by late 1547.[18]

14 Eunice D. Howe, 'Architecture for "Divine hymns"', in McIver, *Art and Music in the Early Modern*, pp. 57–90.

15 Patrizia Melella, 'Vita musicale e arte organaria a Santo Spirito in Sassia nel cinquecento: note e documenti', in Bianca Maria Antolini (ed.), *La musica a Roma attraverso le fonti d'archivio* (Lucca, 1994), pp. 507–519, esp. p. 514.

16 'un organo buono et Perfetto del modo qualita'; and later, 'buono e bello al giudizio di huomini periti et experti di tal arte si come sono suonatori et cantori quali habbino l'una et l'altra virtu': ASR OSS 237 fols 5r–6r. This source has been published in part in Patrizia Melella, 'Vita musicale', and published in full but not translated in Howe, 'Architecture for "Divine hymns"', pp. 57–90.

17 OSS 230 f3v–4r also in Howe, 'Architecture for "Divine hymns"', p. 84. 'Azzuro fino' was probably derived from Lapis lazuli while the pigment of 'smalto' came from copper or cobalt.

18 Payments often appear in the record books monthly or quarterly, paid in arrears.

The documents state that 'the said organ should be of 10½ feet and should be suitable for accompanying singers in plainchant and polyphony'.[19] Howe interprets the phrase 'che sia commodo con li cantori cosi al canto fermo come al canto figurato' as indicating that it was suitable to accommodate singers on either side: in other words, suggesting a singers' gallery or cantoria. Singers may well have been able to stand in a small gallery on either side of the organist, but it would have been a cramped space. However, the phrase 'che sia commodo' may equally refer to the pitch of the instrument being suitable. The disposition of voices in polyphony would dictate a pitch range that would neither be too low for the bottom of the bass range, nor too high for the sopranos.[20] The fact that the organ was later re-tuned and pipes added suggests that it refers to pitch.

The instrument was to have nine registers, of which the Principale, placed at the front, was to be made of tin, while the others that were to go behind, were to be made of lead. Besides the Principale, there were to be eight other registers: Octava, Quintadecima, Decimanona, Vicesimaseconda, Vicesimasexta, Vicesimanona, a flute with the Principale and a second flute in Quintadecima. It was to have a mechanism for pedals, a keyboard of forty-seven keys and four bellows.[21] The specification makes the Santo Spirito organ a typical instrument of its time, and one that was similar to those by the famous Brescian organ builder Antegnati and his followers. At this time, Italian organs generally had only a single keyboard and the pedals were not constructed as a separate 'keyboard' for the feet, but worked on a pull-down mechanism that used the same registers as the main keyboard. These organs had no solo stops but relied on a ripieno chorus contrasting with the Principal. The Principal of a large instrument of this type would have been a 16', thus the ripieno would comprise 8', 4', 2 2/3', 2', 1 1/3' and 1'. The hospital instrument would probably have had a similar specification.

Significant alterations were carried out on the organ between 1603–1605 as a contract with Stefano Blasi, dated 9 December 1603, required him to 'reduce the keyboard to the modern style with the Mi, Re, Ut, but with the same pipes'. It must have become obvious at some point that it was not possi-

19 'detto organo debbia essere piede dieci e mezzo che si còmmodo con li cantorij cosi al canto fermo che al canto figurato', ASR OSS 237 f5.

20 Arnaldo Morelli, *Teatro della vista e dell'udito: la musica e i suoi luoghi nell'età moderna* (Lucca, 2017), p. 23.

21 ASR OSS 237 5r–6r 'Item: sia tenuto fare il registro principale del sudetto organo di stagno, in facciata con li altri che vanno dietro di piombo, quali registri tutti sono gli infrascritti, cioè: 1° il principale; 2° la octava; 3° la quintadecima; 4° Decimanona; 5° Vicesimaseconda; 6° Vicesimasexta; 7° Vicesimanona; 8° Un flauto con le principali; 9° Un alto flauto in quintadecima con le principali. Con la tastadura de tasti 47 tra bianchi e neri; con un somaro a vento di legno buono et secco, acciò sia piu durabile; con li cadenazzi di ferro che fanno giocare li tasti con il suo pedale, et condotto del vento da quattro mantici, quali sono idonei a far suono detto organo'.

ble to do the job without adding pipes, as a second contract with his brother Luca, dated March 1605, indicates that the work needed to be completed differently and refined. At the same time the bellows were moved to make more space for singers.[22] The requirement for the organ to be pitched differently is perhaps indicative of an increased use of complex accompanied vocal music. We can only assume that the other two organs in the Hospital were similarly adjusted. It's hard to imagine that the smaller tribune organ would not have been re-tuned to match the nave organ, even though no documentary evidence has come to light.

The organ in the liturgy

The organ in the hospital ward would have played a crucial role in the celebration of Mass on a daily basis, acting as a substitute for a choir, playing in alternatim with the chant sung by the officiating priest or perhaps, on more important occasions, accompanying a choir. In particular, organ music would have accompanied the most sacred part of the Mass – the Eucharist. At this focal point of the Mass, the transubstantiated bread and wine are raised up by the priest to expose them to worshippers as the body and blood of Christ and for worshippers to kneel in adoration. The gestures of this ritual, or enactment of a mystical drama, offered opportunities for musical accompaniment. In the twelfth century new prayers such as 'O salutaris hostia', 'Verbum caro factum' and 'Adoramus te Christe' were introduced to be used just before and at the moment of transubstantiation. These in turn generated musical settings, effectively surrounding the visible actions with a halo of sound.[23]

In response to the Tridentine statements regarding the Eucharist, a new instrumental genre, the elevation toccata, emerged in the late sixteenth and early seventeenth centuries specifically for this function. The characteristics of the elevation toccata include long note values, dissonance and chromaticism, often creating a lack of modal or tonal focus. Pieces entitled 'durezze e ligature' have similar characteristics and were probably used for the same purpose. Elevation toccatas were intended to create an atmosphere of awe and reverence at the mystery being enacted, and to move the emotions of the congregation to adoration of the host.

Early seventeenth century performance manuals for organists stipulate requirements for the music provided for the elevation. Banchieri emphasises the need to move the emotions. In his instructions to the beginner organist as

22 The rather complicated relationship between Luca and Stefano Blasi and the work on the organ at the Hospital is explained in Furio Luccichenti, 'Luca Blasi (c. 1545–1608): profilo di un organaro', in *L'Organo*, XIX (1981), 113–131, esp. 124–125.

23 Agnese Pavanello, 'The Elevation as Liturgical Climax in Gesture and Sound: Milanese Elevation Motets in Context', *Journal of the Alamire Foundation*, 9 (2017), 33–60.

to where and what to play for Mass, he notes that at the elevation, the organist must play softly and solemnly to move the faithful to devotion.[24] Elsewhere he makes it clear that a variety of styles and moods are required, but the elevation should be serious and tender.[25] The 1611 edition of *L'organo suonarino* contains two toccatas specifically identified as for the elevation, providing a model for the organist as to what was expected at this point in the Mass.

Diruta goes further, noting both the timbre and harmonic qualities required, instructing the organist to choose registrations appropriate to the psalm tone of the music being played. He notes that the second and fourth tones are almost the same, and serve for the elevation of the holy body and blood of our Lord Jesus Christ, imitating with the 'sonata' the hard and bitter torments of the Passion. For Tone 2, which has a melancholic character, he advocates only the Principal plus a tremulant, while for Tone 4, that has the qualities of lament and sadness, the Principal with tremolo gives this effect, with occasional use of the flute.[26] He is however careful to qualify his recommendations by saying that not all organs are the same, with some having more and others fewer registers available, but it is enough to know the harmony created by a particular psalm tone to use good judgement in seeking out an appropriate registration. What is evident in his discussion is the intention that the music move the passions in a manner appropriate to the specific moment in the liturgy. In order for the listener to be receptive to the sacred mystery of the Eucharist and ready to accept the 'medicamentum' of sacrament, it was a matter of priority to move his or her passions.

McClary analysed the 'Toccata per l'elevazione' in the *Missa degli Apostoli* from Frescobaldi's *Fiori musicali* within the context of an argument that one of the achievements of Italian music of the seventeenth century was the simulation of desire by means of manipulating certain musical devices, notably the power of the leading note within incipient tonality, to create particular effects.[27] While her general hypothesis remains controversial, the specific requirement of the elevation to create a yearning for devotion is correct. Mystical or spiritual experiences recounted in hagiographies were often accompanied by angelic music and the association with music that moved the passions of the

24 … si suona alla Levatione, ma piano, & cosa grave, che muovi alla devotione': Banchieri, *L'organo suonarino* (Venice, 1611), facsimile edition, ed. Giulio Cattin, Frits Knuf (Amsterdam, 1969) p. 38. The two toccatas are in the *quinto registro*, pp. 36, 37.

25 1605 edn, p. 143. For the variations between the three editions of Banchieri's *L'organo suonarino*, see Donald Earl Marcase, 'Adriano Banchieri: L'organo suonarino: transcription, translation and commentary' (unpublished PhD thesis, Indiana University, 1970).

26 Girolamo Diruta, *Seconda parte del Transilvano*, lib IV (Venice, 1609), p. 22. Facsimile edition, ed. Edward J Soehnlen and Murray C. Bradshaw (Buren, The Netherlands, 1983).

27 Susan McClary, *Desire and Pleasure in Seventeenth Century Music* (Berkeley, Los Angeles, CA, London, 2012), pp. 6 and 181–187.

soul to ecstatic union with the divine was widely understood. The transformative contemplation of the mystical experience of transubstantiation might also be seen as a parallel to the ecstatic 'fiery prayer' of the Pentecostal moment, in which the divine, in the form of the Holy Spirit, descended and the earthly soul ascended to join it. Music for the elevation had therefore to engender emotions appropriate to this 'mystery.'

Although there are no elevation toccatas that can be traced with any certainty to Santo Spirito, those printed in Frescobaldi's second book of toccatas of 1627 may well have been developed during the time in which he was organist at both the Hospital and the Cappella Giulia.[28] Ercole Pasquini's manuscript 'durezze' too cannot be securely dated, but one might speculate that they present examples of the type of music he would have played for the purposes of the elevation. The two elevation toccatas in Frescobaldi's *Secondo libro* conform to Diruta's suggestion that Tone 2 and Tone 4 are appropriate for elevations, but while Diruta notes their sad or harsh qualities, Frescobaldi confronts the listener with constant transformations of the expected minor triad tonal focus of the D and A modes. In a meantone tuning of the type that would have been used for keyboard instruments in the early seventeenth century, there would have been stark contrasts between the purity of major triads on D and A and triadic sonorities on other scale degrees, especially minor triads that included B flat. Frescobaldi's harmonic language which manipulates and evades tonal closure, combined with an organ registration using a tremulant, creates a sense of hovering that emulates in sound the liminality of the moment of elevation. This effect is further enhanced by successive suspensions that undermine the sense of pulse. In terms of the concept of the music of pulse, the erosion of tactus to the point where the metric impulses are widely separated would further induce calm and stillness.

The sounds of an organ, together with visual splendours of light emanating from numerous candles; colour in paintings and priestly vestments; and the smell of sweet incense; would have created a multi-sensory experience designed to propel the emotions of the worshipper to deeper piety, penitence and devotion. Thomas Mace's somewhat florid description of how organ music can lift the soul, although from the Protestant orbit and distant from Italy, is equally pertinent in this context. In describing its importance, he calls true music 'a certain divine-magical-spell against all diabolical operations in the souls of men.'[29] On an intellectual level, the aspiration was that the musical-visual experience would render the soul susceptible to unity with the divine, but in practice, for the poor layman living a hand-to-mouth existence, it may well have been fairly overwhelming, and indeed akin to something magical.[30]

28 Frescobaldi, *Libro secondo di toccate… d'intavolatura di cimbalo et organo* (Rome, 1627).

29 Thomas Mace, *Music's Monument* (London, 1676), part 1, p. 12.

30 It is perhaps understandable that the words 'hocus pocus' traditionally used in magic

Music as therapy

While the musical adornment of the medicine of the sacrament was one function of the hospital organ, a second use that similarly relied on moving the passions of the soul was as a different kind of therapy, apparently separate from the religious, and firmly within the scope of medicine. This second use of music was as part of a health regimen for the patients in which the organ was played at mealtimes. Although documentary evidence is sparse, the practice was clearly well-established in the first decades of the seventeenth century as the vagueness of the contemporary accounts infer that the reader would be familiar with this type of activity. John Evelyn for example visited the hospital in 1645 and noted that 'The Organs are very fine, & frequently play'd on to recreate the people in Paine'.[31] A similar description in Italian is found in Totti's 1638 guide to Rome, which mentions the beautiful chapel in the hospital ward which had an organ 'on high' that from time to time is played to 'recreate' the patients.[32]

These third-party 'ear-witness' accounts of the practice of playing the organ for the patients are supported by two sources originating within the Hospital administration: the account of the archconfraternity and hospital by Pierre Saulnier printed in 1649, and a manuscript written by Domenico Borgarucci dating from 1623 on which Saulnier's content is based.[33] Saulnier was prior of the hospital and Borgarucci the secretary of the Order of Santo Spirito, thus both are likely to be reliable witnesses. Aside from describing the position of the organ, Saulnier's account notes only that it was played at mealtimes to 'recreate' the patients.[34] Borgarucci's document is equally frustrating, as he notes that 'to alleviate and cheer the sick, each evening and morning a large organ situated in an eminent position in the middle of the ward is played with voice of music to treat the patients until they have finished eating'.[35] The use of

---

shows are derived from the Latin 'hoc est corpus', the words spoken by a priest at the moment of elevation of the transubstantiated bread and wine.

31 E. S. De Beer and R. Strong (eds), *The Diary of John Evelyn* ([Oxford, 1959] Oxford, 2006), p. 148. Entry for 23 January 1645.

32 'con un'organo di sopra, che di quando in quando si suona per ricreatione de gli ammalati': Pompilo Totti, *Ritratto di Roma moderna* (Rome, 1638), p. 41.

33 D. Borgarucci, *Relatione del modo che si tiene da religione di S. Spirito nel governo dell'Archihospedale Apostolico di Santo Spirito… scritto da Fra Domenico Borgarucci Religioso*, 1623. GB-Lwl EPB/B/46633.

34 'Aulaeis permagnis e' figurato inaurato'que corio circumuestiuntur utrimque patrietes, nisi qua' ex editiori pulpito effert se pneumaticum fistularum organum, cuius subinde modulato canto recreantur aegri dum cibum sumunt': *De capite sacri ordinis S. Spiritus dissertatio F. Petri Saunier* (Lyon, 1649) pp. 128–129.

35 'In tanto, che tutte le sopra dette cose si fanno per sollevare, et rallegrare gl'infermi si suona sera, et mattina un organo grande situato in mezzo del'hospidale, et in luogo eminente, et con voce di musica si trattengono gl'infermi finche habbino finito mangiare…': Borgarucci, *Relatione del modo…* 1623, GB-Lwl EPB/B/46633.

the phrase 'con voce di musica' may indicate that there might also have been a singer, although the phrase is vague enough that it may equally imply just the singing quality of the organ music, or even more specifically to a specific organ register such as a Voce Umana or the combination of registers that created a similar effect. If there was a singer, it was perhaps an alternative to the more usual monastic practice of listening to readings while eating. Motets or spiritual songs conveying uplifting or doctrinal texts would have functioned as a substitute for spoken words from suitable religious books. For now, I will continue to explore the therapeutic role of the organ, but I will return to vocal music below.

The similarity of language in the third-party accounts of music in the hospital wards, notably words such as 'recreate' or 'alleviate', reflects the common usage of the time. Derived from the Latin *recreationem* or *recreatio* meaning recovery from illness, the use of the word 'recreate' is a direct reference to music's healing function – to restore or renew the patient.[36] 'Sollevare' or to alleviate implies a 'raising up' – a literal raising of the spirits. It was, in other words, a proto music therapy. The expectation implicit in the sources is that the organ music would effect a change in the listeners; that music would alter the patients' mental state, to cheer them up or soothe them. It can perhaps be inferred from these statements that there was a fear that patients were likely to fall into melancholy, a condition considered serious, and for which music was widely perceived as an active curative.

While Borgarucci's description is vague concerning specifics of the music, it does tell us the times of the meals, which, conveniently for the organist, were just before or after key moments in the daily schedule of Mass and Offices. The main Mass of the day took place after the morning meal, and Vespers was after the evening meal. The two duties of playing for a service and playing for the patients would have been done consecutively so he presumably just moved between the different parts of the organisation to perform his duties. We can build a reasonable picture of what was expected of the organist at Mass and Vespers, especially after 1600, when centralised efforts to reform liturgical practices took the form of printed ceremonials, missals, breviaries and other service books. Any similar documentation of music that might suggest some sort of control over what or how the music should be played at mealtimes however, is completely absent.

We can only imagine the sonic landscape of these hospital wards. The hard stone and marble surfaces of walls and floors and the high ceilings are likely to have made the space quite resonant, even when filled with several hundred beds. Large numbers of patients too would have ensured a constant background hum of activity, no doubt punctuated by sounds of human suffering. Medical treatments administered by barbers and surgeons without anaesthetic were unlikely to have been done in silence. The sound of music from the

36 https://www.etymonline.com/word/recreation.

organ would have been a welcome relief from what may well have been quite an unpleasant aural environment.

Two of the organists, Ercole Pasquini and Frescobaldi, have been mentioned already. As they were also composers in the modern sense that they wrote their music down, their outputs offer a glimpse of the kind of music that might have been played in the ward. Making explicit connections between their surviving music and the job they were doing is however problematic as we have no evidence that identifies specific pieces of music that were played at precise moments in either the church or the hospital. A further hypothesis regarding Frescobaldi's music will be offered below.

The financial records provide us with the names of many organists who worked at the Hospital, though, just as with the maestro di cappella, there are periods in which no organist is listed with the salaried employees. At these times, we can perhaps assume that one of the friars took the role and was not paid specifically for the job. Normally though, the organist was 'secular', that is, someone not associated with the Order of Santo Spirito. This is attested to in a number of documents, but is explicit from 1595 onwards. Among the organists were several major figures on the Roman musical scene: Ercole Pasquini, Girolamo Frescobaldi, Ercole Bernabei, Bernardo Caffi and so on. These men stand out from the others listed simply as 'Tomaso organista' or 'Vincenzo organista' who we may never identify precisely, though we might perhaps guess at a few. Some served for long periods of time, such as Andrea Vespino, who was organist for over a decade, and whose sudden death in 1620 led to the appointment of Frescobaldi.[37] Others appear in the records for only a month or two.

One key piece of information does emerge from documents in the second half of the seventeenth century, and that is that the duties of the organist were divided at some point, probably in the late 1650s. Spada's *Stato della Casa* is probably the most useful document in unpicking this element of the history of the hospital. It is in Spada's account of the hospital that the first internal documentation of an organist in the hospital ward appears, even though third-party accounts of music in the hospital wards reach back to the beginning of the century. He states that following an Apostolic Visitation ordered by Innocent X, the running of the hospital was revised, and new regulations written and printed in 1654.[38] It was around 1660, during his time as commendatore, that the financial records change. At this point, the salary lists for 'servants in the hospital' include not only the barbers, surgeons and carers of various types, but also an organist, thus it appears that the role of organist in the hospital was separated from that of organist in the church. Sadly though, none of the organists

37 The first payment to Frescobaldi was in July of 1620. ASR OSS 1921, *Copie di mandati*, 1620, item 964.

38 ASR OSS 47, Spada, *Stato della Casa*, cap X, p. 568ff describes the many regulations set out following the Apostolic Visitation made by three prelates on behalf of Innocent X. Among others these lay out the minimum requirements for student physicians.

listed among the hospital staff left written compositions. The regular organist continued to be listed with the singers and chaplains in the church, and that role remained as it had been for the previous decades.

Spada describes the hospital organist as a minor servant at a salary of 2 scudi per month, and that he was entitled to eat in the refectory with other low-status hospital staff.[39] One individual, Pietr'Angelo Guidoni is named in this role for three decades, 1670–1700.[40] In the 1660s, several members of the choir doubled up as organist in the hospital and were clearly multi-tasking. In 1663, for example, Pietro Antonio Abrugia and Donato Rafaelli who were both salaried singers in the church also received payments at different times as organist in the hospital, Abrugia for the first half of the year and Rafaelli for the second half.[41] It could be that this pattern is explicit in the records for this year, but that the practice of singers doubling up as instrumentalists had been in operation before this point without it being recorded. However it was dealt with administratively, the importance of the organ in the ward continued throughout the seventeenth century. Indeed, the role of the hospital organist survived beyond the period in which the professional choir was suppressed in the eighteenth century, as it is still mentioned in a printed *Regole* for the hospital issued by the commendatore Buffalini in 1751.[42] This book, published in memory of his predecessor Pallavicini, had the stated aim to reiterate the good practices of running the hospital. To this end it describes the various duties and procedures of each job, rather like a modern job description, and includes the organist as a particular role. It is absolutely clear that the organist played at mealtimes, and no other duties are mentioned. Mealtimes are given a few pages later, thus one can see exactly when that musician had to be in post and working.[43] Canezza, following the model of the nineteenth-century hospital, suggested that the organist was a wealthy amateur who volunteered his services. The accounts of Spada and Buffalini as well as the payment records suggest otherwise.[44]

Organists then, as now, routinely improvised music required for church services. A number of instructional books on playing the organ outline various techniques through which the organist can learn how to perform different

39 ASR OSS 47, Spada, *Stato della Casa,* p. 613.

40 ASR OSS 1966, *Copie di mandati,* 1670, items 255, 617, etc. ASR OSS 1995, *Copie di mandati,* 1700, items 203, 433, etc.

41 ASR OSS 1959, *Copie di mandati,* 1663, items 236, 590, 932, 1290.

42 *Regole da osservarsi nel sacro ed Apostolico Archiospedale di Santo Spirito in Sassia di Roma* (Rome, 1751), p. 13.

43 'Per far la guardia al Portone dello Spedale vi è un Portinaio; e per suonar l'organo quando mangian gl'infermi vi è l'Organistà': *Regole da osservarsi nel sacro, ed apostolico Archiospedale di Santo Spirito in Sassia di Roma* (Rome, 1751), pp. 13 and 26.

44 Alessandro Canezza, *Gli arcispedali di Roma nella vita cittadina nella storia e nell'arte* (Rome, 1933), p. 51.

types of improvisation. Diruta for example demonstrates techniques for elaborating an existing melody with the addition of diminutions as well as how to 'compose out' contrapuntal cadences which, once mastered, can be extended into longer ricercari.[45] The term 'improvisation' is misleading as these are really mental composition techniques and belong with what many other theorists of the time call *contrapunto alla mente*. There is a sizable literature on the subject of oral/aural composition. Suffice it to say that it was a technique absolutely required for the appointment of singers and organists at high status institutions such as St Peter's in Rome, St Mark's in Venice and Toledo Cathedral, just to name three for which there is documentary evidence of the abilities of musicians either employed by them, or applying to work in them.[46] The vestiges of such unwritten practices may be traced in notated pieces such as hymn versetti, variations on popular songs or dances, and toccatas. It is a safe assumption that the organists of Santo Spirito routinely improvised, whether for Mass, or for the purposes of 'recreating' patients. However, it is only via notated music that we can trace vestiges of improvisational practices, thus it is to notated music that we have to turn to investigate the notion of a proto music therapy. Frescobaldi is the only composer whose works for keyboard can securely be dated to a period in which he was employed at the Hospital.

Repertory

In 1624, four years after he started working at Santo Spirito, Frescobaldi brought out his *Primo libro di Capricci* for keyboard. It was printed by Luca Antonio Soldi, whose print shop was located within the Hospital. Frescobaldi had been organist there since 1620, fitting his duties around his job as organist of St Peter's. The volume was popular enough to be reprinted in Venice by Vincenti in 1626, 1628 and 1642.[47] Hammond suggests that their attractiveness was due to the accessibility of the musical subjects on which the pieces were based, and that they have a sense of fun that is not obscured by the contrapuntal

45 Diruta, *Il Transilvano* (Venice, 1593, 1609); Massimilano Guido and Peter Schubert, 'Unpacking the Box in Frescobaldi's Ricercari of 1615', *Music Theory Online: Journal of the Society for Music Theory*, 20:2 (2014), https://mtosmt.org/issues/mto.14.20.2/mto.14.20.2.guido_schubert.html; Massimiliano Guido, 'Counterpoint in the Fingers. A Practical Approach to Girolamo Diruta's Breve & Facile Regola di Contrappunto', *PhilomusicaOnline*, 11:1 (2012), 63–76.

46 Bonnie J. Blackburn & Edward Lowinsky, 'Luigi Zenobi's Letter on the Perfect Musician', *Studi musicali*, 22 (1993), 61–114.

47 The Venice edition of 1626 brought together the 1615 *Ricercari et Canzone francese* and the 1624 *Capricci* in a single volume and was clearly popular enough to be reprinted twice.

mastery – elements that perhaps evoke a courtly environment.[48] I would like to offer an alternative reading.

For Frescobaldi, whose previous prints included high quality engravings, Soldi was an odd choice of printer. He was neither the best known nor most skilled printer in Rome at the time. As Darbellay has pointed out, changes had to be made during the production of the *Capricci* as the order of items is different across surviving examples of Soldi's print.[49] The tiny proportion of instrumental music within Soldi's output, only four books out of fifty-four suggest that his interests lay in vocal music.[50] Of these four, two were prints of Ricercari by Cifra, and the third of Ricercari by Cava. As will be seen, Soldi's connection with Cifra is easily accounted for, but for Frescobaldi, who usually took immense care with the music that he committed to print, intervening in correcting and revising his work, the connection with Soldi demands further investigation. The *Capricci* are generically for keyboard, playable on either organ or harpsichord, and not specifically for liturgical use. They could therefore have been played in various environments prior to being captured in print. I will argue that several of the *Capricci* fit with the broad notions of healing within a pre-Cartesian humoral framework.

Four of Frescobaldi's *Capricci* are based on popular songs of the time, a fifth uses the call of the cuckoo as its musical starting point. Several other compositions in the collection set specific compositional challenges and may well have been worked out at the keyboard in a semi-improvisational way as outlined in the didactic treatises of Diruta and Banchieri. One might imagine that from the composer's point of view, the provision of music to lighten the mealtimes of patients in a hospital was an ideal environment for experimentation with various compositional workings – a non-critical, not very attentive audience just glad of some entertainment.

The simple fact of creating music around melodies that would have been recognisable suggests a strategy that could be understood within the unique hospital environment as 'cheering'. The repeating harmonic patterns of the 'Ruggiero' even if not specifically recognised or familiar to the poor folk in the hospital, would have been easily accessible. In similar fashion, the evocation of nature by means of a bird call may have entertained the immobile patients, most of whom would have occupied the insalubrious 'inner city' streets of the Borgo, and for whom a bird such as a cuckoo was probably a rare sight.

[48] Frederick Hammond, *Girolamo Frescobaldi: An Extended Biography* (online), paragraphs 14.10 and 14.22. Hammond also provides a brief analysis of each capriccio, https://girolamofrescobaldi.com/14-diversi-tempi-variationi-the-capricci-of-1624/.

[49] Étienne Darbellay, 'L'Énigme de la première édition (1624) des *Caprices* de Girolamo Frescobaldi', *Canadian University Music Review*, 3 (1982), 123–157. There is evidence of printing errors in other books issued by Soldi, for example, Kapsberger's *Poematia et carmina* discussed below.

[50] These figures are derived from the listings in RISM.

As noted in Chapter 2, the somatic effects of the imagination as a cause of disease due to the unity of body and soul were well understood in pre-Cartesian thought. For the same reason, the contemplation of nature and of art were deemed therapeutic. Burton articulated these ideas about the contemplation of nature in his *Anatomy of Melancholy* (1621). Contemporary with Burton, the physician Giulio Mancini who worked at the Hospital from 1593 to 1623 wrote a treatise on painting in which he suggests that for those who are unable to wander in gardens or the countryside, walking in a gallery in which landscape paintings are hung and contemplating each one, mentally wandering in the environment depicted, had the same curative effect as walking in a real landscape.[51] For Mancini, landscapes generated a healthful and temperate optical exercise and a corresponding sensation of physical perambulation.[52] Another contemporary of Mancini and Burton, Grazio Uberti, described the power of natural sounds to alter the physical state of man: 'If someone is tired from travel, if he sits by a stream, he is without doubt comforted by its murmuring; if he rests in a shady place, he is certain to be consoled by the chirping of the birds; if he stops in an open place, he is sweetened by the whispering of the breeze…'[53] In the context of these widely held notions concerning the somatic effects of sound, the *Capriccio sopra il cucho* could be understood very differently as a musical manifestation of the notion of contemplating nature as a promoter of health.

Beyond the effect of the physical sound of the bird call, the cuckoo is associated with the arrival of spring and all that it represents in the natural cycle of rebirth and renewal. In religious terms, spring is the season of Easter, representing the ultimate moment of salvation and new life in Christ. In addition, there is a common symbolism of birds generically as representing the soul, especially in religious imagery. Birds also represent the element of air.[54] In humoral theory, spring and the element of air together indicate the hot and moist humour, blood, that directly opposes the cold and dry humour of black bile, the cause of melancholy. This composite of physical sonic characteristics

[51] Frances Gage, 'Exercise for Mind and Body: Giulio Mancini, Collecting, and the Beholding of Landscape Painting in the Seventeenth Century', *Renaissance Quarterly*, 61:4 (2008), 1167–1207, esp. 1168. Mercuriale, *De arte gymnastica* (Venice, 1601), ed. Concetto Pennuto (Florence, 2008), p. 265, discusses the benefits of walking in the outdoors.

[52] Frances Gage, *Painting as Medicine in Early Modern Rome: Giulio Mancini and the Efficacy of Art* (University Park, PA, 2016), pp. 85–86.

[53] 'Stanco, che sia alcuno per lo viaggio, per lo corso, per lo moto, se siede appresso un rio, non ha dubio, che si conforta al dolce mormorio. Se in luogo ombroso si posa certo è, che si consola al garrirre del gl'augelli. Se si ferma in luogo aperto, vero è che s'addolcisce al sibillare dell'aure…': Grazio Uberti, *Contrasto musico: opera dilettevole*, 1630. Facsimile edition ed. Giancarlo Rostirolla (Lucca, 1991), pp. 81–83, 85.

[54] James Hall, *Hall's Dictionary of Signs and Symbols in Art* (London, 1974), p. 48.

and symbolic associations aligns this music with the intellectual notions of physical and spiritual wellbeing of the time.

The call of the cuckoo is heard around seventy times in the course of the piece. The predominance of the motif in an upper voice repeating the same pitches (D-B) is almost hypnotic as it is heard against an apparently static harmonic backdrop. The G-natural tonal type sets up the cuckoo call as sol-mi in the hard hexachord, but by shifting the hexachord, Frescobaldi ensures that there is ample contrapuntal interest.

The seven sections delineated by metrical changes are marked by cadences in which the pitches of the D-B cuckoo motif are, with only two exceptions, the chordal root and third respectively of the two chords forming a perfect cadence closing on G. The other two cadences are elided. At the end of the first triple section, the D functions as the chordal root and the B as the chordal fifth in a stepwise progression from an implied minor triad on D (at the actual point of closure the chordal third is absent) to a major triad on E. The D (sol) in the upper voice at the point of arrival is the first note of the cuckoo motif. The B (mi) of the motif starts the following section where it functions as the chordal fifth of an E major triad. This progression is continued by harmonic movement through a short cycle of fifths, E-A-D-G provided by the lower three parts, which subsequently break into rapid contrapuntal interplay using the descending minor third. The playful exploitation of the hexachordal sol-mi in the third section of the piece is typical of the kind of compositional strategies one might expect in Frescobaldi.

While the display of compositional virtuosity in this piece invites an intellectual appreciation of skill and engages with the potentially somatic effects of the imagination, at the same time, the music exhibits characteristics that align with the acoustic cues identified by Spitzer as signifying agape.[55] These include a slow harmonic rhythm, lack of variability and absence of extreme dynamics or articulation. While Spitzer, following Juslin and Timmers, equates agape to tenderness, in religious terms it refers to the love of God.[56] The *Capriccio* could thus be understood not just as an aural aid to the imagination of a therapeutic landscape, but as a sonic representation of the cosmic harmony of man and nature, or man and God.

Other capricci in Frescobaldi's collection can also be understood differently in the hospital context. While the *Capriccio sopra il cuchu* exhibits acoustic cues that might signal cosmic harmony through reference to the natural

55 Michael Spitzer, *A History of Emotion in Western Music: A Thousand Years from Chant to Pop* (Oxford, 2020), p. 88; Patrik Juslin and Renee Timmers, 'Expression and Communication of Emotion in Music Performance', in Patrick N. Juslin and Justin A. Sloboda, *Handbook of Music and Emotion: Theory, Research, Application* (Oxford, 2010), pp. 453–492.

56 The separation of agape and eros, divine and erotic love, reaches back to Augustine and is also pertinent to the sense of yearning expected in the elevation toccata.

world, the *Capriccio di durezze* and the *Capriccio cromatico con ligature al contrario* offer cues to a different sort of alignment. The *Capricco di durezze* is constructed using continually overlapping suspensions and dissonances within contrapuntal textures. These create harmonic tension and resolution, or, tension and evaded resolution, that undermine the sense of tonal closure. The harmonic vagueness thus created affects the perception of pulse, suggesting a different therapeutic aspect to this music. The striking of dissonance followed by resolution effectively imitates a strong-weak or diastole-systole movement, that coupled with a slow musical tactus may have been intended as calming or slowing the agitated pulse of patients.

The *Capriccio cromatico* adds a dense use of linear chromaticism to the mix of suspensions and dissonance with a slow overall tactus. Frescobaldi further intensifies the effects by restricting the resolution of dissonance to the opposite of the expected direction of movement, 'al contrario', thus creating successions of ascending resolutions. While contrapuntally a masterpiece, affectively, the mix of ascending resolution and melodic chromaticism successfully winds up the sense of tension and the subsequent relief in resolution and release. The diastole-systole of dissonance and resolution on the one hand, and the overall erosion of the sense of rhythmic movement on the other, seems to distil the essence of Aristotelian time, of stillness and motion.

At a different level, both the *Capriccio di durezze* and the *Capriccio cromatico* allude to the elevation. Frescobaldi adopts Tone 2 and Tone 4 respectively for these pieces, that is, those recommended by Diruta as appropriate for eliciting the necessary feelings of awe and devotion, and both use the multiple suspensions, dissonances and chromaticism usually found in elevation toccatas, to engender a sense of yearning. These capricci, played in the hospital environment, perhaps intended to channel something of the 'medicamentum' of the sacrament, slowing or suspending activity to absorb its spiritual medicine.

Some of the capricci on hexachordal subjects may also be viewed differently. While the solmisation syllables of the hexachord were the bread and butter of music education for the better part of six centuries, they could also substitute for words and infer linguistic meaning or even take on symbolic meanings. Josquin's Mass on la-so-fa-re-mi making explicit reference to the dismissive 'lascia far a mi' of a patron unwilling to pay his musicians is just one famous example. The same syllables could also have lascivious meanings as noted by Holford-Strevens.[57] More pertinent in the context of the Hospital is the 'spiritual singing' developed by Jean Gerson noted in Chapter 3. The spiritual change, or ascent of the soul toward the divine, articulated through hexachord syllables, aligns with the Christian Neo-Platonism embraced by Cirillo and other leaders

[57] Leofranc Holford Strevens, 'Fa mi la so la: The Erotic Implications of Solmization Syllables', in Bonnie J. Blackburn and Laurie Stras (eds), *Eroticism in Early Modern Music* (Aldershot, 2015), pp. 43–58.

of the Hospital of Santo Spirito in the years prior to and around the time of Frescobaldi's employment.

There is plenty of evidence in Frescobaldi's music of intricate playing out of hexachordal subjects, using *inganni* and hidden complexities in his contrapuntal writing.[58] It seems possible that the hexachordal subjects identified in his *Capricci* could refer in some way to Gerson's 'song of the heart'. If a capriccio on the descending theme la-sol-fa-re-mi were translated to Gerson's internal meaning, it might signal the listener to contemplate love and joy (la and fa) in relation to fear (sol) and the hope (re) inspired by pity and compassion (mi). The ascending ut-re-mi-fa-sol-la might represent the journey from pain or sorrow through hope and compassion to joy.

As Connolly has shown, the journey from sorrow or mourning to joy, and notions of spiritual transformation, are deeply embedded in much medieval mystical devotion and are especially played out in devotions to St Cecilia.[59] A compositional representation of the transformation of the soul, if attached to a cantata or oratorio text, would be commonplace, so I would argue that an abstract representation through hexachordal solmisation may stand as a substitute. The subject of Frescobaldi's *Capriccio sopra ut-re-mi-fa-sol-la*, heard as a simple ascending scale, might therefore 'translate' as the emotional journey from sorrow, through hope and compassion, to joy and love, or, in a parallel reading that reflects Neo-Platonic cosmology, from the physicality of the body to the joy of union with divine love. Corroborating evidence of the use of an ascending scale as representative of movement heavenward is also found in music by Frescobaldi's student Froberger. In the autograph manuscript of his 'Lament on the death of Ferdinand IV', the final ascending scale ends in a drawing of cherubs and clouds, suggesting the ascent and arrival of his soul in heaven.[60] For those who wished to hear it, the message of the ascending scale of the hexachord was immediately audible, while those who simply enjoyed the contrapuntal dexterity of the composer working with a simple subject could delight in the healthy *allegrezza* it provoked.

The combined concerns that were the primary functions of the Hospital enable new interpretations of instrumental music of the period that may appear to have no specific liturgical or courtly function, such as the Frescobaldi *Capricci*. Such music may fulfil the objectives of humoral medicine in allevi-

58 John Harper, 'Frescobaldi's Early Inganni and Their Background', *Proceedings of the Royal Musical Association*, 105 (1978–1979), 1–12.

59 Thomas Connolly, *Mourning into Joy: Music, Raphael, and Saint Cecilia* (New Haven, CT and London, 1994).

60 Froberger, 'Lamento sopra la dolorosa perdita della Real M.sta di Ferdinando IV', *Partita* FbWV 612, Libro Quarto, 1656. For a facsimile of this image, see Froberger, ed. Siegbert Rampe, *Neue Ausgabe sämtlicher Clavier- und Orgelwerke*, vol. 2, (Kassel, 1995), p. xxxviii.

ating the negative passions, regulating the pulse and at the same time, address the Christian desire for greater devotion and piety.

There is of course no hard evidence as to how Frescobaldi might have come across these ideas. The extent to which he understood affect within medical theory and theology beyond the normal early modern mindset is impossible to prove. He would certainly have been aware of mottos commonly used in harpsichord decoration that underscored music as a cure for sorrow as well as a companion of pleasure.[61] In addition, the prefaces to several of his books indicate his deep awareness of the power of musical affect and the role of the performer in ensuring the affective impact of his music. What we can assume is that Frescobaldi's 'way of knowing' the world was similar to anyone else of his social status and of his time. He probably did have some awareness of popular health regimens such as those of Castore Durante, and as a church musician, would have sat through hundreds of homilies, some of which may have been drawn from popular books on preaching by authors such as Pietro da Lucca.

It is also impossible to reconstruct oral transmission of ideas through circles of friendship, preaching, academic discourse and the many day-to-day interactions of normal working people. Discourse about music was a high-status activity. The social chasm between the likes of Giovanni Battista Doni, whose erudite theoretical writings encompassed discussion of the power of ancient music, and a practical musician such as Frescobaldi, was substantial.[62] Doni's scathing criticism of Frescobaldi as a man whose 'knowledge was in his fingers' and his antagonism towards him may have been triggered by the musician's grasp of topics deemed above his social station.[63] We will never know.

While he may not have been able to interact with high status courtiers in their elite discourse about music, there is compelling proof of Frescobaldi's acquaintance with intellectuals who navigated the social territory between the aristocracy and 'mere' artisans, and these men are likely to have transmitted medical, philosophical and religious ideas. Aside from Mancini who was contemporary with Frescobaldi at the Hospital, Frescobaldi also knew Johann

61 For example, 'musica laetitiae comes et medicina dolorum' is a motto used on Flemish virginals and harpsichords and is also featured in paintings of the same period such as Vermeer's 'music lesson'. Roger Harmon, '*Musica laetitae comes* and Vermeer's Music Lesson', *Oud Holland*, 113:3 (1999), 161–166.

62 The social interactions of music theorists and the world of learning, in contrast with dealings with practical musicians, is discussed at length in Eric Bianchi, 'Bad Latin, Bad Manners: Giovanni Battista Doni, Marin Mersenne and Literary Style in Seventeenth-century Music Theory', *Music & Letters*, 92:2 (2015), 167–184; 'Scholars, Friends, Plagiarists', *Journal of the American Musicological Society*, 70:1 (2017), 61–128.

63 'on peut dire qu'il ait toute sa science aux bouts des doits': Letter from Doni to Mersenne, 22 July 1640. Cornelius de Waard, *Correspondence du P. Marin Mersenne*, 9 (Paris, 1965), p. 488.

Faber.[64] Beyond the Hospital, Frescobaldi, Mancini and Faber all enjoyed the patronage of the Barberini family.

Frescobaldi's friendship with Lelio Guidiccioni, a poet and intellectual virtuoso who acted as a go-between for artists, musicians and patrons, is also beyond doubt. Guidiccioni wrote the Latin dedication for Frescobaldi's 1627 motet collection and owned a harpsichord that Frescobaldi had called 'la Gioia' and a portrait of the composer.[65] He, like Mancini and Frescobaldi, moved in the same patronal circle. Guidiccioni wrote a treatise on music that draws on Neo-Platonic concepts of harmony, but his other writings are also saturated with references to Platonic cosmography and suggest more than a passing familiarity with the Christian Neo-Platonism of Marsilio Ficino, demonstrating an understanding of the power of music, including music in the service of God.[66] That Frescobaldi was familiar with Neo-Platonic notions of cosmic harmony is evident in his adoption of an emblem containing a hexachordal puzzle canon with the motto 'discordia concors'.[67] Might Guidiccioni also have been familiar with the mystical musical ideas of Jean Gerson and have shared them with Frescobaldi? Or might the transmitter have been Banchieri, a monk resident in Bologna, also known to Frescobaldi, and who used the same 'discordia concors' emblem? As noted in Chapter 3, Gerson's thought was transmitted in Italian by the popular preacher Pietro da Lucca whose books were reprinted multiple times in Bologna and other cities.

Proving the specific influence on Frescobaldi of Mancini, Faber or Guidiccioni is simply not possible beyond stacking up the circumstantial evidence. To this end, the wider output of his printer, Luca Antonio Soldi, offers further support to bolster evidence of ways in which the *Capricci* might have aligned with a specific purpose within the Hospital of Santo Spirito. As Soldi's output was primarily of vocal music, the puzzle of what Borgarucci's comment that the organ was played 'with voice of music' might mean, first needs to be addressed.

64 Faber acted as a go-between for Friedrich Fugger and Frescobaldi in commissioning a motet. The letter survives in the Academica dei Lincei, Fondo Faber. See Hammond, *An Extended Biography*, 8.13, https://girolamofrescobaldi.com/ and pp. 18, 24.

65 Arnaldo Morelli, 'Un amico di Frescobaldi: Lelio Guidiccioni, uomo di lettere, connoisseur d'arte e di musica', in *A fresco: Mélanges offerts au Professeur Étienne Darbellay*, ed. Benno Boccadoro and Georges Starobinski (Bern, 2013), pp. 51–67.

66 *De Musica*, V-CVbav Barb. Lat. 3879, trans. Andrew Dell'Antonio, in *Listening as Spiritual Practice in Early Modern Italy* (Berkeley, CA, 2011), p. 150; and *Discourse on eloquence*, V-CVbav Barb. Lat. 2960, fol. 182v.

67 Naomi J. Barker, 'Mottos and Metaphors: Toward an Interpretation of the Emblems in Frescobaldi's Primo Libro d'Arie Musicali', *Journal of Seventeenth-Century Music*, 25 (2019), https://sscm-jscm.org/jscm-issues/volume-25-no-1/barker-mottos-and-metaphors/.

Singing for the sick

The health-giving properties of liturgical music was a common topos in music-theoretical writing throughout the medieval period, thus singing religious music for the sick in the wards of the hospital is not in itself surprising.[68] It is however, vocal music beyond that of the daily Mass to which Borgarucci appears to be referring. There are plenty of possible candidates for vocal music suitable for use in the hospital ward. For a start, we know that the sound of Litanies would have been a constant presence in the Hospital. Every day after Terce, the Litanies were sung, probably by the duty chaplain. On Saturdays, the Litanies of the Madonna were sung with organ in front of the altar of the Madonna in the church, and the commendatore and friars were expected to say Litanies every evening.[69] The daily recitations were probably of the Litany of the Saints, the oldest and most commonly used version of the Litany. This form was adaptable to include local saints or saints for specific needs such as invocations to St Sebastian at times of plague.[70] As devotional singing was understood as a means of combatting illness, the Litanies were an integral part of the healthcare regime. The integration of sung prayer and caring for the sick is even suggested in a miniature painting in the fifteenth-century copy of the Rule in which the decoration of the initial letter shows members of the order caring for the sick and distributing the sacrament, while at the foot of the page there is an image of five men in various vestments standing around a lectern in the way in which a choir would sing from a choirbook.[71]

The sources are ambiguous about where the daily Litanies were sung, but as the Saturday Litanies are always noted specifically as in front of the altar of the

68 Peregrine Horden, 'Religion as Medicine: Music in Medieval Hospitals', in Peter Biller and Joseph Ziegler (eds), *Religion and Medicine in the Middle Ages* (York, 2001), pp. 135–154, esp. pp. 151–153.

69 'Finita Prima ad hora compa[gn]a si suona la messa grande, si dice Terza, si cantano le litanie, e poi la messa conventuale con musica, et cosi si osserva ogni giorno... Tutti li sabati finita compieta si cantano le litanie della Ma[donn]a avanti il suo altare con musica et organo... Tiene sei cappellani quali anco servono per cantori...' ('Prime ended, at the appropriate time the main Mass is played, Terce is said, the Litanies are sung and then the Conventual Mass with music, and so it is observed every day... All Saturdays after Compline, the Litany of the Madonna is sung in front of her altar with music and organ... Six chaplains who also serve as singers are retained for this'): *Stato temporale delle chiese di Roma fatto nel pontificato di Urbano VIII l'anno 1625*, ASV. Misc.Arm VII /77, fol. 643.

70 Chiu has noted that the iconic sound and common musical thread of public devotions such as processions at times of plague was the Litany. During the plague in Milan in 1575 Cardinal Borromeo issues specific instructions to the public to sing Litanies and prayers at the sounding of the bells. Remi Chiu, *Plague and Music in the Renaissance* (Cambridge, 2017), pp. 55 and 103.

71 ASR OSS 3193, f49r. http://www.cflr.beniculturali.it/Preziosi/preziosi.php?lar=1600&alt=900.

Madonna, it seems likely that the daily Litany may have been sung in the hospital chapel. If this were the case, the patients could take part, either passively or in singing or reciting the responses. On Saturdays the Litany of the Madonna is specified. As the organist, – an external hired professional – was also required to play for the Litanies, these were no minor part of the religious observation of the Order. The fact that four singers were paid for the Litanies suggests that they were sung in falsobordone at the very least, and for feast days possibly in polyphony. During the 1640s, a named singer, Pietro Peschio, was hired for singing the Litanies at a set rate of 40 baiocchi per week which suggests he was employed only for this specific duty.[72]

The Litany of the Madonna had become popular as a vehicle for musical settings around 1600. In the approximately 300 collections of liturgical music printed between 1601 and 1700, there are nearly 600 settings of the Litany.[73] Multi-voice settings of the Litany of the Madonna by at least one composer-singer employed by the Hospital have survived.

A key part of the Litany in the context of the Hospital is the invocation to the Madonna as 'health of the sick' (*salus infirmorum*).[74] The view that the maternal compassion of the Madonna was a powerful intermediary on behalf of those suffering is an enduring one. It is evident also in other Marian texts that predate the formalisation of the Litany of Loreto. These prayers to the Madonna in the form of non-liturgical devotional songs may also have been performed in the wards. A setting of the medieval sequence 'Benedicta es, caelorum regina' from the mid- to late-sixteenth century in the Regensburg choirbook, BH 6003, is one likely example. The first verse of this text invokes Mary as medicine for the sick.[75]

Benedicta es, caelorum regina,	Blessed you are, queen of heaven,
Et mundi totius domina,	And ruler of the whole world,
Et aegris medicina.	And medicine for the sick

In addition, in the wake of Fillipo Neri's Oratorians' devotional practices, collections of laude praising or petitioning the Madonna were printed. Paolo Papini, who was a longstanding member of the Order of Santo Spirito, contributed to

72 *ad 40 p[er] lett[anie]*: ASR OSS 1938, *Copie di mandati*, 1640, item 66. By 1646, Peschio was singing in the Cappella Giulia. See Rostirolla, *Musica e Musicisti nella basilica di San Pietro: cinque secoli di storia della Cappella Giulia* (Vatican City, 2014), vol. 1, p. 427.

73 David Blazey, 'The Litany in seventeenth-century Italy' (unpublished PhD thesis, University of Durham, 1990), vol. 1, p. 2.

74 For a full text of the Litany see Michael Martin, *Thesaurus precum latinarum*, https://www.preces-latinae.org/thesaurus/BVM/Laurentanae.html (accessed 30/09/2022).

75 For the full text see https://www.cpdl.org/wiki/index.php/Benedicta_es_caelorum_regia.

at least two of these, thus we might infer that during his time in the Hospital in the last quarter of the sixteenth century, such songs were also sung there.

It is in another of the Regensburg choirbooks containing works by Papini that there is perhaps further evidence of liturgical music being sung in the hospital or sung with a view to its healing properties. D-Rp BH 6009 is a lavishly illuminated choirbook, the frontispiece of which bears an inscription noting its presentation to the commendatore in 1603, and the name of the scribe.[76] The initial letters of each section of the Masses written in the first half of the book are decorated with botanical paintings along with miniatures of the emblem of the Order of Santo Spirito and symbols of Pentecost. Although they are badly ink-damaged, quite a few of the illustrations are recognisable as plants illustrated in common text books on botanical medicine, such as Mattioli's commentary on Dioscorides' *Materia Medica*.[77] That this was indeed the intention, and they are not generic decorations, is attested to in the payment made to Domenico Aniboni, a singer in the choir, who copied the music and text as well as painting the illustrations, which indicates that the capital letters were illustrated 'from the boxes in dispensary'.[78] I understand this to refer to the round wooden boxes in which herbs would have been kept alongside other vessels such as the ceramic apothecary jars or *albarelli* used for extracts, distillations and other herbal remedies, and for which there is ample iconographic evidence for such uses.[79] In the manuscript, plants such as the rose, olive, laurel and wheat are all identifiable. While some of these plants also have religious symbolic meanings, their oils and extracts were crucial to the medicines of the period. The book thus makes an explicit connection between liturgical music and health: the health of the soul and the physical health of the listener. It perhaps also served as a reminder to the singers using it that what they were doing was essential to the care of the patients for whom they were singing.

One further category of vocal music that might fit Borgarucci's description is the motet. A large quantity of seventeenth-century motets from the Santo Spirito music library have survived in manuscript. The majority are for multiple voices and so presumably would not be for mealtime 'entertainment'. A few are for solo voice and organ and therefore would be practical for this purpose,

[76] D-Rp BH 6009. The commendatore was Girolamo Agucchi and the scribe, the singer Domenico Aniboni.

[77] Petri Andreae Matthioli Senensis, ... *Commentarii denuo aucti in libros sex Pedacii Dioscoridis Anazarbei de medica materia...* (Lyon, 1563).

[78] 'Domenico Aniboni 12 di moneta è dato ne debito apartene et alquale li paghano per havere notare le noti et le parole in un libro grande di cinque messe per la nostra chiesa e per haverne fate le lettere maiuscole alle scatole della drogheria': ASR OSS 1910, *Copie di mandati*, 1604, item 41. Domenico Aniboni had been employed since at least 1595, as payments to him are noted in ASR OSS 1905, *Copie di mandati*, 1595, e.g. item 2125, but he cannot be traced earlier due to the lacunae in the financial records.

[79] An overview of the uses of such jars and boxes is given in Leah Clark, *Courtly Mediators* (Cambridge, 2023) pp. 196–209.

but printed collections of devotional songs are equally likely candidates. Identifying specific items that might have been sung is impossible, but perhaps the small-scale solo motets in Frescobaldi's *Liber secundus sacrarum modulationum* published in 1627 were tried out in this setting. Compositions printed in his first book of motets, although now lost, were presumably also in circulation during the time in which he was employed at the Hospital. The consideration of the role of motets and Masses in the hospital brings us back to the printer of Frescobaldi's *Capricci*, Luca Antonio Soldi.

Luca Antonio Soldi at the Hospital

In the jubilee year of 1625, Soldi brought out a reprint of Palestrina's *Hymni totius anni*, the title page of which explicitly states the location of his shop as in the building of the Hospital of Santo Spirito: 'in aedibus Sancti Spiritus in Saxia'. Unlike the first edition printed in 1589 in splendid choirbook format, Soldi's reprint is of poorer quality and in cheaper partbook format.[80] Franchi notes differences in the content of the book when compared to the original: it includes some hymns on texts which post-date Palestrina's death, and therefore cannot be by him, unless they are contrafacta.[81] Soldi's title page also indicates the existence of an organ bass part, but none has survived, although there is a manuscript copy in Hanover.[82]

Among the items of liturgical organ music in Frescobaldi's *Secondo libro di toccate* of 1627, there are hymn versetti. Annibaldi has demonstrated that the contrapuntal reworkings of a number of hymns in a rare Frescobaldi autograph manuscript, R-Vat MS Chigi Q.IV.19, use Victoria and Palestrina as models, and that the Palestrina models were taken from the *Hymni totius anni*.[83] This manuscript was compiled in the mid-1620s, the period in which Frescobaldi was working at both the Hospital of Santo Spirito and at St Peter's. Annibaldi assumed that Palestrina's 1589 print was used, but I would argue that the smaller partbook format of Soldi's print, and presumably easy access to it given

[80] *Hymni totius anni secundum sanctae Romanae ecclesiae consuetudinis necnon hymni religionum* ('Hymns for all the year according to the use of the holy Roman church as well as hymns of the religious orders) (Rome: Apud Iacobum Tornerium, & Bernardium Donangelum, 1589).

[81] Saverio Franchi and Orietta Sartori, *Annali della stampa musicale romana dei secoli XVI–XVIII*, vol1/1 (Rome, 2006–2012), vol. 1, p. 503.

[82] The Hanover manuscript is noted on the Printed Sacred Music database http://www.printed-sacred-music.org/manuscripts/00000000002506.

[83] Claudio Annibaldi, 'Palestrina and Frescobaldi: Discovering a Missing Link', *Music & Letters*, 79:3 (1998), 329–345. The Chigi keyboard manuscripts belonged to Leonardo Castellani, one of Frescobaldi's students, who also served as organist at Santo Spirito 1638–1641.

that it was printed at the Hospital, make it a more likely contender. One might even speculate that Frescobaldi could have had a hand in creating the organ bass that Soldi apparently printed and advertised on the titlepage.

Palestrina dedicated the 1589 first edition of his collection of hymns to Pope Sixtus V. Soldi's print is dedicated to Giuseppe Anselmi, the commendatore of the Hospital at the time. There is no evidence of a new collector or editor for the volume. It would thus appear that Soldi was responsible for choosing to reprint this music, which was by then more than thirty years old; and the authorial voice of the dedication is his.

> Antiquity was accustomed to call the entire mass of creation, which coalesces from the harmony of diverse bodies differing unanimously, a volume of music; where, whether gems in the sea, flowers on the earth or stars in the sky, Augustine, that most perfect interpreter of the truth, acknowledges to be like the notes of divine voices. Without doubt this is an outstanding work of divine Love, who teaches music: nay rather, if I may speak with Pythagoras, it is in the numbers of things that the melodious smith expresses himself.[84]

One might easily dismiss this dedication referring to the common topos of the power of music as rhetorical posturing, but it is not an isolated example and follows a trajectory that starts from Soldi's first print issued from the Hospital, a reprint of psalm settings by Cifra dated 1619. This book includes a dedication that, referring to Plato, suggests that 'those who sing to God, reside in the celestial bodies, indicating that song is shown to the Godhead in the movement of the spheres'.[85] It continues with further references to Macrobius' 'The Dream of Scipio' and to Pythagoras, before directly addressing the dedicatee in a passage that indicates a belief that music opens the way for unity with the divine.

> You are delighted by music, as by something divine: not because the soul had brought into the body a memory of the music which it knew in heaven, as the Pythagoreans related, but because that thing pleases profitably in this life, which is the eternal occupation of the best. I believe that you cannot believe that anything is utterly vile, which is the most venerable study of the greatest office. Let them therefore be praised who seek some fruit of the hoped-for beatitude from the good muses – and let the enemies of the heavens be

84 'Universam hanc rerum molem, quæ ex diversorum corporum unanimiter discrepantium consonantia coalescit, Musicum volumen appellare consuevit Antiquitas; ubi, sive gemmas in Mari, sive flores in terra, sive in Cęlo sydera, veluti divinarum vocum Notas agnoscit veritatis interpres integerrimus Augustinus; nimirum hoc divini Amoris, qui Musicam docet, Egregium est opus; imò seipsum, ut cum Pythagora loquar, in rerum numeris canorus faber expressit': Palestrina, *Hymni totius anni* (Rome, Soldi, 1625), translated by Shelagh Sneddon.

85 'Sirenas, hoc est, Deo canentes, orbibus cælestibus insidere Plato tradidit; significans sphærarum motu cantum Divino Numini exhiberi...'

damned: and let that true saying not be thought empty, that great men by this pleasure can even open a return to heaven for themselves.[86]

Although this dedication appeared in the first printing issued by Robletti in 1609 and addressed to a different dedicatee, Soldi may well have been an associate in the Robletti firm at that time. Franchi rather cynically suggests that Soldi dedicated this book to Giacinto Petroni, the papal official responsible for overseeing printing and bookselling in the city, and deliberately used these elevated intellectual references in order to cast himself and his fledgling business in a positive light.[87]

In the same year, 1619, Soldi printed a volume of Cifra Masses, his *Missarum liber primus*. Unlike much of Soldi's output which appeared in partbook format, this volume is a large choirbook of high quality. The dedication to Prince Carlo de Medici refers to the sympathetic resonance of well-tuned lyre strings and infers Neo-Platonic notions of attunement.[88] Beyond the Neo-Platonic references, the decorative capital B that is used as the initial letter of two voice parts of the Benedictus in each of the six Masses in the book contains a miniature of the Holy Spirit, in the form of a dove descending on the head of a haloed but veiled figure presumably representing the Madonna. Above it, the motto 'Beatum medicent' – blessed medicine – reinforces the notion of the Madonna as 'medicine for the sick' and the sacrament as a medication.[89]

Further, Soldi's 1621 print of Allegri Motets for two, three and four voices dedicated to Pietro Dini, archbishop of Fermo, expresses notions relating to Platonic conceptions of music as reflecting and affecting the disposition of the soul.

86 'Tu musica delectaris, ut re divina: non quod in corpus deferat anima memoriam musicæ, cuius in cælo conscia fuerit, ut Pythagorici fabulabantur; sed quia utiliter in hac vita placet, quæ sempiterna optimorum occupatio est. Te arbitro, nihil infimum credi licet, quod studium augustissimum est summi officii. Laudentur igitur, & cælestium æmuli censeantur, qui speratæ beatitudinis fructum aliquem petunt à bonis musis: neque inane veri dictum putetur, magnos viros hac oblectatione sibi posse etiam reditum in cælum sperire [*r.* aperire]': Cifra, *Psalmi septem qui in vesperis ad concentus…* (Rome, Soldi, 1619), translated by Shelagh Sneddon.

87 Franchi and Sartori, *Annali*, p. 309.

88 'Est enim ea rerum musicarum cognatio, atque natura, ut si una testudo resonet, altera consentiens, quamvis minor, e regione respondeat' ('For there is that kinship and nature of musical things that, if one lyre resounds, the other in harmony, although lesser, responds from the same region'): Cifra, *Missarum liber primus* (Rome, Soldi, 1619), translated by Shelagh Sneddon.

89 The same set of letters is used in Cifra's *Missarum liber secundum* (1621), and Soriano's *Passio secundum Mattaeum* (1619). It is unlikely that Soldi's set of decorative letters was unique to him, but his choice of that image at that point in the Mass seems to be making a deliberate statement as to the sacrament as 'medicamentum'.

... I might hope that these measures might fall most pleasingly upon the ears, just as the plentiful sweetness of your ways wonderfully attracts and holds the minds and eyes of all. And certainly with Plato, the perfect philosopher in all numbers, music is in a certain way an imitation of habits: so that it seems that music which imitates the wicked, should be rejected, but that which imitates the good, should be approved. I might undoubtedly have a reason to exult gloriously, if I might attain your habits, that is, the best ones, in melody.[90]

One further print can be added to this list, containing devotional, rather than specifically liturgical music, that is, Kapsberger's settings of devotional poetry written by Maffeo Barberini before he was elected Pope Urban VIII. The small-scale solo motets in Kapsberger's book can be added to the list of likely compositions that fit the description of 'con voce di musica' performed in the wards at mealtimes. This volume, entitled *Poematia et carmina*, includes a dedication that again references the power of music, but in addition alludes to the pontiff as a modern parallel of David, the musician king. While overtly and obsequiously flattering, the dedication encapsulates the mix of religious and secular authorities of antiquity that underscore music's power.

For the city could not previously hear the Pindaric spirit thundering in the Latin tongue, even from the Prince of Lyric Poets himself. My care, on seeing David's glory flourish again in the erudition of our Supreme Pontiff, was to set those poems to musical numbers, which embrace their worthy thoughts with Pontifical piety, and always either pursue the triumphs of the saints, or lay open the oracles of human wisdom.[91]

The comparison of Urban with the biblical figure of David by implication suggests that Urban's music had the power to heal, just as David's music had cured King Saul. Further, there is an inference that Urban's poetic texts were as powerful as those of David, that is, the psalms.

It seems highly unlikely that Soldi penned these Latin dedications. While little is known of his background or early career, his social status was not suf-

90 'Enimvero sperarem modulos hosce iucundissime auribus accidere posse, quemadmodum animos, atque oculos omnium allicit mirifice, detinetque morum tuorum numerosa suavitas. Et certe cum Platoni numeris omnibus absoluto philosopho, morum quędam imitatio sit Musica: ita ut quę malos imitetur, reiicienda: quæ verò bonos, approbanda videatur; haberem profecto cur gloriose gestirem, si tuos, hoc est optimos mores modulatione consequerer': Allegri, *Motecta binis, ternis... vocibus* (Rome, Soldi, 1621), translated by Shelagh Sneddon.

91 'Pindaricum enim spiritum latino ore tonantem, neque ab ipso Lyricorum Principe Urbs olim potuit audire. Mihi, qui Davidis gloriam in Maximi Pontificis eruditione reflorescere video, curæ fuit musicis numeris ea carmina modulati [*r.* modulari], quæ dignas Pontificia pietate sententias complectuntur, semperque aut Sanctorum triumphos persequuntur, aut humanæ pandunt oracula sapientiæ': Kapsberger, *Poematia et carmina* (Rome, Soldi, 1624), translated by Shelagh Sneddon.

ficiently elevated to include a Latin education. The range of Neo-Platonic, Pythagorean and other ancient references to the power of music indicate a well-educated writer and perhaps points to a single author, probably one that was familiar with the Hospital and its mission.[92] Table 6.1 summarises the books in Soldi's output that refer to the power of music.

Table 6.1 Sacred music with dedications referencing the power of music printed by Soldi.

Composer	Title	Date	Dedicatee
Cifra	Psalmi septem, qui in vesperis ad concentus... opus septimum	1619	Giacinto Petroni
Cifra	Missarum liber primus [a 4,5,6 vv]	1619	Carlo Medici
Pace	L'ottavo libro di motetti a una, due, tre e quattro voci...	1619	Marco Sitico Altemps
Allegri	Motecta binis, ternis, quaternis, quinis, senisque vocibus	1621	Pietro Dini
Palestrina	Hymni totius anni... cum basso ad organum	1625	Giuseppe Anselmi
Palestrina & G. F. Anerio	Messe a quattro voci	1626	Francesco Soderini
Kapsberger	Poematia et carmina	1624	Francesco Barberini

Aside from the intellectual affinity with the work of the Hospital expressed in the Neo-Platonic dedications, Soldi's output also includes collections of music connected to the Hospital through the composer, collector or dedicatee, the details of which are summarised in Table 6.2. Giovanni Boschetti, for example, was maestro di cappella at the Hospital between 1620–1622. His third book of *Sacrae cantiones* printed by Soldi in 1620 was dedicated to the then commendatore Evangelista Tornioli. The volume contains motets for one to five voices with organ bass, all of which were functional within the liturgy.

Francesco Samaruco, a singer at the Hospital in 1623–1624, published his *Sacri affetti* with Soldi in 1626. This collection of sacred music includes pieces by several composers employed at various times at the Hospital though not necessarily at the time of the publication, including Frescobaldi; Cesare Zoilo, maestro di cappella 1610–1623; Vincenzo de Grandis, maestro di cappella 1604–05; and Gregorio Allegri who would become maestro di cappella briefly in 1628; and himself, Samaruco. The title, *Sacri affetti*, 'sacred affects', in itself is indicative of musical intent to move the affects or passions of the soul. At least

92 Soldi's career, printing business, circle of patrons and likely author of his dedications is the topic of ongoing research.

one of the pieces in Samaruco's collection does have an identifiable use within the Hospital that is attested to in documents, and that is his own setting of the Litany of the Madonna. As already noted, singing Litanies for the sick was an established tradition that was documented as part of the daily religious observance at the Hospital.

An even stranger reference to the Hospital is found in Agazzari's *Eucharisticum melos* (1625). In this print, the bass part contains a woodcut image of Veronica holding the veil on which the face of Christ was imprinted. The veil of Veronica was a relic of great importance to the Hospital. Innocent III was the first of many popes to process with it from the Vatican to the Hospital every year, and for a time in the fourteenth century the relic was actually housed in the church of Santo Spirito. In the jubilee year of 1625 it was displayed at St Peter's for pilgrims to venerate. Agazzari's motets are all on Eucharistic texts, so would also have been suitable for veneration of the Sacrament in the *Quarantore* celebrations that became popular in post-Tridentine Rome, and furthermore, align with the notion of the sacrament as medicine for the sick.

Table 6.2 Music printed by Soldi, associated with the Hospital by composer, dedicatee or content.

Composer	**Title**	**Date**	**Dedicatee**
Boschetti	Sacrae cantiones... liber tertius	1620	Evangelista Tornioli
Samaruco	Sacri affetti	1624	Carlo Madruzzo
Agazzari	Eucharisticum melos	1625	Blessed sacrament
Palestrina	Hymni totius anni... cum basso ad organum	1625	Giuseppe Anselmi
De Grandis	Sacrae cantiones	1621	Giuliano della Rovere
De Grandis	Salmi ad Vesperis	1624	Francesco Barberini

Sacred music accounts for 70% of Soldi's output (thirty-seven of his fifty-three prints), seven of which include dedications referencing the power of music. The reconciliation of Platonic teaching to Christian doctrine was a significant challenge to the intellectuals of the fifteenth and sixteenth centuries. Marsilio Ficino's commentaries on Plato, Plotinus, Porphyry and Iamblichus demonstrate the difficulties of explaining such problems as the descent and ascent of the soul. Christian Neo-Platonism aligned to some extent with the Tridentine rhetoric that positioned the reform of the Church as bringing back a purer form of liturgy that reached back to a period closer to that of the Church Fathers. Soldi's dedications reference a broad range of these complex philosophical points either directly or indirectly by mentioning an ancient author's name, but offering no obvious didactic explanation, allowing the reader (most obviously the dedicatee, but no doubt owners of the books) to draw their own conclusions. These prints seem to take on the doctrinal challenge of Christian Neo-Platonism by presenting music that promotes Tridentine Christian doctrine with its purer liturgy bolstered by ancient authorities, while at the same time using other classical references to the likes of Plato and Pythagoras to endorse its power to bring soul and body into harmony and to promote good morals.

Even if the dedications and contents of Soldi's prints indicate their suitability and functionality in the Hospital, they are not proof that they were actually used. It might be inferred that those items dedicated to one or other of the commendatori would be put to use, but they may equally have ended up in their private libraries. Fortunately, there is solid evidence that at least some of Soldi's prints were in the music library of the church of Santo Spirito. There is a record of payment to Soldi in September 1622 for two books for the choir, though sadly the books are not identified.[93]

Further, a rare survival in the British Library of all nine partbooks of Annibale Orgas's *Sacrarum cantionem* printed by Soldi, complete with their paper covers, provides unassailable proof that this copy belonged to Santo Spirito. On each cover, the title has been written along with the double cross symbol of Santo Spirito, and, in the upper right-hand corner, a number that indicated its position in the Santo Spirito library, similar to those on some of the manuscript items.[94] As it was printed it 1619, it may have been one of the books paid for in 1622. There is no named dedicatee of this volume. Instead, it is dedicated to the Holy Nativity, thus we have to assume that Soldi himself, or someone within the Hospital, wrote the dedication that refers to the angelic choirs that announced the birth of Jesus and the harmonious responses of the shepherds.

The contents include motets for up to eight voices in two choirs. Some of the texts such as 'Tantum ergo' and 'Benedicam dominum' appear regularly in various liturgical contexts, while others are more explicitly associated with Christmas. While the text content of the book is eminently usable within the

93 '... a luca Antonio Soldi libraio per due libri sciolti haverti da lui il coro': ASR OSS 2820, *Libro mastro giornali*, 1622. There is a cross reference to mandato 1264, but the *Copie di mandati* for 1622 are no longer extant.

94 L-Bl, D.118. This hand is evident in I-Rsc G.MS.796–805. For the organisation of the music library of Santo Spirito see Laurence Feininger, 'Membra disjecta riperta', *Acta Societatis Universalis Sanctae Ceciliae*, 3 (1964); Clemente Lunelli, *I manoscritti polifonici nella Biblioteca L. Feininger* (Trento, 1994). This is the first piece of surviving seventeenth-century printed music from the Santo Spirito music library that can be securely identified. One other item, an incomplete copy of De Grandis, *Salmi ad Vesperas*, 1624, that survives in the Biblioteca del Conservatorio di Santa Cecilia may possibly have been from Santo Spirito. Its five surviving partbooks have old paper covers similar to the British Library partbooks, and the cantus primus part bears a library number.

liturgy, from a practical point of view, Soldi had to explain the disposition of the various parts across the partbooks in the contents list so that the user could locate some of the parts. For example, the additional voice part in the five-part motets is noted in the contents by 'doi soprani' or 'doi tenori' so that the user can find the correct partbook, while the music for the four-part 'Jesu rex mirabilis', for example, is noted as located in the partbooks for choir two. Whether the contents listing suggests Soldi's experience as a practising musician or is simply an expedient for simplifying the printing process is impossible to tell. One thing is certain, and that is that in 1619, Santo Spirito employed the forces required for singing this music.

Soldi and Tridentine reform

Soldi issued a significant quantity of music within a relatively short space of time between 1618 and his death in 1627. The proportion of music within his output that points to a use within the broad environment of the hospital and church of Santo Spirito raises questions about Soldi himself. Facts about Soldi's life are scanty and there are anomalies in the biographies. The record of his death in the Hospital of Santo Spirito notes that he was seventy years old and from Pisa, thus born around 1557–1558, and a 'musico' at Santo Spirito.[95] The term 'musico' is ambiguous as it sets him apart from the singers, usually referred to as 'cantore', but implies a practising, rather than theoretical musician. However, his name does not appear in the payment records for salaried musicians. In the dedication of a 1609 print of Cifra's third book of motets that he collected and edited for the Robletti press, Soldi states that Cifra was his teacher. Cifra, born in 1584, was a choir boy until 1596, so Soldi could not have been his pupil until around 1600. He would thus have been some twenty-five years older than his teacher, and studying music in his fifties. Cifra died just two years after Soldi in 1629.[96]

The preponderance of Cifra's music within Soldi's output may be explained as a kind of homage from Soldi to his teacher. It also invites the question as to whether Cifra had a personal connection to the Hospital, perhaps as a member

[95] 'Luc'Antonio Soldi del quondam Pietro di Pisa, stampatore et musico in S. Spirito morì alli nobili del nostro ospedale di età 70 anni incirca doppo havere ricevuti li santissimi sacramenti di Santa Chiesa, fu sepolto sotto la nostra chiesa di S. Spirito': I-Rvic, Santo Spirito in Saxia, *Morti*, (parish record of deaths).

[96] Saverio Franchi and Orietta Sartori, 'Luca Antonio Soldi', in *Dizionario biografico degli Italiani*, vol. 93, 2018, https://www.treccani.it/enciclopedia/luca-antonio-soldi_%28Dizionario-Biografico%29/; Rostirolla, *Musica e musicisti nella Basilica di San Pietro*, Appendice VII, Dizionario dei cantori, pp. 342–343; Jerome Roche, 'Antonio Cifra', *Grove Music Online*, https://doi-org.libezproxy.open.ac.uk/10.1093/gmo/9781561592630.article.05775.

of the lay Confraternity. It is highly likely that Cifra and Frescobaldi knew each other as they had a common friend in Lelio Guidiccioni who owned portraits of both composers.[97] More importantly though, Cifra's style conformed to the requirements of Tridentine reforms: polyphony that allowed for intelligible texts, and that was not overly complicated nor overloaded with chromaticism or dissonance. A manuscript copy of Cifra Masses for four, five and six voices in a large choirbook format was gifted to the Hospital in 1636 by Vitale Bianchi. It contains four of the masses from Cifra's *Missarum liber secundus* printed by Soldi in 1621, and is further evidence that Cifra's music was used at the Hospital, almost certainly having been copied from that print.[98] A second choirbook of Palestrina motets was copied in 1625 by Paolo Troiano, the maestro di cappella that year, which suggests not only that manuscripts were still in use even though Soldi was printing the same kind of music at the same time, but also that it was this style of music that was needed.[99]

For all that Soldi's titlepages advertise his presence at the Hospital of Santo Spirito, there is little documentary trace of him there. The Hospital was a complex institution that by the mid-1620s housed over 2,800 people. It also owned a large number of domestic, agricultural and other properties. So far, I have been unable to find any record of rental agreements for any of the Hospital's many properties situated in streets close to the Hospital complex in the Borgo, or indeed, for any of their properties in other areas of Rome. This would suggest that his shop was indeed as the 1625 title page suggests, in the Hospital buildings. However, the *Stato temporale delle chiese di Roma* for 1625 doesn't mention him or a print shop as either generating income or requiring payment.[100]

There must have been a commercial or ideological reason for Soldi to set up his print shop at the time and location that he chose to – late in his life and in a place that was not a commercial centre. My guess at this stage is that as the Hospital apprenticed orphan boys to tradesmen once they reached a certain age, Soldi's print shop might have been an on-site training enterprise that also generated income for the Hospital from the sales. Boys from the orphanage could have learned the trade, thus enabling them to go on to support themselves when they left the Hospital in their early to mid-teens. The patchy quality of Soldi's prints might then be explained away as the work of apprentices. This scenario might also part-explain the preponderance of reprints in his output, as there would have been extant models for apprentices to copy.

97 Morelli, 'Un amico di Frescobaldi', p. 64.

98 D-Rp BH 6001. The date of the gift and donor are noted on the flyleaf of the book. Bianchi was a priest in the church who was paid for various roles, notably sub-sacristan, from the mid-1630s through the 1640s.

99 D-Rp BH 6007.

100 V-VCaav Misc.Arm VII / 77 *Stato temporale delle chiese di Roma fatto nel pontificato di Urbano VIII l'anno 1625.*

The majority of Soldi's prints would have had a use in the Hospital and its church, whether in the form of motets (for the adoration of the Eucharist, singing for the sick, or for the liturgy), hymns, psalms for Vespers or instrumental music for the hospital ward. What they have in common is that the music they contain conforms closely with Tridentine reforms. Concerns regarding correct liturgical practice that aligned with the reforms may well have been the reason for Soldi's choosing to print or reprint the music of so many composers from the Roman milieu, and especially those who had worked in either the Cappella Giulia or Cappella Pontificia at St Peter's, such as Palestrina, Soriano, Anerio and Agostini, and of course, Frescobaldi. The geographical proximity to St Peter's as well as the patronal and administrative ties to the papacy probably drove some anxiety for conformity in liturgical practices. In the intellectual climate of 1620s Rome, at least a façade of religious orthodoxy was essential, especially if the scientific activities of the physicians in the hospital were starting to undermine long-held beliefs.

A small group of Soldi prints also have connections to the Barberini papacy. Kapsberger's settings of Maffeo Barberini's *Poemata* in particular suggest a close link to Urban VIII, but he also printed two other volumes of music by Kapsberger. In the 1630s Frescobaldi was to join Kapsberger as part of the musical entourage of Cardinal Francesco Barberini, but as organist at St Peter's, he would have been known to the Barberini pope and his cardinal nephews before then. The connection is probably co-incidental but is indicative of intersecting spheres in the artistic and intellectual circles of 1620s Rome.

There is, of course, a gap between intellectual discourse about music and the actual day-to-day practice of working musicians. The oral and aural is lost, and notated music can only hint at what might have happened. The cluster of books, the location in which they were produced, the personalities involved are all perhaps indicative of big philosophical ideas on the one hand, but compliance with Church politics on the other. Soldi's volumes contain functional items that were usable within the context of the Hospital's liturgy, but simultaneously suggest that this music is able to improve the morals and spiritual health of the listener. We will probably never know the full story of Soldi's career. What does seem beyond doubt is that the man himself had a commitment to the cause of the Hospital and its mission to cure body and soul.

7

Stefano Vai: the 1644 Decree and Retrospective Reforms

Music therapy in the great wards of the Hospital reached across boundaries of status. The organist was the medium through which mere mortals, whether brothers of the Order or the sick poor, were enlivened by intangible intimations of the celestial. When it came to providing music in the church, it was a different matter, as the reformed liturgy had to be strictly observed. From the time of Urban VIII Barberini and throughout the seventeenth century, the Hospital of Santo Spirito, like all hospitals and churches in Rome, was subjected to the increasing scrutiny of Apostolic Visitations. Surviving documents indicate that conduct and procedures in various parts of the institution, from the dispensary to the church, were tightened.[1] This chapter will consider papal attempts at control in general, before evaluating a decree from the mid-seventeenth century and a backward-looking eighteenth-century iteration of it.

Spada's *Stato della Casa* written in 1660 makes multiple references to Apostolic Visitations, and to the ways in which the institution had made changes to comply with instructions issued after such visits.[2] The directives concerning the hospital were primarily targeted at ensuring that there were sufficient priests on hand to hear the confessions of patients, to teach them correct doctrine and to perform the last rites as and when necessary.[3] Beyond that, the behaviour of the personnel caring for the sick was to measure up to the standards of Christian charity set out in the Rule of the Order of Santo Spirito. On the actual practice of medicine or the conduct of physicians, there is comparatively little, and most of it concerns standards of hygiene and dietary rules.

Paolo Zacchia was employed by the Hospital in the decade prior to Spada's incumbency (1648–1659), and presumably had to ensure these standards were met. Zacchia had by that stage in his career already published a significant number of books, including those on observing a Lenten diet without damag-

1 There are multiple volumes of edicts and Bulls issued by various popes through the century, many of which remain in the Archivio Apostolico Vaticano in various collections, such as Misc. Arm IV–V, Misc. Arm VII.

2 The records of a number of these visits have survived in ASR-OSS 901, *Sacra visita, Atti diversi relazione 1592–1734.*

3 A list of parish churches who were to supply priests on a daily rota to the four hospitals of Rome can be found in V-CVaav Misc. Arm IV–V/9 fol.27.

ing one's health, and on 'hypochondriac diseases'.[4] The latter includes a chapter on the passions of the soul – a topic that remained important in medical practice. However, it was not just internal orders that controlled the activities of the Hospital. For the popes of the seventeenth century, the Hospital continued to be a means of demonstrating both political power and Christian charity, just as it had been for their medieval predecessors. The papacy was both a source of charitable funding and a regulatory body that ensured adherence to the Christian Rule that bound the members of the Order. There can be no doubt that the Church saw healthcare as part of its remit. Whether it was part of a broader political initiative to exert temporal power over the city and its population, or a response to the increasing population which inevitably brought with it higher levels of poverty and disease, by the seventeenth century, successive popes were making edicts about caring for the sick.

Urban VIII had ordered Apostolic Visitations to all the hospitals of Rome during 1624–1625, the observations of which were recorded in greater or lesser detail. The visit to S. Giacomo dei Spagnoli resulted in lengthy instructions, while visits to other institutions merited little more than an acknowledgement of how many beds they had and the number and nature of the personnel who attended the sick.[5] Following his visitations, Urban VIII issued a general order to be observed by the hospitals of Rome in 1627, that instructed all hospitals to keep a certain number of beds for the poor, and obliged them to accept such patients, even if they had scabies or other such diseases. An order such as this was likely to have had a practical purpose, aiming to reduce the number of poverty-stricken sick folk on the streets of a city that was a hub for travellers from all over Europe. The order required anyone finding a sick person out in the streets to find the portable beds which were located at specific points in each parish, which were listed, and to take that person to the nearest appropriate hospital. The list of hospitals indicated those that were managed by communities of other nationalities, such as the Spanish and Germans, and suggested that if the patient was a foreigner, they should be cared for by those who spoke their language.[6] Along with the list of locations of beds and hospitals was an indication that for those paying for the transport of a patient, reimbursement would be made for the cost of the carrier. The pragmatism which made a payment available speaks to the social hierarchy at which the edict was aimed. It was not an empty order, but one that had been thought out from a practical point of view.

4 *Il vitto quaresimale di Paulo Zacchia medico romano* (Rome, 1636); *De' mali hipochondriaci libri due di Paolo Zacchia medico romano* (Rome, 1639).

5 V-CVaav Misc. Arm VII /113, fols 107–186.

6 V-CVaav Misc. Arm IV-V/ 9, fol. 16. *Ordine generali da osservarsi nelli ospedali di Roma, per sovvenimento de'poveri ammalati*, Roma nella stamperia della Rev. Camera Apostolica 1627.

The general instruction issued by Urban VIII as a printed broadsheet, suitable to be displayed in public places, presumably stemmed from reviewing the records of the visits to all the hospitals. It is indicative of the authority of the Church over the jurisdiction of what today would be an entirely separate secular matter. An identical edict was issued by Urban VIII's successor in 1644, with the printer simply changing the names, stemma and date on the broadsheet print. Others followed at various times throughout the seventeenth century, with similar changes to the names and heraldic symbols. These general instructions were not the only indications of efforts on the part of the Church to control the activities of medical practitioners. Bulls and edicts addressed to physicians, barber-surgeons, apothecaries and midwives were issued with regularity from the mid-sixteenth century onwards, in attempts to control costs of medications, licensing of physicians and irregular practices of all sorts.[7]

By 1677, when Innocent XI issued his instructions to hospitals, the document suggested that he wanted a more unified approach to the care of the sick across all the hospitals of Rome. However, the most evident concern is for the religious care rather than the practical needs of treating, housing or transporting patients.[8] He instructed clerics to visit the sick regularly, to hear their confessions, teach them Christian doctrine and to find out their condition from doctors in order to assess whether to offer them the sacraments of the dying. While care of the soul had always been a part of the hospital regimen, there seems to have been a shift towards making it overt, public and politicised, no doubt as part of the post-Tridentine attempts to reclaim ground lost to Protestantism.

The church of Santo Spirito and its liturgical practices were evidently subject to considerable scrutiny in the 1640s, though it was probably not alone, given the number of printed edicts concerning the correct observation of Mass, feasts, processions and so on, that have survived. A telling comment is Spada's defensive point that the church had upheld the decrees of commendatore Stefano Vai, issued in 1644. During his eighteen years as commendatore of the Hospital of Santo Spirito, Vai oversaw restoration of the buildings, including the refurbishment and decoration of the sacristy; creating additional windows in the church to let in more light; introducing better iron beds to the hospital wards; and, as noted previously, renovating (and probably moving) the tribune organ.[9]

7 V-CVaav Misc. Arm IV–V/68 is an enormous collection of broadsheet edicts aimed at medical practitioners dating from the mid-sixteenth to the early eighteenth centuries.

8 V-CVaav Misc. Arm IV–V /9, fol. 28. 'Instruttione formata d'ordine della santità di N. S. PP Innocentio XI per li religiosi ripartiti alla visita quotidiana degl'infermi nelli spedali di Roma, acciocché, si come il fine, & oggetto di questo pio essercitio è il medesimo à tutti, così fra la diversità de sacri operarii sia uniforme il modo di praticarlo.'

9 For information on Vai's career, see Stefano Tomasetti, 'Stefano Vai', *Dizionario Biografico degli Italiani*, vol. 97 (2020); Giulio Negri, *Istoria degli scrittori Fiorentini* (Fer-

Vai was a zealous manager and the minute books of the Order document a number of decrees formulated during his tenure. According to Spada, many of these were issued in response to an Apostolic Visitation of 1643–1644.[10] If the papal inspector had found that the institution was not operating efficiently or according to either its own Rule or to the standards expected for all Catholic churches and institutions, the commendatore would have been responsible for ensuring that the necessary changes were made internally for the correct running of the institution. In 1644 Vai issued a decree on the correct observation of services in the Hospital and its collegiate church.[11] The need for such a decree probably stemmed from Urban VIII's edict concerning the revision of feast days, issued in September of 1642.[12] However, there is also plenty of evidence to suggest that undisciplined behaviour among priests, singers and even members of religious Orders in monasteries and convents was cause for concern, and had been, throughout the sixteenth century. Discipline was a focus of several of the canons and decrees of the Council of Trent. Even the papal choir was not exempt from criticism for poor discipline, neither was it the epitome of high standards of vocal performance of liturgical music.[13] Perhaps discipline at Santo Spirito too had become lax.

The 1644 decree

The decree of 1644 signals Vai's intentions to realign the hospital with the ideals of the incumbent papacy and post-Tridentine reforms, and perhaps also hints at how the revisions to the liturgy instigated during the reign of the Barberini pope, Urban VIII, notably Urban's revised breviary, were imposed on churches that did not conform. As Kurtzman has noted, the successive papal Bulls issued in 1657, 1687 and 1692 requiring all music performed in churches in Rome to use only prescribed texts from the breviary, missal or scriptures indicate that churches were by no means compliant in conforming to the new service

rara, 1722), p. 507; Franceso Trucchi (ed.), *Poesie Italiane inedite di dugento autori* (Prato, 1847), pp. 259–267; Moroni, 'Commendatore di S. Spirito', in *Dizionario di erudizione storico-ecclesiastica*, XV (Venice, 1842), p. 74.

10 ASR-OSS 47, Virgilio Spada, *Stato della Casa dell'Archiospedale di S. Spirito di Roma l'anno 1661.*

11 ASR-OSS 134: *Spedizioni e decreti, Rubricella atti, 1642–1645*, 'Decreta observanda in Ecclesia S. Spiritus circa Sacras Functiones', fols. 129r–133r.

12 A printed broadsheet suitable for display in churches survives in V-CVaav Misc. Arm IV–V/7, fol.48.

13 Marco Gozzi, 'Liturgical Music and Liturgical Experience in Early Modern Italy', in Daniele V. Filippi and Michael Noone (eds), *Listening to Early Modern Catholicism* (Leiden, 2017), pp. 55–78; Richard Sherr, 'Competence and Incompetence in the Papal Choir in the Age of Palestrina', *Early Music*, XXII:4 (1994), 606–630.

books.[14] Vai's decree raises the question as to whether it was issued because the Apostolic Visitation discovered that at Santo Spirito, an institution that was both physically, and in terms of patronal relationship, in the pope's backyard, the Tridentine service books were not being followed.[15] The references in the decree to both the *Breviarum Romanum* and the *Caeremoniale Episcoporum* are indicative of Vai's desire to reinforce the use of the still relatively new service books that emerged from the Tridentine reforms. The references to the *Breviarum* and *Caeremoniale* were probably deliberate, in order to satisfy the authorities of the correctness of the procedures the decree outlines. The decree may also have served to correlate and bring together information from older practices and to align them with the new service books, especially the revised list of feast days recently issued by Urban VIII. Sadly, the old liturgical books from the Santo Spirito library have yet to come to light, so comparison is not possible.

In itself, the document seems unremarkable, but the frequency with which the decree was copied in both the vernacular and in Latin and reissued by the successive leaders of the Hospital is indicative of its significance and validity over a long period of time. The numerous iterations perhaps also indicate continuing concerns over compliance with the revised liturgy. As it may also have wider relevance for comparison with other Roman institutions, the decree is given in full in Appendix B.

The decree, apparently agreed by the leading officials of the Order, first and foremost asserts the need for correct and devout observation of Mass and the Offices. Vai refers to the founder of the Order, Innocent III, as well as to the decrees of the Council of Trent and of Pope Urban VIII to reinforce the authority of his instructions. That Vai was concerned with correct procedures and behaviours is attested to elsewhere. He had a window opened up in a gallery of the commendatore's palazzo to provide a view over the hospital ward to make sure the patients were being cared for according to the Rule, which included both physical and spiritual care. According to Spada's history, when he was at the window the staff in the hospital continued their work with fear.[16] Another

14 Jeffrey Kurtzman, 'Motets, Vespers Antiphons and the Performance of the Post-Tridentine Liturgy in Italy', in E. Rodríguez-Garcìa and Daniele Filippi (eds), *Mapping the Motet in the Post-Tridentine era* (Abingdon, 2019), pp. 36–56, esp. p. 37. These edicts followed an Apostolic Visitation regarding music issued by Urban VIII with a number of reiterations thereafter as noted by Kurtzman. These edicts survive in V-CVaav Misc. Arm IV–V/7, fols 101–106.

15 Although Vai's decree predates the death of Urban VIII by a few months, he continued to serve under Innocent X whose policies were more conservative and cautious.

16 'Per tenere svegliati i serventi dell'Hospitale, fece fare un finestrino che risponde in una galleria dell'appartamento de commendatori; et essendosi in una testa del gran hospitale, lo domina tutto, e non potendo i serventi scorgere, quando il commendatore sia al finestrino, se segue, che continuamente stanno in timore': Spada, *Stato della casa*, 1660, ASR OSS 47, p. 595. The window still exists, hidden behind the bookshelves of the Biblioteca Lancisiana, and offers a commanding view of the entire length of the wards.

window from the commendatore's private chapel opened into the church so that he could observe and hear services, which similarly served to keep in fear those who sang, not knowing or seeing when he was there.[17]

From a musical point of view, read carefully, his instructions are such that they allow for quite a wide range of practice, thus the phrases 'sung or said' or 'with song' for example, are vague enough to encompass a variety of music. There is so little specific mention of musical style that one has to conclude that correct texts and observation of the details of liturgical rites were more important than the music. The decree is far from user-friendly and relies on a fair amount of knowledge on the part of the reader as to what was normal for various levels of solemnity for feast days. The instructions are vaguely grouped, so instructions for the Offices are mostly in one place, directions as to who should celebrate the various Masses on specific feast days in another.

After a preamble invoking precedent authority, specific instructions are given in order of the Offices, starting with instructions for Matins, then Lauds and so on, for ferial days and each of several named feast days (Christmas, Epiphany, Easter, Pentecost and so on). As Urban VIII had at that date only recently reduced the number of feast days to thirty-six in the Bull *Universa per orbem*, presumably some clarity was needed as to which were the correct feasts to be celebrated, and the nature of the solemnity of each.[18] This Bull initiated a further reduction in feast days following the cutback already imposed with the reformed liturgies issued in the Tridentine breviary (1568) and missal (1570). These feasts are outlined in a way that was presumably comprehensible within the daily life of the Hospital, though reading it today, without the experience of life there, it is hardly a straightforward set of instructions.

Following the preamble, Vai commences his guidelines for the Offices, with a statement that hints at the sound that punctuated and ordered the daily routine: the bell. Rung at sunrise, the bell signalled the start of Matins. Thereafter there is a brief description as to how the friars and chaplains were to enter the choir at the sound of a particular sequence of bells following the first Mass. The day starts with the prayer 'Aperi Domini os nostrum' ('Open Lord my mouth') that Vai notes was recently published in the 'daybook', that is, the revised breviary of Urban VIII, then Matins commences, led by the prior.[19] At this date, we know the prior was none other than Pierre Saulnier who was to publish his history and description of the Order five years later, in 1649. Vai's instruction for the Office is both revealing and vague. There is an assumption that the reader

17 '... serve anche per tenere in timore i salmeggianti non sapendo, ne vedendo quando siano ivi': Spada, *Stato della casa*, ASR-OSS 47, p. 124.

18 Universa per orbem, 13 Sept., 1642. *Catholic Encyclopedia*, The New Advent, CATHOLIC ENCYCLOPEDIA: Ecclesiastical Feasts (newadvent.org) (accessed 25/10/2021).

19 ASR OSS 134, *Spedizioni e decreti, Rubricella atti, 1642–1645*, fol.129r, Appendix B, pp. 210, 215.

knows the physical actions required and whether the Office should be recited or sung (presumably depending on the specific day).

> ... the Office should be begun, reciting or singing clearly and gently, and with the interpunction in the middle of the verses of Psalms and Canticles very recently restored in the Roman breviary; the appropriate order of standing, sitting, genuflecting, raising the head, and inclining it is to be observed.[20]

Perhaps the significant point here concerns the psalms and canticles. One of the reasons for the Tridentine reform of the breviary was to remove accretions, abuses and local variants in order to return the daily cycle of Offices to a more original form and thus to resemble more closely the practice of the early Christians, the rhetoric of restoration aligned with the Barberini political strategy of fashioning a triumphant Christian Rome on a par with its Imperial past. In this passage, Vai was essentially instructing the Order to follow the reformed breviary reissued by Urban VIII, and not older practices or institutional habits that did not conform to the Tridentine directives.

If the general instruction that Matins should be recited or sung clearly and gently is vague, a more specific instruction follows, indicating the feast days for which Matins should be sung: Christmas (and the two feast days following); Epiphany; from Holy Thursday through to two days after Easter; Ascension Day; Pentecost and the two following days; the Assumption; and All Saints. The question as to what singing actually meant is more problematic. It would be safe to assume at least plainchant, but as we shall see, it may have been falsobordone or even polyphony. If the preceding instruction is read knowing that Matins was sung only on specific feast days, the assumption would be that it was said on the remaining days.

Vai's instruction is further complicated by a paragraph that adds comment about when the Office of Matins is to be performed at certain times of the year. For certain feasts, not necessarily coinciding with the previous list, Matins is observed after Compline on the day before. Of these, the *triduo* of Holy Week and the second day of Pentecost coincide with the list of sung Matins, but the Feast of St Mark, the second Sunday after Epiphany and the whole Octave of Corpus Domini and the Commemoration of All Souls are identified as special exceptions but not necessarily sung.

The decree continues with the days on which Lauds is sung. The list starts with all feasts of precept, but then adds to that days when Matins has been sung. A directive about the use of three pluvials – a type of semi-circular cape, often richly decorated – obscures the clarity of the instruction.[21] It would seem to mean that Lauds is sung for all feasts of precept and the feasts on which Matins is sung. A further addition of feast days to the list already given for sung

20 ASR OSS 134, *Spedizioni e decreti, Rubricella atti, 1642–1645,* fol.129v, Appendix B, p. 210.

21 Surviving inventories in ASR-OSS 29 and ASR-OSS 237, indicate that the Hospital owned a significant number of pluvials that were kept in the sacristy.

Matins includes the feast of St Augustine (28 August) and of the consecration of the church (9 May), neither of which appear on Urban VIII's list of feast days, but would fall under the category of feast days special to the church or location.

The instructions for Prime that follow are ambiguous, not due to the lists of requirements, but to the way in which it is described.

> Prime is said with song when nocturnal Matins have also been sung, and also on Christmas Eve, for the solemnity of the martyrology, and on the feast of Holy Trinity, when the creed (*simbolo*) is also sung.[22]

The phrase 'Prime is said with song' (*Prima cum cantu dicitur*) seems to blur the distinction between singing and speaking and again raises the question as to what singing means in this context. The instruction does seem to connect sung Prime to sung Matins observed the night before the feast day. It is only in comparison with other material that the probable meaning of this passage emerges, as we shall see below. Terce is a little more straightforward in that this Office is to be sung for all feasts of precept, though the style of singing is not specified. The minor hours of Sext and Nones are said before or after the Conventual Mass, and Vai refers the reader to the rubrics of the missal for the prescriptions of these Offices.

As noted previously, Vespers was the most important of the Offices celebrated at the Hospital, but Vai's instructions do little to clarify his somewhat perplexing description of the Offices up to this point. They start with who is responsible for leading the Office, followed by directives about the number of pluvials to be worn. The first Vespers of major feasts warrant five pluvials while the second Vespers of those feasts, seven. Other feasts of precept warrant three pluvials and more ordinary feasts along with Sundays, only one. While apparently of little musical interest, the quantity of decorative clothing worn by the priests hints at the visual splendour of the services for major feasts – a splendour that was almost certainly matched by the music. Although there is nothing specific about the music, the comment that the friars in the choir should be forewarned about the tone of the versicles presumably refers to the need for them to know the correct psalm tone to be used in singing the Office. This comment also hints at the fluidity of the personnel involved.

> If the number of brothers in the choir is small, there may be added the vice-curate and the master of the school, and in greater feasts, beyond the four aforesaid, two from the chaplains of the hospital of the infirm who are not prevented by service at the time may be included. All of whom the ceremoniary should forewarn at the right moment about the tone [*tonus*] of the versicles, the Benedicamus and the other rites.[23]

22 ASR OSS 134, *Spedizioni e decreti, Rubricella atti, 1642–1645*, fol.130r, Appendix B, p. 211.

23 ASR OSS 134, *Spedizioni e decreti, Rubricella atti, 1642–1645*, fol.130v, Appendix B, pp. 211–212.

Having a full complement of singers for Vespers was clearly desirable. This comment aligns with the quantity of Vespers music from the musical archive that has survived, and further underlines the importance of the observation of this Office, noted in Chapter 5.

A further hint regarding musical activity is hidden in the instruction for Compline. This Office should be sung for feasts of precept, unless there were sung Litanies. The Litany of the Virgin was sung every Saturday evening and for the Marian feasts when they fell on a Sunday. In the latter case, the Litanies were followed by versicles and responses sung by the musicians. The pattern for the Litanies followed by versicles and responses is also to be followed for the celebration of the *Quarantore*.

Vai's instructions about the Offices seem rather like a rehearsing of the theoretically correct observation of each service, a presentation of what should be done. It is therefore hard to imagine it as a working document that was understandable in terms of day-to-day performance of the Offices. It is perhaps significant that it was issued just two years after a new edition of Guidetti's *Directorium chori* was published. The *Directorium chori* was first printed in 1582, commissioned by Gregory XIII to be used in conjunction with the revised breviary of 1568. Following Urban VIII's further revisions to the breviary, Florido de Silvestris revised it, and it was printed by Andrea Fei in 1642. Florido was subsequently employed at Santo Spirito for more than a decade from 1646, and was active as a collector and editor of sacred music. He had already had anthologies of sacred music printed by Fei, the contents of which demonstrate his alignment with composers active on the Roman circuit at the time, and whose music features in the musical archive of Santo Spirito.

The *Directorium chori* is addressed to the hebdomadary or maestro di cappella and is designed as a practical handbook outlining all the chants, antiphons, responses etc. required for each feast day. It essentially eliminated the need to memorise hundreds of chants in their entirety. Vai's decree follows a similar pattern in that it presents all the Offices in daily order, with their variants for ordinary days and feast days. Perhaps the lack of detail is because he assumed the availability of the *Directorium* to supply missing information. If one were to use Florido's edition of the *Directorium* as a companion to Vai's decree, it would enable a reimagining of the Offices with their associated chants; however, we probably do not know enough about actual performance practices to recreate what they really would have sounded like.[24]

Vai's instructions for the correct procedures for Mass are less concerned with the 'how' of procedure than with the 'who'. In particular, he notes which of the officers of the Order (prior, deacon, master of the school etc.) should carry out specific roles in celebrations as well as the various degrees of solemnity of

[24] For more on how chant was taught and performed, see Michele Chiaramida, *Manuale di canto fermo: Modelli e consuetudini nella prassi didattica tra XVI e XVIII secolo* (Lucca, 2020).

the celebration depending on the importance of the feast day. The more senior officers – the preceptor or commendatore, the prior and the school master – were all expected to conduct services at certain times. The parish priest too was identified as required to carry out certain duties, but with the proviso that he was also a professed brother. This last point is perhaps significant in that it indicates that some of the clergy in the church were not necessarily members of the Order. The instruction that Communion when celebrated by the preceptor should be only for the brothers, not the general congregation, similarly suggests a separation between the regular clergy and the Order.

It is in the context of these various instructions about personnel and solemnity of feasts that Vai provides an instruction regarding the organ and music more generally:

> The organs: in Solemn Masses, Vespers, Matins and Lauds and Litanies of the Blessed Virgin let the larger or the smaller be played, according to the custom of our church, except Sundays removed in the Caeremoniale Episcoporum.
>
> Let Gregorian chant and music be used in the holy Offices according to the discretion of the seasons from the prescribed ceremonial.[25]

The wording of this instruction reinforces the impression that a wide variety of music was acceptable so long as it conformed to the *Caeremoniale Episcoporum*. The *Caeremoniale* was issued in 1600 and was, like the revised breviary and missal, intended to align practices in churches in the post-Tridentine Catholic world. The book offers a glimpse into the physical actions of the celebration of Mass, its sensory experiences, whether visual, such as the appropriate ecclesiastical garments, or olfactory, indicating correct use of incense and of course sound, though explicit information about music is scarce. The Sundays on which organ music was excluded were those of Lent and Advent, but there were exceptions when major feast days fell during those periods.

Vai's description of processions follows on from this brief instruction about music. He does not stipulate specific feast days, but as noted previously, we know that there was a long-standing tradition of processions that included those during which unmarried girls who had been cared for by the Hospital were offered dowries in order to marry and leave the care of the institution. The Pentecost celebrations were the most elaborate and while the details of this ritual do not seem to originate in the Rule, the Rule concerning the observation of Pentecost is lengthy compared to many of its other instructions. Much of the detail concerns the solemn duties of various members of the Order and meetings of the council that took place on that feast day.

The instruction for the singers to be near the cross at the head of the procession is perhaps a pertinent one. Music led the procession, thus sound signalled to the surrounding area the approach of what must have been an

25 ASR OSS 134, *Spedizioni e decreti, Rubricella atti, 1642–1645*, fol.132v, Appendix B, pp. 213–214.

impressive sight. The hymn 'Veni Creator Spiritus' and the Psalm 'Emitte spiritum tuum' (Psalm 104), both items proper to that feast day, marked the start of the processions. These are the only musical items identified by Vai, and both are also specified in the Rule. Vai's directive simply confirms an existing practice. The musical sources however suggest that it was 'Veni Sancte Spiritus' that was sung by the choir, kneeling in front of the altar in the hospital during the Pentecost procession, probably reflecting changes instituted in the reformed missal.[26]

It is impossible to evaluate the immediate impact of Vai's decree, since it deals with procedures rather than specific details. As such, the scope for musical styles is not restricted so long as the rites are observed correctly, and behaviour is disciplined. Indeed, the surviving financial records for the 1640s support the impression that Vai accorded a certain importance to sung feasts and that at least some of these were celebrated with substantial musical embellishment. While Vai may have had to impose stricter control on music and on the Hospital more widely, there is no evidence that he cut back expenditure on music.

In 1644, the year of the decree, there was a regular choir of six voices, including the maestro di cappella, Antonio Carpani, plus the organist, Ercole Bernabei, who started working there in May.[27] Indeed, throughout the 1640s, six adult singing chaplains in addition to the maestro di cappella and organist were employed at the Hospital.

[28] Carpani was given an extra payment of 4 scudi in January of 1644 for providing music for Christmas. Given the singers' monthly salary was 3.40, 4 scudi would have paid for several musicians, probably singers and instrumentalists. Perhaps the music might have included his motet 'Exsultata filia Sion' for five voices and organ, a manuscript copy of which survives in the Biblioteca del Conservatorio di Santa Cecilia.[29] For Pentecost in 1644, Carpani was given 17 scudi, indicative of a substantial number of additional musicians for the processions. Manuscripts of music by Bernabei, Carpani and Benevoli survive in the musical archive. These include settings for eight voices of texts associated with Pentecost, such as 'Loquebantur variis linguis', as well as Magnificats and Vespers psalms. Although they may be copies of earlier works, it seems probable that they do in fact date from the 1640s. The organ in the hospital was also serviced and tuned as there is a payment of 8 scudi to Ennio Bonifatio in the

[26] I-Rsc G.MSS. 796–805; I-TrFeininger FP 121/1–10, etc.

[27] OSS 1943, *Copie di mandati,* 1645, items 340, 571 etc.

[28] In February 1640 these singers were Francesco Ronconi, Giovanni Filippo Torti, Pietro Paulo Valerano, Giovanni Battista Violino, Pietro Paulo Peschio, Simone Borgio. Antonio Carpano was maestro di cappella and Leonardo organist. This Leonardo was probably Leonardo Castellano who had been organist in 1638. ASR OSS 1938, *Copie di mandati,* 1640, items 161, 424.

[29] I-Rsc G.MS.0148.

records for 1644 that details that work, presumably done ahead of the Pentecost celebrations.[30]

The surviving manuscript scores provide ample evidence that polyphonic music was performed regularly. We can only guess at the extent of what might have been regarded as 'ordinary'. As noted in the previous chapter, the music printed by Soldi, dominated by music in the Palestrinian style, notably by Cifra, fulfilled a function within the Hospital as well as being a commercial venture. Given that during Vai's tenure, Carpano was paid for buying books of music, including a copy of Victoria's *Hymni totius anni* in 1641 and, in 1642, books by Vitali and Pacelli, it is probable that most Masses that demanded something more elaborate than plainchant continued to use the kind of music evident in the 1582 inventory, and music for larger forces was limited to major feast days.[31] If this were the case, music for four to six voices by Palestrina and the generation following him, for example Vincenzo de Grandis, Paolo Agostini and G. F. Anerio, would have remained in a prominent position, with larger eight-voice settings confined to Pentecost or Vespers on important feast days.

While in one sense, Vai's decree is useful as an indicator of the localised use of post-Tridentine service books, on the other, it is frustratingly vague. It is about correct procedure and discipline, not about music per se, thus one has to read between the lines to evaluate its musical content. The decree, however interpreted, was clearly the 'gold standard' for how the Offices and Masses should be observed in the church well beyond Vai's tenure as commendatore. The fact that Spada refers to this decree in his defence of music in the church and provides a copy of it indicates that it was still operational in 1660. While Spada's defence of music seems to have been on the grounds of finances, there were perhaps other issues brewing concerning lack of discipline, or perhaps more dangerously, for the continued use of music that did not conform to the reformed breviary and missal.

In the years after Spada, there must have been continuing problems, as further copies of the decree were made in the eighteenth century. The most important of these dating from the 1740s followed another inspection by the papal authorities that resulted in the dismissal of the professional musicians.

30 ASR OSS 1942, *Copie di mandati*, 1644, item 567.

31 ASR OSS 1939, *Copie di mandati*, 1641, item 585; ASR OSS 1940, *Copie di mandati*, 1642, item 908. Meloncelli has suggested that the Pacelli book was probably one of his collections of *Sacrae cantiones* published in Rome in 1597, 1599 and 1608, and the Vitali his *Sacrae cantiones sex vocibus* (Venice, 1625) or *Hymni Urbani VIII* (Rome, 1636). Raoul Meloncelli, 'Musica nell'arcispedale di Santo Spirito', *Il Veltro*, XLVI:1–4 (2002), 263–277.

Eighteenth-century 'copies'

A decree issued in the early 1740s appears to have been the final turn of the screw of papal scrutiny and control of liturgical practice at the Hospital, especially with regard to music. The outcome was a rubric, copied into a larger collection of documents dated 1745 on its cover that also includes Vai's decree, dated 1743 by the scribe, extracts from Spada's book and Campori's 1611 instructions, all of which indicate a period of change and tightening of control.[32] I will refer to this document by its callmark OSS 1298. The most complete and clear copy of the rubric survives in a small booklet entitled *Rubrica da osservarsi... nella chiesa collegiale e parochiale di Santo Spirito in Sassia di Roma copiata dal suo originale autentico che si conservava nella Sagrestia della medesima Chiesa dell'Anno 1644* (henceforth simply the Rubric).[33] The final page of the document is signed and dated 1752. The second part of the title suggests that it is a direct copy of Vai's decree, but this is not quite true. Beneath this title are the words 'And reduced to the method that is presently observed according to the reform made by the Apostolic Visitation of the year 1738'.[34] This is a crucial piece of information as will be seen below.

The information in the two versions of the Rubric matches, but the Italian wording is often slightly different, suggesting that there was a common Latin original, either Vai's original decree or a later copy of it, such as the one in OSS 1298. Although they are fundamentally the same document, there are some different annotations and details. The 1752 version is somewhat sparser, for example, leaving out asides about the donation of relics and abbreviating some of the text incipits that are spelled out in the OSS 1298.

The eighteenth-century scribes seem at pains to emphasise that the Rubric does not deviate from the decree of 1644 nor that of 1611, and, broadly speaking, it doesn't. As the 1611 decree gives only general instructions for decorum and devotion in the singing of Mass and the Offices, there are no specifics from which to deviate, and, at the level of matching feast days and instructions for Offices in the 1644 decree, there is no conflict.[35] What the Rubric does give is some remarkable detail not in Vai's original. It is from these details that specific elements of what by then were musical practices of the past come to light.

[32] ASR OSS 1298, *Scritture concernenti interessi della Chiesa collegiale di S. Spirito.*

[33] 'Rubric to be observed throughout the year for the feasts which happen in the venerable collegiate and parish church of S. Spirito in Sassia in Rome copied from its authentic original which has been kept in the sacristy of the same church since the year 1644.' The booklet is separate and unnumbered within a large busta of papers: ASR OSS 1299, *Chiesa di S. Spirito, Ordini e istruzioni.*

[34] 'E ridotta nel Metodo, che presentemente si osserva, secondo la Riforma fatta dalla Santa Visita nell' Anno 1738': ASR OSS 1299. The Apostolic Visitation actually started in December 1737, but the resulting reports and decrees started emerging in 1738.

[35] ASR OSS 1299, *Chiesa di S. Spirito, Ordini e istruzioni, Ordine per la chiesa, p.o di novembre 1611 da Mons. Campori.*

Whoever compiled the Rubric appears to have done all the cross-checking of ceremonial books that might have been required to fill in the gaps in Vai's instructions. In addition, Vai's confusing lists of feasts of various degrees of solemnity for each Office are collated into a more readable and user-friendly order. Thus the Rubric presents the instructions for each feast day in chronological order, starting from January, including the various different requirements depending on level of solemnity for each one, in order, through the year. It also includes the details of the physical aspects of ritual such as vestments and the use of incense and which are noted by Vai in relation to the type of feast with reference to ceremonials, thus relying on the reader's familiarity with them, rather than spelling out the requirements. Most importantly for this study, it also identifies a number of musical items either by text, or by text and composer, as well as noting aspects relevant to performance practice. For this reason, it is given in full in Appendix C.

Where Vai leaves chant or polyphony to the discretion of the time and *Caeremoniale Episcoporum,* the scribe of the Rubric notes Offices that use Gregorian chant (*canto gregoriano* or *canto fermo*), those which are sung in falsobordone, those which are sung in polyphony (*canto figurato*) and others which are said. Furthermore, it also stipulates where the mass is 'con risposte d'organo', that is, sung in alternatim with organ. These details clarify Vai's vague phrases and eliminate the need to consult other sources. The only musical detail that Vai does give, for the music to be sung at the start of processions to St Peter's during the celebration of Pentecost, is missing in the eighteenth-century Rubric.

Any attempt to correlate the date of the Rubric, the date of the document it purports to copy and the dates of the musical items to which it refers, which range from the 1550s to the turn of the eighteenth century, is useless in one sense, but raises questions about the target readers of the Rubric, and about the implications of the practices it describes. The reason it was written is given in the instruction for 1 January, the feast of the Holy Circumcision:

> Holy Circumcision: Low Matins; Te Deum, sung Lauds, Benedictus falsobordone. Mass and Vespers with organ. Here it is observed that since the Apostolic Visitation in 1737, the polyphony with organ has been reduced to Gregorian chant in the choir.[36]

Almost every subsequent entry indicates some element of the Office or Mass to be read, sung in falsobordone, or plainchant. The instruction for Mass for a significant number of feasts indicates it should be sung in alternatim with organ. For example, shortly after Epiphany, the feasts of St Antony Abbot and Saints Fabian and Sebastian simply say 'Organ response to the sung Mass without incense'. The general thrust of the Rubric is that the music was reduced to simple formats with limited items in polyphony. The additional information

[36] ASR OSS 1299, *Rubrica da osservarsi...*, fol. 3r. Appendix C p. 222.

about the use of incense is a further indicator of stripping away some of the extravagant embellishments used for many feast days.

The historical context of the Rubric

The reasons for the changes outlined in the Rubric can be explained by looking at the historical context. 1737 was something of a tumultuous year for the Hospital of Santo Spirito. Pietro de Carolis, who had been commendatore since 1729, resigned his position, just before the Apostolic Visitation made by Cardinal Leandro Porzia that started in December 1737. De Carolis had been profligate, living a princely lifestyle in the commendatore's palazzo, and no doubt left before he was publicly ousted. His successor Antonio Maria Pallavicini had to deal with the inspection instead.[37] Porzia, to reduce costs, made drastic changes to the institution, including the abolition of the procession of maidens at Pentecost, and the removal of the professional choir and the maestro di cappella, Don Francesco Bonanni. Bonanni had been in post for nearly twenty years, having succeeded Cannicciari when the latter took up the prestigious position of maestro di cappella at Santa Maria Maggiore in 1709. Porzia's view of the choir was that it was made up of mediocre subjects who promoted boredom rather than devotion.[38] Ultimately, Pallavicini had to deal with what became eleven years of continual visitations, but after the death of Clement XIII, and under Pope Benedict XIV, he managed to restore and rebuild elements of the Hospital following Porzia's draconian economising. The version of this rubric in OSS 1298 appears to date from Pallavicini's tenure, as does a copy of Vai's decree in the original Latin dated 1743 that presumably was the point of reference for it.[39] The 1752 copy is signed by his successor, Giovanni Ottavio Bufalini. The decree then was aimed at a body of chaplains not used to providing music to any great extent, as they had previously had professionals to do that job for them.

To put this into a wider historical context, Benedict XIV, born Prospero Lambertini, was a highly esteemed scholar, a supporter of both the arts and sciences, who on his election determined to see through the reforms instigated by the Council of Trent. The conclusion I draw from this is that Pallavicini was making an effort to rebuild liturgical-musical practice at Santo Spirito based

37 The history of the Apostolic Visitation and its impact on all aspects of the Hospital are given in Maura Piccialuti, *La Carità come metodo di governo: istituzioni caritative a Roma dal pontificato di Innocenzo XII a quello di Benedetto XIV* (Torino, 1994), chapter 4, especially pp. 107–129.

38 '... di mediocri soggetti che promuovevano più la noia che la divozione'. Cited in Piccialuti, *La Carità come metodo di governo*, p. 121.

39 ASR OSS 1298, *Chiesa di S. Spirito, Scritture concernenti interessi della Chiesa collegiale di S. Spirito*, pp. 21–28.

on models from a century or more earlier, sticking closely to the ceremonial of the period of post-Tridentine reform. This late Rubric offers a unique view of the reception history of the reforms as it is a step removed from Vai's initial document, written a century earlier, and impelled by the different motives of its own time. While superficially the eighteenth-century Rubric might appear to give us a better idea of the way in which music was used in the previous century than the vague documents that actually date from that period, such as Vai's decree, what it does better is demonstrate the development of post-Tridentine notions of appropriate music in a specific environment: perhaps not incidentally, one close to the papacy. More than a century after the event, this attempt to return to 'pure' post-Tridentine styles and practices may well be more idealistic and follow Tridentine reforms more closely than any actual practice of the late-sixteenth or early-seventeenth centuries ever did.

The suppression of the professional musical establishment at the Hospital forced the use of only the chaplain-singers who were members of the Order of Santo Spirito without the support of professional singers. The large polychoral musical settings with instrumental accompaniments that were a feature of celebrations of feast days in the seventeenth century were therefore no longer possible. The music, even for important feast days, had to be stripped back to settings for four to six voices either unaccompanied or with just organ. Only Pentecost is identified as having music for four choirs, and only four feasts are identified as having music for two choirs – Ascension, Assumption of the Virgin Mary, All Saints and Christmas. As the professional choir had been dismissed, presumably singers were hired just for these occasions and needed to know what to do. The absence of Vai's specific instruction for the music at the start of the Pentecost procession is explained by the abolition of the procession itself.

The Rubric allows a glimpse into the physical theatre of the religious observations of the Hospital as it outlines some details of visual elements and, for some of the feast days, also physical movement around the space of the church or surrounding area. It also mentions styles of singing more often than specific pieces of music. It is these that are perhaps more telling about the drastic changes made following Porzia's visit, especially when they are set in the context of named items or composers.

The instruction for the Feast of the Circumcision cited above is the first of many such cases. The very specific 'low Matins', the use of falsobordone rather than polyphony and Mass and Vespers with organ suggest it was a pretty low-key affair, potentially only needing a minimal number of celebrants who could sing both in alternatim with the organ, and in falsobordone. As Kendrick has pointed out, falsobordone was, and is, an improvisatory practice using a fixed pattern of consonant harmonisation of a melody, usually sung by an inner voice, with two simple cadential formulae at the half-verse and verse endings. Although evidence of notated falsobordone appeared around 1500, it was immensely popular in monastic Offices and used by more than just clerical or monastic singers.[40] Falsobordone is probably what Vai meant in the phrases 'with song is said' and 'gently reciting or singing'. It would be a logical way of describing the practice if one did not have a musical vocabulary to be more specific. This document is testament to the long survival of the practice and perhaps indicative that other oral practices such as *contrapunto alla mente* – a style of improvising counterpoint following specific fixed rules to create a harmonious result – also continued into the eighteenth century.[41]

Throughout the Rubric, falsobordone is connected to either the 'Gloria Patri' or to the 'Benedictus', usually contrasting with an instruction for sung Lauds or 'Te Deum'. The juxtaposition of falsobordone and singing suggests a contrast between the loosely improvised harmony of the former and a more formally composed setting of text in the latter. Lack of a choir seems to have been compensated for by increasing the use of the organ. The substantial role of the organist is indicated in parallel with notes about styles of singing. This too demonstrates the longevity of the old style of performance in alternatim and equally the necessity for improvisational skills in playing versetti. For Epiphany for example, the organist had to provide cadences for the falsobordone of the 'Gloria Patri' and responses to the verses of the 'Te Deum' for Matins, then responses to each verse of the 'Benedictus' which was also sung in falsobordone. The latter was to allow time for the altar to be incensed, so presumably relied on the skill of the organist to keep the music flowing until the liturgical actions were complete. The considerable number of available printed versetti for all sorts of common hymns, Magnificat versetti in various psalm tones and organ Masses would have provided an organist with limited improvisational skills, such as one of the brothers of the Order, with a sufficient repertory of items to fulfil these tasks.

The repertory: prescription and description

The Rubric identifies specific musical items for several of the important feast days. Some of these are no more than text incipits and could indicate falsobordone or plainchant just as easily as they might a polyphonic setting. However, a list of music can be extracted from the Rubric and matched with the printed and manuscript musical sources known to have been in the Santo Spirito music library.

40 Robert Kendrick, 'Orality and Sacred music in Early Modern Italy', in Stefano dall'Aglio, Brian Richardson and Massimo Rospocher (eds), *Voices and Texts in Early Modern Italian Society* (London and New York, 2017), pp. 229–240, esp. pp. 234–235. The written-out falsobordone 'Veni sancti spiritus' in I-Rsc G. MSS 796–805 and the various settings by Papini in D-Rp BH 6005 indicate that the style was well-established at S. Spirito at least as far back as the last quarter of the sixteenth century.

41 The literature on *contrapunto alla mente* is large. See Massimiliano Guido (ed.), *Studies in Historical Improvisation: From Cantare super Librum to Partimenti* (Abingdon, 2017) for a collection of essays by key scholars in the field.

The first mention of a specific text incipit is for the Purification of the Blessed Virgin Mary on 2 February, also known as Candlemas.

> Purification of the Blessed Virgin Mary: Matins is read. Te Deum and Lauds sung, Benedictus falsobordone, Terce is sung then the blessing of the candles at which time versetti are sung in plainchant in the choir, 'on the book' and one does the procession after the distribution [of the candles]. On the streets 'Responsum accepit Simeon' is sung, which is in the booklets. The procession finished, Mass is sung and Vespers with organ, low Compline, Litanies with organ, and Ave Regina.[42]

The detail here for the music sung on the streets 'Responsam accepit Simeon' and specifically where to find it – that is, in the 'libretti' – refers to a set of partbooks. This reference is crucial, and I will return to this source below.[43] The phrasing of this instruction seems to present the material as if to someone inexperienced or unfamiliar with the environment. Prior to this, the description of the musical styles suggests familiarity with common musical practices. Although the phrase 'ut in libro' used to describe the singing of versetti during the blessing of the candles ('nel qual tempo si cantano in coro li versetti in canto fermo, ut in libro') is sometimes used to suggest *contrapunto alla mente,* it is more likely to indicate plainchant sung from a book.

For the Feast of the Annunciation on 25 March, the Rubric not only gives instructions about style, but also about locations and times of observations of the Offices.

> Most Holy Annunciation: Benedictus falsobordone, after Terce Mass with organ; when finished return to say Sext and Nones and then the ferial Mass a cappella; when finished, one goes to sing another Mass at the oratorio of the brothers past the hospital; after which one returns to sing Vespers with organ at 20 hours.[44] Compline is also sung with organ; when finished, the sermon is said, then one sings the Litanies and Ave Regina.[45]

The Confraternity (as opposed to the brothers of the Order of Santo Spirito) had an oratorio that over its long history was located in various parts in the hospital precincts and outside of it. The oratorio moved as changes to the buildings, such as extensions to the hospital, convent and orphanage, happened over a period of time. Eventually, in 1744–1746, a new oratory was built. This building survives and is situated on the corner of Borgo S. Spirito, opposite the end of the Sistine ward, facing the River Tiber. Prior to the building of flood defences

42 ASR OSS 1299, *Rubrica da osservarsi...*, fol. 4r. Appendix C p. 222.

43 I-Rsc G.MSS 796–805.

44 Pre-Napoleonic Italy used a unique way of recording time, known as *Ore Italiane*, counting from sunset of the previous day. Conversions from *Ore Italiane* to modern time in this study are reliant on Michael Talbot, 'Ore Italiane: The Reckoning of the Time of Day in Pre-Napoleonic Italy', *Italian Studies*, 40 (1985), 51–62.

45 ASR OSS 1299, *Rubrica da osservarsi...* fol. 5r. Appendix C, p. 223.

which started in 1875, it was probably on the main route between Santo Spirito and the Castel Sant'Angelo.[46] The location described as 'past the hospital' confirms that it was to this new building that the procession moved. There is evidence of a longstanding relationship between the choir and the oratorio, as the rector of the Assumption (*rettore dell'assuntione*) was listed with the chaplains and singers in church for a substantial period in the early seventeenth century.[47]

Holy Week

As might be expected, the instructions for Holy week are particularly detailed. Of these, the Rubric for Palm Sunday is one of the most comprehensive.

> Palm Sunday: Benedictus falsobordone, sung Terce then Mass. Before [the Mass] Asperges is sung in the usual way in the choir, then the blessing of the palms, and the choir comes singing in plainchant Hosanna. The Sanctus in polyphony, at the distribution of the palms Pueri Hebreorum by Victoria is sung; when finished, the deacon says Procedamus in Pace, the choir responds in Nomine Christi – Amen and the procession begins and the chaplains sing Turba multa which is in the booklets. Arriving at the door of the church two of the chaplains sing from inside while the others who are outside sing in polyphony Gloria Laus[48] and those who are inside sing in plainchant the verses that are in the ritual, and they sing in alternatim until the sub-deacon strikes the door of the church with the rod of the cross, the door opens and Ingrediente Domino is sung. The procession ended, the introit begins Domine P[ater] then Kyrie Eleison 'alla Palestrina' after the Epistle, its gradual, Tract and versetti in plainchant, then the Passion by three canons and the responds of the crowd in 4 voices in polyphony by Victoria. The Passion finished, the Credo is sung, the Offertory *Improperium* with Sanctus and the motet for 6 voices at the elevation. Agnus Dei as usual, post Communion.[49]

The musical items, instructions and accompanying actions for Palm Sunday given in this Rubric are summarised in Table 7.1.

46 For a history of the Confraternity and of the building, decline and rescue of this church, see *La Chiesa di S. Maria Annunziata in Borgo, L'Arciconfraternità di S. Spirito, l'opera pia di S. Michele Arcangelo*. A cura di M. B. (Rome, 1973). For the flood defences see Jeffrey Carlson, 'The Past, Present and Future of Flood Control in Rome', *Engineering Rome*, http://engineeringrome.org/the-past-present-and-future-of-flood-control-in-rome/.

47 In 1610 and for many years thereafter, for example, this post was occupied by Giovanni Andrea Condelli, ASR OSS 1913, *Copie di Mandati*, 1610.

48 The hymn 'Gloria, laus et honor' which has a response between each verse.

49 ASR OSS 1299, *Rubrica da osservarsi*... fols 5r–5v, Appendix C, p. 223.

Table 7.1 Musical items and instructions for Palm Sunday.

Item	Musical instruction	Action
Asperges me	In the usual way	
Hosanna	Canto fermo (plainchant)	Choir enters
Sanctus	Canto figurato (polyphony)	
Pueri hebreorum	By Victoria in 4 voices	Distribution of palms
In nomine patri	Choir responds	
Turba multa	5 voices in the 'libretti'	Procession begins
Gloria laus	2 chaplains sing plainchant the verses in the ritual inside the door in alternatim with 2 outside in polyphony	Procession arrives at church door
Ingrediente Domino	Sung (si canta)	Subdeacon opens the door, procession ends
Introit Domine	(Domine ne longe facius / Domine pater et deus?)	
Kyrie eleison	'alla Palestrina'	
Epistle		
gradual, Tract and versetti	Plainchant	
Passion	3 canons responding to turba of 4 in polyphony by Victoria	
Credo, Offertory with Sanctus		
Motet for elevation	For 6 voices	
Agnus dei	As usual	
Post communio	As usual	

The pieces by Victoria identified in this instruction almost certainly refer to printed items. They are absent from Rostirolla's list of music manuscripts once owned by Santo Spirito but the description of the Passion as 'in four voices in polyphony' matches the settings in Victoria's *Officium Hebdomadae Sanctae* (Gardano, 1585) which includes two Passion settings (St Matthew and St John).[50] The St Matthew Passion is proper to Palm Sunday and the St John

[50] Giancarlo Rostirolla, 'L'Archivio musicale della chiesa annessa all'ospedale di Santo Spirito', *Il Veltro* XLVI:1–4 (2002), 279–343.

proper to Good Friday. We know that Victoria's music had considerable longevity in Rome as it was heard by Mendelssohn in the Sistine chapel on Good Friday 1831. In addition, the antiphon 'Pueri Hebreorum' is the first item in the same collection. Further evidence that supports the conclusion that it is Victoria's *Officium* that is intended for use in this celebration is an instruction for Holy Wednesday that notes that the responses of the second and third nocturnes are sung 'in the book by Victoria'. These items too are also included in the 1585 volume.

The Kyrie is identified as 'alla Palestrina', that is, in the style of Palestrina. There was ample material by Palestrina and his followers available in the Santo Spirito library. The 1582 inventory and nineteenth-century list previously discussed in Chapter 4 provide evidence that the Hospital owned a number of sixteenth-century prints and copies of prints.[51] Those volumes were predominantly publications by composers such as Morales, de Kerle, Ortiz and Palestrina and includes Palestrina's first three books of masses (1554, 1567 and 1570) as well as Victoria's *Officium Hebdomadae Sanctae*. It seems highly likely therefore that a Palestrina Mass would have been used. Only the Kyrie is specified, but is it possible to assume that the rest of the same Mass setting was followed for the Credo, Sanctus and so on? As books are mentioned in the Rubric, an affirmative answer to this question is justified on the grounds that singers would be using books and not singing from memory. The fewer books required, the easier the transition from one item to another and the required processional movement of the choir. Although the Regensburg choirbooks contain a number of Palestrina Mass settings, and Feininger identified a further eight-voice Missa 'Iste confessor', now a disputed work, it seems just as likely, if not more so, that whatever Mass was chosen, it was from a printed collection.[52]

Copies of Palestrina's first two books of Masses bearing an inscription indicating that they were the gift of Pompeo Cannicciari ('Pompeus Canniciarius donavit') are now in the library of the Conservatorio di Santa Cecilia in Rome along with a substantial number of manuscripts from the Santo Spirito archive.[53] Cannicciari was maestro di cappella of S. Spirito between 1694–1709

51 ASR OSS 29, fols 27–28; see also Patrizia Melella, 'Vita musicale e arte organaria a Santo Spirito in Sassia nel cinquecento: note e documenti', in Bianca Maria Antolini, Arnaldo Morelli and Vera Vita Spagnuolo, *La Musica a Roma attraverso le fonti d'archivio: Atti del convegno internazionale, Roma, 4–7 giugno 1992* (Lucca, 1994), pp. 507–519, esp. p. 518; Rostirolla, 'L'Archivio musicale', pp. 287–88; Lorenzo Feininger, 'Membra disjecta conjuncta', *Acta Societatis Universalis Sanctae Ceciliae*, 4 (1966), 31–32.

52 A further Missa 'Iste confessor' (I-TRfeininger FP 9/1–10) includes an Agnus dei that is by Palestrina, but the authorship of the rest of it is disputed. See Lorenzo Feininger, 'Membra disjecta riperta', *Acta Societatis Universalis Sanctae Ceciliae*, 3 (1964); Clemente Lunelli, *I manoscritti polifonici della Biblioteca musicale L. Feininger* (Trento, 1994), p. 116.

53 The inscription does not say who the books were given to, but Feininger and Rostirolla assume Santo Spirito.

before moving to Santa Maria Maggiore and, in addition to his prolific compositions, owned a large collection of music books.[54] For the purposes of reimagining the celebration described in the Rubric, the Palestrina Masses in these books are a good fit.

The other named items in the Rubric for Palm Sunday, that is the 'Turba multa', 'Gloria Laus' and 'Ingrediente Domino' can also be traced, thanks to the work of Feininger and Rostirolla, to the same set of partbooks that contains 'Responsam accepit Simeon' noted above, now in the Biblioteca del Conservatorio di Santa Cecilia.[55] These partbooks form two collections of thirty-two and thirty-six motets respectively, for use in processions. The contents of the two collections are largely the same, and the items follow in the exact order in which they are described in this Rubric.[56] The words 'In Domenica palmarum' appear at the top of the pages on which 'Turba multa' is written in each partbook. On the following page 'Gloria Laus' is laid out so that the texts of the verses are given below the polyphonic setting, each line starting with an enlarged capital letter. This would facilitate the alternating chant and polyphony described in the Rubric. In the cantus partbook, a pencilled attribution to Palestrina is given for this item. Feininger asserts that this attribution is incorrect, and the music is by Cannicciari.[57] 'Ingrediente Domino' follows, exactly as per the Rubric. The introit described as beginning 'Domine' may well be 'Domine pater et deus' by Palestrina, also in this motet collection.

Both motet collections contain music in four and five voices dating primarily from the late sixteenth century by Palestrina, Lassus, Felice Anerio and similar composers, plus some anonymous pieces. The contents of the books appear to have been collated at two different periods.[58] The first half, a miscellany of twenty-six motets of the late sixteenth and very early seventeenth centuries is largely in one scribal hand characterised by rounded upright letters. Inside the cover of the altus part of the first collection (G.MSS 796–800) is a list of contents in the same hand. The second part of the book, that is the items that match the Rubric, are not listed. These are in a different hand, a more elegant cursive style of text and flowing musical notation. The pages are also less

[54] Maria Caraci, 'Cannicciari, Pompeo', https://www.treccani.it/enciclopedia/pompeo-cannicciari_%28Dizionario-Biografico%29/.

[55] I-Rsc MSS. G.796-805.

[56] Items 12, 16, 18, 27 and 28 in the collection of thirty-six motets are the only items that are either different or additional.

[57] Rostirolla follows Feininger in this attribution. 'L'Archivio musicale' items 66–68 Cannicciari in 32 Motets for Processions, I-Rsc G.MSS.796–805. All three are for four voices. Feininger, 'Membra disjecta conjuncta', pp. 12–16.

[58] O' Regan suggests that the collection was compiled around 1600, and has identified within it five motets from Palestrina's printed Offertory collection of 1592. Noel O'Regan, 'Palestrina's Mid-life Compositional Summary: The Three Motet Books of 1569–75', in Esperanza Rodrìguez-Garcìa and Daniele V. Fillippi (eds), *Mapping the Motet in the Post-Tridentine Era* (Abingdon, 2019), pp. 102–122, esp. p. 114.

damaged by ink, suggesting that they may be more recent, though there are no visible watermarks that might give a clue as to the date of copying. The bindings are a commonly used type of cream parchment that are attached to the old paper covers. It is only where the two covers have come apart, notably in the altus part, that the old table of contents is visible. In one of the parts of the second collection, where the two papers of the cover have separated, the double cross symbol of the Order of Santo Spirito is visible, confirming indisputably the provenance of the collection. Feininger noted that the binding included 'tongues' of paper to which additional pages could be attached, thus enabling the collection to be expanded after the date of binding.[59]

The second set of partbooks (G.MSS 801–805) includes a further setting of 'Turba multa' and 'Ingrediente Domino', both anonymous, placed before 'Responsam accepit Simeon'. This music has the appearance of being hastily written – a rather scruffy, scratchy, sloping music notation and text that is quite a contrast to the rest of the book. In one sense, the composer is unimportant, as it is the alignment of the musical source with the Rubric that is striking. The detail of this Rubric identifying the uses of some specific processional motets goes some way to filling the gap noted by O'Regan: that we don't know exactly when these motets were sung in processions.[60]

The only remaining musical item identified in the Rubric is the motet in six voices for the elevation. Given the music identified up to this point, it seems highly likely that the six-voice 'O Domine Jesu Criste' from Victoria's *Officium hebdomadae Sanctae* would fit the description. A summary of the music now identified is given in Table 7.2.

Table 7.2 Reconstruction of printed and manuscript musical items for Palm Sunday.

Item	**Musical instruction**	**Musical reconstruction**
Asperges me	In the usual way	
Hosanna	Canto fermo (plainchant)	Plainchant
Sanctus	Canto figurato (polyphony)	Palestrina *Liber primus / secundus / tertius*
Pueri hebreorum	By Victoria in 4 voices	Victoria *Officium hebdomadae sanctae*
In nomine patri	Choir responds	
Turba multa	5 voices in the 'libretti'	Palestrina / Cannicciari

59 Feininger, 'Membra disjecta conjuncta', p. 12.

60 O'Regan, 'Palestrina's Mid-life Compositional Summary', pp. 102–122, esp. pp. 114–115.

Gloria laus	2 chaplains sing plainchant the verses in the ritual inside the door in alternatim with 2 outside in polyphony	Palestrina / Cannicciari
Ingrediente Domino	Sung (si canta)	Palestrina / Cannicciari
Introit Domine	Domine pater et deus	Palestrina
Kyrie eleison	'alla Palestrina'	Palestrina *Liber primus / secundus / tertius*
Epistle		
gradual, Tract and versetti	plainchant	Plainchant
Passion	3 canons responding to turba of 4 in polyphony by Victoria	Victoria *Officium hebdomadae sanctae*
Credo, Offertory with Sanctus		Palestrina? *Liber primus / secundus / tertius*
Motet for elevation	For 6 voices	Victoria 'O Domine Jesu Criste' *Officium hebdomadae sanctae*
Agnus dei	As usual	Palestrina? *Liber primus / secundus / tertius*
Post communio	As usual	

For the days following Palm Sunday, the Rubric gives a fair amount of detail for the various Offices and Masses, although the scribe does get somewhat muddled in places. For Tuesday, a Passion, presumably for three voices, should be sung by three chaplains of the first choir. Holy Wednesday required another Passion in three voices, this time sung by chaplains of the second choir. Solemn Matins for Holy Thursday is sung without organ. However, the passage that follows suggests that the choir probably had two sets of books to hand for Matins, one of which was Victoria's *Officium Hebdomadae Sanctae*: 'The first responses are sung in the booklets, the responses of the second and third nocturnes are sung from the book by Victoria, Benedictus and Miserere of the same'. The phrasing suggests that the first responses came from elsewhere, although Victoria's collection does contain them.

For the minor Offices of Maundy Thursday, the Rubric simply instructs that they are 'to be sung as in the breviary', and the scribe concentrates on the details for Mass. This is a strange mix of instructions that simultaneously infers certain knowledge and provides quite specific detail. There is further reference to music 'in the libretti', this time to Palestrina's 'Cenatibus illis' in four voices, the first item in G.MSS. 796–805. Named items after that are intoned, chanted or recited while the altar is stripped. The evening Offices are given 'as yesterday' or 'as in the breviary'. Proceedings for Good Friday once again reference Victoria's *Officium Hebdomadae Sanctae*, this time the Passion of St John and 'Vere languores' for the adoration of the cross.

The Rubric for Holy Saturday describes the procession outside the church for the blessing of the candles and the return to the church for the Lumen Christi. Once all the candles are lit, there is a further procession to the font which is accompanied by the singing of 'Sicut cervus', and after the blessing of the font, the Litany is sung while returning to the choir. A setting of 'Sicut cervus' follows the music for Palm Sunday in G.MSS 796–800. The music is headed by the note 'In benedictione fontis', once again making the collection an exact match to the Rubric. Further chants that may have been sung at the blessing of the font can be traced back to an even earlier source, as the fifteenth-century *Liber annualium* contains several chants copied on two pages, the first of which is headed by the text 'ad processionem a fonte in tempore pascali' – to be sung in the procession to the font at Easter.[61] The first of these chants is 'Isti sunt agni novelli qui'. We therefore have both a pre-Tridentine and a post-Tridentine source for music for the celebration of this moment in the liturgical calendar in this specific location.

Following the blessing of the font, the Kyrie (and presumably the rest of the Mass) was sung a cappella in polyphony. The final part of the Rubric for this Mass reads like a 'step-by-step' set of instructions as though for singers unfamiliar with the sequence of events: 'The first Alleluia after the epistle the celebrant intones and then the choir responds, two tenors chant Confitemini and two sopranos chant Laudate, two basses Quoniam confirmata est'. The apportioning of voice order here is worth noting. It is the bass that starts the Alleluia, but there is an inference that he must first take Communion. The texts follow exactly that of the 1570 *Missale Romanum* up to 'Vespere autem Sabbati'.[62]

> After taking the sacrament, the bass intones Alleluia, the rest is sung in counterpoint, Laudate Dominum in falsobordone, finishing with a repeat of Alleluia as above, then the Celebrant intones Vespere autem Sabbati, the choir respond to that which follows.[63]

The implication is that the singers will know what follows, but in fact the scribe probably intends that it is the Magnificat that is sung in response, as that is the section that follows 'Vespere autem Sabbati' in the *Missale Romanum*. The sentence that follows would then make more sense: 'The Magnificat of Morales is sung and the organ responds for every verse'. A Magnificat by Morales had been in the library of the church since at least 1582, as noted in Chapter 4, so this part of the Rubric is again drawing on much older repertories.

61 ASR OSS 72, *Martirologio*.

62 *Missale Romanum* (Rome, 1570), p. 274.

63 ASR OSS 1299, *Rubrica da osservarsi…* fol. 6v, Appendix C, pp. 224–225.

Throughout the Rubric there are hints at the unwritten performance skills of the organist; for example, playing a little before the beginning of the Gloria when 'the organ is played somewhat and bells are rung'. As is so often the case, the organ provides appropriate music to accompany the physical actions of the ritual.[64]

After the detail of music given for Palm Sunday and through Holy Week, Easter itself has less detail.

> Solemn Matins with organ responses, Te Deum in polyphony, Lauds embellished the same as Vespers, in place of the Capitolo, Haec dies in polyphony a cappella, Prime and Terce sung and a solemn organ Mass in the fifth tone is played, then Sext and Nones in the choir. At 19 hours: Vespers is sung, in place of the hymn Haec dies is sung in 8 voices. Compline is sung because there is no longer the usual sermon.[65]

There are any number of settings of the 'Te Deum' in seventeenth-century printed collections of music and three that have been identified in the library of manuscripts from Santo Spirito. A 'Te Deum' by Festa was in the library from at least 1582 as noted in the inventory discussed in Chapter 4. 'Haec dies' too is a commonly set text. Both items appear in the collection of motets for processions, G. MSS. 796–805, that has already featured a great deal in this discussion. These settings are by Felice Anerio and Nanino for the 'Te Deum' and 'Haec dies' respectively. The eight-voice setting stipulated for Vespers, though, is harder to identify, as the surviving settings in manuscript are for three to five voices.

Aside from the information about specific music for Holy Week, one other feature stands out in these instructions, and that is the stipulation of specific psalm tones. On Holy Wednesday, the lesson is to be sung in the *tono prophetiae* and the epistle in the *tono epistolae*. In one respect this seems remarkably archaic, but on the other is perhaps indicative of the level of competence of the intended readers of the Rubric. In the same vein, the instruction for Easter notes that a solemn organ Mass in the fifth tone is to be played. The specificity of the psalm tone might suggest that by this date, familiarity with the psalm tones was waning as major-minor tonality was becoming the norm. An alternative possibility is that the author of the Rubric was aware of modal affect, and it was the affective nature of Tone 5, that is of joy, appropriate to the occasion, that was required. Tone 5, correlating to the Lydian mode, is perhaps not coincidentally associated with blood and the sanguine temperament according to humoral theory, and also to spring (and therefore rebirth).

64 ASR OSS 1299, *Rubrica da osservarsi...* Appendix C, p. 224.

65 ASR OSS 1299, *Rubrica da osservarsi...* fol. 7r, Appendix C, p. 225.

Pentecost and Corpus Domini

For Pentecost, the patronal feast day for the Hospital Order of Santo Spirito, the celebrations took place over several days and apparently with the possible participation of the pope. The Rubric notes that the procession of maidens, as in January, had been discontinued following the Apostolic Visitation of 1738. Music for the blessing of the font during the vigil of Pentecost and the accompanying procession is identified as the same as that for the same purpose on Holy Saturday, that is, 'Sicut cervus'. The anonymous setting headed 'In benedictione fontis' in the Santa Cecilia motet collection may well have been reused.

> Monday at an appropriate hour without onlookers and without music the Holy Sacrament is exposed. When the papal and general procession is finished one goes to the choir and says the Hours of low Prime, Terce and one sings Mass with the organ, a short one for being late, after which one returns to the choir and says Sext and Nones. Solemn Vespers for the feast day of the church, Compline and low Matins for the following day and then at the Ave Maria the Tantum ergo is sung in cantus firmus or polyphony with organ and the blessing is given to the people. At the procession of the maidens that goes to St Peter's on the Tuesday the musicians of St Peter's choose and take motets to sing in the street. On the return the Te Deum is sung as it is in the libretti. When they arrive in church, the organist plays the organ until all the dowries are given to the maidens and then one goes into the choir and says low Prime. Terce is sung, and after [Terce] the solemn Mass in four choirs. When it is finished, Sext is said, and Nones. Solemn Vespers in four choirs, Tantum ergo from the musicians of the first choir, Benediction and low Compline. Said on solemn Tuesday as for Monday.[66]

This instruction seems particularly pared down for what was probably the most important celebration at the institution, apart from Easter. The items for which text incipits are given are those in common use and are sung at regular points throughout the liturgical year – the 'Te Deum', 'Tantum ergo' and 'Ave Maria'. However, a setting of the 'Te Deum' by Felice Anerio and of 'Tantum ergo' (attributed by Feininger to Palestrina) are once again to be found in the Santa Cecilia collection of motets. If the music really had been stripped back to the bare essentials, a core repertory from a single source, or a handful of readily available sources, may well have been what the now musically untrained chaplain-singers relied on to provide the more elaborate services. It is worth noting that in the motet collection, the final item, the prayer 'Veni Sancte Spiritus', in some of the partbooks separated from the rest of the music by some blank pages, is written out in what is essentially falsobordone, followed in the cantus partbook by 'Emitte Spiritum tuum' in plainchant, with the instruction that that section is to be sung by two sopranos, and preceded by an additional aide memoire that it was to sung in the hospital in the Pentecost procession (See

66 ASR OSS 1299, *Rubrica da osservarsi…* fol. 9r, Appendix C, p. 226.

Example 5.1). As this text was so crucial to the Order of Santo Spirito, having it accessible to inexperienced chaplains along with a core repertory would make this motet collection of significant importance if used alongside the Rubric.

If the assumption of a small core repertory is correct, and the four and five-voice polyphony of the manuscript motet collection is what provided the nucleus of music for the most important feast days, it would explain the number of times the type of Mass for minor feast days is stipulated as 'Organ Mass' or 'Mass with organ'. Such a directive, presumably indicating that the celebrant would chant the Mass in alternatim with the organ, would eliminate the need for a choir. Even for the Pentecost celebration, the role of the organist seems to be more important. The explanations for having a short organ Mass rather than a high Mass suggests a considerable reduction of forces in comparison with what might have been done previously. The Mass for four choirs is restricted to one Mass on the Monday. It is also the organ that provides music until the dowries are distributed, perhaps indicative of a further change from elaborate choral or even polychoral music at this point in the celebration.

The details of the rubrics for Corpus Domini reinforce the importance of the sacrament as a holy medicine discussed above. The feast of Corpus Domini was instituted in the thirteenth century to celebrate the body of Christ in the sacrament. It was, and still is, marked by processions in which the sacrament is paraded along a route around the parish for the public to gaze at and worship. The 1752 Rubric appears to be somewhat muddled at this point.[67]

> Thursday Corpus Domini: When the papal procession from St Peter's is at St Giacomo Scossacavalli, *our church* starts to play then one enters in the choir and says Prime, Terce and low Sext, Nones is sung.
>
> The hymn is sung on Hymn of the Madonna = the Psalm Mirabilia is sung in the tone of the choir book, Mass with organ, when finished the parts of the Pange lingua are distributed and the procession begins. When the foot of the hospital is reached where there is an Altar placed, the blessing is given to the castle, after firing [the canons], one comes singing the Tantum ergo, and returns to the hospital, pausing at the altar and once more singing the Tantum ergo and with the versetto Panem de Coelo from the sopranos, and the blessing is given to the patients. From there one goes to the nuns and maidens and one does the same at the church of St Tecla. At the door of the conservatory the same blessing is given, the maidens first singing the Tantum ergo, one then returns to the church singing the Tantum ergo in the same way with the versetto from the sopranos as above, prayers are said and the blessing given, the Holy sacrament is exposed until the last Mass and then one retires.[68]

67 Variants in OSS 1298 are clearer, given in italics.

68 ASR OSS 1299, *Rubrica da osservarsi…* fol. 10r–10v, Appendix C, p. 227.

First, the arrival of the papal procession is noted along with the moment at which the organist needs to start playing, that is, when the procession reaches San Giacomo Scossacavalli.[69] It then gives the instructions for the lesser hours, before continuing with the description of elements of the Mass and then the procession. It is worth noting that the Mass is with organ, which might suggest an alternatim mass rather than one sung in polyphony, especially as the parts for the 'Pange lingua' are distributed afterwards for the procession to begin. Might these parts once again be the partbooks of G. MSS. 796–805 given that the set contains both the 'Pange lingua' and 'Tantum ergo'? The psalm 'Mirabilia' must mean 'Mirabilis facta est', verse 6 of Psalm 138.[70] The comment regarding the psalm tone 'in the tone of the choirbook' is somewhat puzzling, but I would suggest that it intended to send the reader to a known reference text, probably Giuditti's *Directorium chori*, that gives the chant incipits for all the major feast days. What it means by the hymn of the Madonna is less obvious, as it could be one of several Marian hymns, or indeed a Magnificat.

The description of the processional route also relies on the assumed knowledge of the reader. It clearly processed the length of the hospital towards the river, pausing at certain points, before returning through the hospital complex, including the orphanage and conservatory. The furthermost stopping point must have been the Castel S. Angelo, as it describes blessing the castle and the firing of the cannon in response before returning to the hospital. It is on the return to the hospital that the detail is given regarding blessing the patients and the singing of 'Tantum ergo' and 'Panem de coelo', the latter by the sopranos alone. As the Rubric does subsequently qualify the instruction stating that these two items are to be sung in plainchant after Matins, perhaps one might infer that during the main procession at least one of them would have been in polyphony. It seems likely that a similar practice to that described for Pentecost with the sopranos responding in chant with 'Emitte tuum' to the choral 'Veni Sancte spiritus' is what is required here. No polyphonic settings of 'Panem de coelo' have survived in the manuscript collection, but as noted previously, there are several of 'Tantum ergo'. The scribe could of course have used a remembered phrase to identify a motet such as 'Ego sum panis vivus', of which there are settings in printed sources, for example by Palestrina and G. F. Anerio, or 'Hic est panis de coelo' by Gombert.

At this point in the Rubric, there is no cross-reference to the observation of the *Quarantore* which is described in the document ahead of the individual feast days of the liturgical calendar. Conversely, the description of the *Quarantore* does reference Corpus Domini:

69 The church and piazza of San Giacomo Scossacavalli was located approximately 100 metres from the main entrance to the Church of Santo Spirito but destroyed in the 1930s when the new Via della Concilazione was built.

70 'Mirabilis facta est scientia tua ex me; confortata est, et non potero ad eam': 'Though the Lord is exalted, he looks kindly on the lowly; though lofty, he sees them from afar.'

> At the time of the forty-hours devotion one observes that which is noted below: After Terce, the conventual Mass of the saint or ferial [Mass] is sung by a canon or chaplain, according with the Office, then Sext is said and Nones is sung. When Nones is finished, the Organ Mass is sung, all as in the day of Corpus Domini. After Mass is ended, one returns to the choir and the parts for the Pange Lingua are distributed which is sung in the procession. Having returned to the church two of the chaplains come on foot to the High Altar and wait there until the Master of ceremonies advises, then the Litany of the Saints is sung.[71]

The observation of the forty hours of devotion to the sacrament, known as the *Quarantore,* was instituted in Milan in the late 1520s. By the seventeenth century it was an occasional celebration in any individual church, but in some cities, such as Rome, it was treated as a prayer cycle, moving from church to church throughout the liturgical year. During the *Quarantore,* the consecrated Host was placed in a monstrance that may have in addition been adorned with elaborate stage settings known as *apparati,* and exposed for forty hours (three days) as a reminder of the time Christ spent in the tomb following his crucifixion. The exposition of the sacrament was accompanied by music, sermons, extra Masses and opportunities for public devotion.[72] The celebrations of the *Quarantore* in some churches in the first half of the seventeenth century were extraordinarily elaborate and costly, with stage settings commissioned from the likes of Bernini.[73] There are some odd survivals of the *Quarantore* celebrations at Santo Spirito in the form of numbered lists of personnel, including singers, presumably noting the order for the procession for the *Quarantore* for 1619 and 1622–1624.[74]

The music cited in the Rubric for the *Quarantore,* 'the parts for the "Pange Lingua"' and the Litany of the Saints, is all material that saw frequent use. It is perhaps worth noting though that the Litany of the Saints was associated with praying for the sick, its pairing with the adoration of the sacrament places the celebration of the *Quarantore* at the nexus of medicine and religion that was so important in the context of the Hospital. Music supplied suitable adornment, perhaps in the form of Eucharistic motets such as 'O salutaris hostia' or 'Adoramus te Christe', to inspire and move the affects of the participants to piety, and to spiritual and therefore bodily health.

71 ASR OSS 1299, *Rubrica da osservarsi...* fol.2v, Appendix C, p. 221.

72 Marc S. Weill, 'The Devotion of the Forty Hours and Roman Baroque Illusions', *Journal of the Warburg and Courtauld Institutes,* 37 (1974), 218–48, esp. 218, 221.

73 Jennifer Tonkovitch, 'Two Studies for the Gesu and a "Quarantore" Design by Bernini', *Burlington Magazine,* 140 (1998), 34–37.

74 These are on separate pages in the same file of miscellaneous documents relating to the church of Santo Spirito that contains the Rubric, ASR OSS 1299 *Chiesa di S. Spirito, Ordini e istruzioni.*

The combination of assumed knowledge and precise detail expressed in the Rubric suggest that its target reader was one experienced in a range of liturgical matters, but lacking in skills in specific areas, notably music. If the reader had, alongside the Rubric, a small collection of liturgical music made up of tried and tested printed materials and manuscript collections collated for in-house use, he would have been able to follow correct procedure and provide adequate musical celebration that was both economical and within the grasp of singers with limited skills. It would also render obsolete a large library of sacred music amassed over the previous two centuries, and no doubt facilitated its dispersal. Given the preponderance of instructions for Offices to be sung in falsobordone, it seems possible that the style of Papini that was evidently prevalent in the years following the Tridentine reforms during the last quarter of the sixteenth century was the model for this renewed effort to impose a 'purer' form of liturgical music.

The Rubric does raise questions about why such a radical, perhaps even reactionary emphasis on practices and styles that were more than a century old was required. Spada's defence points to financial concerns about the cost of music, but no attempts were made to curb spending in the years that followed his tenure, so presumably money was not an immediate concern at that point. There must have been some serious infractions of post-Tridentine, probably post-Urban VIII directives that triggered Porzia's draconian cuts, but music was obviously reinstated only a few years later.

If the Rubric is read as a series of instructions that revise previous norms, it would explain why some elements are spelled out and others are left vague, with phrases such as 'as usual'. The absence of professional musicians who could have led the singing of liturgical music would have forced priests and chaplains who were not professionally trained to fulfil those musical duties. Roles and routines that had perhaps been unchanged for decades, traditions handed down from one maestro di cappella to another or through generations of priors and chaplains had to be relearned in the aftermath of the Apostolic Visitation.

Faced with communicating to priests and chaplains who were not musically trained how to ensure that all the necessary services were provided with appropriate music, the scribe of the Rubric may well have been reconstructing from memory the way in which things had been done during his time in order for it to be recorded, and perhaps adjusted, to what was practical under the new regime. There is perhaps a hint of the modern phenomenon of the employee who has been made redundant having to train his/her successors, telling them where to find key documents (or in this case music) and some important duties ('the procession on that day is done in this way'). One might also read into the Rubric an element of 'what it might have been like' set against a new norm for how to do things under the new restrictions, whether they were restrictions in terms of personnel or practice, or both.

Although it was essentially based on a seventeenth-century document, the rational presentation of liturgical calendar in an understandable order with references to specific music and liturgical books marks the 1752 Rubric out as fundamentally different from its seventeenth-century predecessor. While the rationalisation of Vai's complex decree is understandable in terms of making the rituals and procedures it describes workable in the 'modern' context of the middle decades of the eighteenth century, the specific references to musical styles and precise identification of composers and music render it inflexible and archaic.

The new norm of the 1740s appears to have been an attempt at 'purer than pure' attention to Tridentine reforms, while the older practices were more flexible, allowing for the kind of celebration that generated huge public interest and encouraged charitable donations to the institution. It perhaps also signals a tightening of the noose of control of the Church over liturgical matters within the day-to-day operation of the Hospital of Santo Spirito, separating religious observation from medical practice. Indeed, similar rules concerning the dispensary, the wetnurses, the women's conservatory and the hospital were issued following the Apostolic Visitation. From the vantage point of today, we can see it as the centuries-old partnership of religion and medicine being stretched, moving away from the humanist past towards the post-Cartesian future of Enlightenment. It is perhaps also symptomatic of the cultural environment that would ultimately shift music as an agent for moving the affects and therefore the soul towards a more defined therapy in the realm of mental health.

Epilogue

By the last quarter of the seventeenth century, various scientific and specifically medical academies were emerging in Rome. These were to a large extent operating beyond the reach of the established medical faculty of La Sapienza, turning away from old fashioned 'book-learning' to carry out experiments and real-life observations in the city's hospitals. The importance of practical teaching both in the form of dissection to understand anatomy and at the bedside with real patients was understood by these informal groups of physicians and scientists. The Hospital of Santo Spirito was at the heart of this new trend, led to a large extent by Giovanni Maria Lancisi.

Lancisi was appointed as a physician at Santo Spirito in 1676 before rising to high status positions at La Sapienza and as the pope's private physician. In 1714 Lancisi opened a library at the Hospital of Santo Spirito, followed shortly thereafter by the establishment of an academy for the study of medicine. Lancisi's library survived and provided the core of what has become the Biblioteca Lancisiana, which still houses some key documents from the early history of the Hospital such as manuscript volumes of Cirillo's letters, but it was Lancisi's mission to make medical learning and practice more scientific. The use of music as a curative was still acknowledged by the presence of an organist in the hospital through the eighteenth century, but of course it was the study of anatomy that gradually emerged into the foreground, leaving behind the more holistic elements of medical care.

Benedict XIV Lambertini, who was to become known as the pope of the Catholic Enlightenment, had worked with Lancisi for twenty years while he was the canon lawyer responsible for interrogating claims of miraculous healing, the *Promotor Fidei* (1708–1728). Lambertini's books and especially his critical examination of the process of saint-making, *De servorum Dei*, are deeply indebted to Lancisi. In them, the visionary nature of baroque religiosity is subjected to critical investigation; the imagination and its powers are separated from the new knowledge of the circulation and the nervous system; and the passions are shifted from their traditional Galenic seat in the heart, to the brain.[75] This period marks the beginning of study of the newly discovered nervous system and early awareness of what we now call psychosomatic conditions. While the provision of music to relieve the patients in the hospital wards continued unaffected by Benedict XIV's enlightened doctrinal policies, his moves to contain and reduce superstitious piety, extravagant celebration of saintly relics and above all, to emphasise adherence to post-Tridentine liturgy are all borne out in the 1752 Rubric.

Lancisi's efforts in creating both a library and an academy for the study of medicine were supported by the pope.[76] Thus, the apex of religious authority funded and protected the fledgling study of scientific medicine. Religious authority that post-Trent had unflinchingly imposed doctrines that punished thinkers such as Galileo and Bruno now supported the study of medicine. At this moment and in this place, reason and enlightenment were supported by religious authority.

However, it appears that at the same time, observation of correct liturgical practices was becoming more tightly controlled. The Apostolic Visitation of 1737 seems to mark a point of no return. Within the walls of a single institution, science was making advances while the doctrines of the Church were entrenched in the ways and practices of the past. While the institution continued to employ an organist to play in the hospital, the professional singers in the church were disbanded. About the former, we know virtually nothing except for the status of the person concerned as a minor employee on a par with the porter or concierge, but the benefits of music, however understood, continued. About the latter, we have ample documentation. Medicine moved on, rapidly developing with new discoveries, but in the same institution, religion reached back to old practices, and reinforced conservatism.

75 Fernando Vidal, 'Modernising the Miraculous Body in Prospero Lambertini's *De servorum Dei*', in Rebecca Messbarger, Christopher Johns and Philip Gavitt (eds), *Benedict XIV and the Enlightenment: Art, Science, and Spirituality* (Toronto, 2016), pp. 151–174.

76 Maria Conforti et al, 'Ospedali, accademie, esperimenti: Giovanni Maria Lancisi e l'ospedale di Santo Spirito in Sassia', *Medic*, 15:2 (2007), 31–38.

There are documents dating from well into the eighteenth century attesting to the faith placed in doctrine (not scripture) as a source of healing. A manuscript fascicle on the care of the sick in the Hospital archive which bears a pencilled date of 1759 is indicative of the continuing demand on those within the hospital to conform to religious requirements. It states that there must always be at least the same number of religious as doctors on duty, of which no less than eight have the duty of care of the souls of patients.[77] The same document includes a section on the sacrament of extreme unction which contains the phrase 'the sacrament of extreme unction as it was instituted by our Lord Jesus Christ not only as a celestial medicine for the soul but also as a salve for the body may be administered to those patients who are in danger of death.'[78] The notion that the sacrament is a celestial medicine for the soul as well as a salve for the body is a clear indication that for all the advances in medicine that, given the importance of the hospital as a leader in the medical field, were presumably practised in the wards, the role of the sacraments was still foregrounded.

By the final decades of the nineteenth century, the organ that had provided solace and relief to the patients in the great Sistine wards of the Hospital of Santo Spirito was deemed too church-like and was removed. Yet, when the Hospital of Santa Maria della Pietà came under the jurisdiction of the Hospital of Santo Spirito in the 1870s, music continued to be part of the care and treatment of the mentally ill patients recovering at that hospital. At that time, Stanislao Lucasi was the music master. He taught several of the inmates and brought them together to play in a band on Thursday afternoons and to give concerts on Sunday afternoons.[79] The ambiguous nature of music and what it does in the minds of listeners enabled its continuity in the medical context. Even though the benefits of music to mental health were not scientifically understood, music continued to be used in a variety of institutional contexts not just in Rome, but across Europe.[80]

77 'Il numero de religione dovrà essere non minore di medici de quali il più degno dovrà l'impiega e titolo di presidente, due saranno destinati per confessore e uno per sagrestano e otto per raccomandatori d'anime e un laico per il servizio…' ASR OSS 1296, *Chiesa di S. Spirito, Scritture varie*. This document is a later copy of the edict issued in 1751 concerning the conduct of activities in the hospital. It references Pope Pius VI (r. 1775–1799), indicating the continued observation of the earlier decree.

78 'il sagramento dell'estreme unzione come che istituito dal nostro signor Gesù Christo non solo come medicina celeste dell'Anima ma ancore per salve del corpo si deve amministrare a quelli'infermi che sono in pericolo di morire …' *Regolamenti per il padre Presidente e Cappellani*, ASR OSS 1296, *Chiesa di S. Spirito, Scritture varie*, separate unnumbered fascicle.

79 Pietro De Angelis, *Musica e musicisti nell'arcispedale di Santo Spirito in Saxia* (Rome, 1950), pp. 30–31.

80 See for example, Rosemary Golding, *Music and Moral Management in the Nineteenth-Century English Lunatic Asylum* (London, 2021).

While this study has demonstrated that in the Hospital of Santo Spirito, music was used as a therapy, broadly conceived, that drew on the deeply rooted collaboration of medicine and religion to prevent and cure ill health, there is much that we will never know. Just as today we don't question our ontology or make notes about it, we will never know the unwritten ways of knowing the world, the orally transmitted information, the practices learned by copying, by rote and by doing, all of which informed what music was used, and how. There are also unanswered questions as to the extent of musical training in the orphanage at the Hospital. We know of named individuals who appear sporadically in the records, but was music routinely used as a teaching resource? Was Soldi's enterprise a social rather than a musical and commercial one? If so, where did the funds come from that supported its establishment? It is unlikely we will ever know.

Music as part of religious practice in the Hospital can be more thoroughly investigated as the trail of evidence is considerable. This study has only shown the tip of the iceberg as far as the musical repertory is concerned. There are sufficient surviving musical sources to support detailed study of genres such as the motet; of institution-specific style; and of particular liturgical functions such as Marian devotions.[81] Given the range of documentary material and the surviving musical archive, a study of the use of motets in the Hospital of Santo Spirito would potentially provide useful insights into the way the genre was used in Rome. Much of the surviving music that carries a composer attribution suggests that Santo Spirito was very much part of the wider Roman musical environment. As such, it should be included in studies of the music of the period of the generations following Palestrina, alongside other major Roman institutions such as Santa Maria Maggiore and S. Giovanni Laterano. The close affiliation to the papacy, and exchanges of singers from the Cappella Giulia and Cappella Pontificia with Santo Spirito add to its importance in the wider field of Roman sacred music.

Sadly, the dispersion of the music manuscripts in five different libraries and the need for a significant amount of transcription is a barrier to easy analysis of the musical sources, of which over 500 survive. In addition, the materials are fragile, especially as many consist of single-page vocal parts not bound into partbooks. Although the collection of administrative documents in the Archivio di Stato is substantial, it too is increasingly fragile, and already some materials such as the large *libri mastri* that potentially contain important financial information are too damaged to be consulted. Regardless of the difficulties, the Hospital of Santo Spirito still has a story to tell that is relevant to the modern world.

As this study was being written, the world was gripped by the Covid-19 pandemic. Bizarre parallels with our early modern ancestors emerged. While ambulance sirens replaced plague bells as a sound-mark of the time, the ben-

[81] An article on the sixteenth-century repertory is in preparation.

efits of music have been widely recognised as the 'go to' resource for crossing physical boundaries and helping deal with both isolation and wider community issues.[82] As human beings we respond to music, but neuroscience and cognitive medicine still cannot fully explain why. Maybe the commendatore of the Hospital of Santo Spirito who had the vision to build an organ in the Sistine wards realised this, and had the resources to make it a practical reality for the patients. The holistic treatment of mind, body and soul practised in the Hospital of Santo Spirito perhaps had merits that should be revisited under the lens of modern science.

82 Videos that went viral on social media of residents of Siena and Rome singing from their balconies, and the use of song to get important messages across to communities are just two examples, http://www.bbc.com/travel/story/20200325-italys-inspiring-response-to-the-coronavirus; https://www.goodthingsguy.com/lifestyle/dont-panic-buy-sa-artists-join-forces-in-a-song-to-keep-our-nation-calm/.

Appendix A
Virgilio Spada, 'Discorso sopra la musica della Chiesa'

Source: Spada, *Stato della Casa dell'Archiospedale di Santo Spirito di Roma*, Chapter 5, Appendix N. ASR-OSS 47, pp. 229–240.

Scribal abbreviations have been silently expanded but the spelling, capitalisation and punctuation of the original are retained. The translation attempts to convey the meaning, rather than giving a literal rendering of the original. There is, therefore, punctuation in the translation that is absent or inferred in the original.

Discorso sopra la musica della Chiesa

li 11 Aprile 1660

La Chiesa di San Spirito, ordinata al servigio di questa casa hospitio d'Infermi, di Proietti, di Monache, di Zitelle, di Balie, di Frati e di Ministri per l'azienda di beni, fondamento temporale di tante opere pie, che si fanno, ha annessa la cura d'anime, quale è appoggiata ad uno di essi frati, e questo ha sotto di sé un sacerdote secolare con titolo di sotto curato, e la cura ascende a circa 2,000 anime.

Il vaso[1] della chiesa è grande competentemente, ma con una sola nave, e senza bracci di croce et oltre l'altare maggiore ha 9 cappelle eguali e bene ornate, in figura di semicircolo con porta laterale incontro ad una cappella, provvista abbondantemente la chiesa di suppellettili sacre preziose, ed ogn'altra cosa desiderabile, riposte in un bel vaso di sacristia, ornato anch'egli più che decentemente.

L'altare maggiore è conforme all'uso antico, posto in Isola fra il corpo di detta Chiesa, et il Choro con quattro pilastri e colonne, che sostengono una cuppoletta.

Non solo vi è il materiale del Choro ma vi è anche il formale, dovendo i frati in virtù delle loro regole fra le funzioni spirituali, a che sono astretti, recitare anche tutte le divine laudi in Choro ogni giorno, ma perché questa Casa si è

[1] The word 'vaso' is not in common modern use. It is defined as the interior part of a hall, theatre church or similar space in relation to its capacity. *Dizionario Treccani* online c.f. vaso, https://www.treccani.it/vocabolario/vaso/ (accessed 27/10/2022).

ridotta a poco numero de frati, non passando hoggi il numero di 23, de' quali 12 solo sono in Roma, e questi havendo il governo degli Infermi, delle Zitelle, delle Balie, delle Dispense, della campagna, e di tante altre cose che derivano da Casali, Castelli, Vigne e simili, non possono per lo più nelle hore debite ritrovarsi in Choro, e dal Priore di Chiesa in poi che non manca mai; pochi altri vi si trovano, eccetto che le feste per le messe cantate, et altre fra settimana, fuori delle Conventuali, quali si cantano da uno di essi à vicenda, anzi cantavano anche le Conventuali una settimana per ciascheduno, mà coll'abbondanza dei cappellani soprannumerarij si sono scaricati di questo peso.

Siccome per l'avanti per mantenimento del Choro havevano introdotto Preti estranei sotto titolo di cappellani ordinarij, e perché li Vespri, e le Messe Solenni si cantavano ogni giorno con canto figurato, et anche le laudi nelle feste solenni, si stipendiavano perciò, oltre i Cappellani, anche i Musici Laici.

Ma nel tempo della sancta Memoria di Urbano VIII sotto Monsignor Anselmo Commendatore fu stimato più utile della Casa che i Cappellani medesimi fossero Musici, e però levati i musici laici si sono poi sempre presi cappellani Cantori, benchè di Classe assai mediocre, e per haverli pronti si alimentano in casa, et oltre la tavola si li dà il salario di scudi 3. e b.40 il mese per ciascheduno, ma con obbligo di 26 messe il mese, stante che la chiesa ha obbligo di messe 5204 l'anno fra piane, e cantate, e li frati suppliscono ad una picciola parte, cioè a 50 basse l'anno per ciascheduno, e qualche volta anche fino a 70, oltre le messe che cantano per turno.

Ma da pochi anni in qua si sono presi altri cappellani suprannumerarij sino al numero di 6, benché hoggi siano solamente 4, a quali si dà la Tavola e scudi dui il mese per salario, e sebbene al bisono della chiesa bastano li duoi Confessori, cioè il Curato e sotto Curato, nondimeno perché questi quattro non stiano fissi, sono stati deputati duoi di essi alle Confessioni.

Vero è che nell'ultima Sacra Visita, benché ci fossero questi cappellani soprannumerarij, nonne fu data nota, come che vi stavano per modo di provvisione, che però ho dato ordine che si licenzino per sgravare questa casa di Scudi 384 l'anno, che tanto importavano.

Hoggi dunque la Chiesa resterà con sette cappellani ordinarj Musici, che risiedono, et alimentano in casa.

Uno soprano non sacerdote, stipendiato a mese senza tavola.

Un'organista stipendiato a mese senza tavola

Un sotto sagristano, che ha tavola, e salario.

Un'aiutante di sagristia, quale hoggi è sacerdote.

Un Sotto Curato.

Oltre il Priore della Chiesa, et il Sagristano in capite che sono frati.

E fra questi, et altri 7 frati sacerdoti che risiedono in questa casa di Roma con impiego in altre faccende, si dicono ogni giorno molte messe in Chiesa.

Oltre sei altri sacerdoti, che servono l'hospitale, e si alimentano ivi, duoi de' quali celebrano nell'Hospitale ogni giorno e 4 hanno le Messe libere.

La spesa del vitto, e Salario di Cantori, Cappellani, et altri stipendiati per la Chiesa in numero di 12 senza li frati e senza li Cappellani soprannumerarij, fu figurata nella Sacra Visita scudi 1450; ma fu calcolata troppo rigorosamente, non passando à creder mio, scudi 1131.60.

Hoggi dunque si è posto in essame, se la spesa de i Musici si possa, e convenga resecare[2], o minorare. Il che pare, che dipenda da due punti, cioè:

1. Se sia espediente mantenere il Choro.
2. Se sia espediente mantenere la Musica.

In quanto al primo punto. Per il mantenimento parmi che si possino addurre duoi motivi:

Il primo perché è conforme alle regole dell'ordine al capitolo 36:

Il secondo perché la chiesa è in questo possesso.

All'incontro pare, che si possa dire:

1. Che niuna Religione in quei Conventi dove i frati sono impediti dal potere andare in Choro, prendano Preti per supplire;
2. Che il possesso deve operare che i frati vadano, se possono, ma non si supplischi per altri, anzi ch'è cattivo esempio per l'universale di tutte le Religioni, potendo con tale essempio i Monachi, et altri Luoghi ricchi lasciare d'andarvi Loro, e far supplire da Preti.

Tuttavia trattandosi del Capo dell'Ordine, dubiterei che fosse d'un cattivo essempio, si li levasse in tutto l'andare in Choro.

Massime che si bene hoggi quei sono pochi frati, nondimeno potrebbero col tempo crescere in numero, anzi si va discorrendo di fare un poco di Novitiato di quattro o sei soggetti, col non occuparli in altro che nel Choro, et Hospitale; ma si levasse affatto il Choro una volta, mai più si rimetterebbe, benchè crescessero di numero i frati, et a fine con conservare, dicono i Sacri canoni, che *Congratio sit ex tribus, sed conservatur in uno* e però crederei che si dovesse mantenere il Choro, anzi che si procurasse che tutti quelli frati che vi possono andare, vi andassero, chi al Vespero, chi alle hore, e chi alla messa cantata, secondo che da i proprij offizij li viene permesso, e particolarmente il sottosagristano.

Il secondo punto circa la Musica ha anche esso ragion per l'una, e per l'altra parte.

[1.] Contro la musica si può dire che *omne gens agit propter finem*, ma che la musica di questa Chiesa non ha fine alcuno, essendo introdotta per allettare la gente al Culto Divino; ma l'essere questa Chiesa (si può dire) fuori della Città, et in una parte hoggi dishabitata e ripiena di povera gente, molti de' quali non possono andar a messa neanche i giorni di festa per mancanza di habiti, nonché i giorni feriali, non serve la musica à cosa alcuna, e de facto si vede che pochissimi né i giorni di lavoro la frequentano; massime essendovi la traspontina, che è in strada più frequentata, e la Chiesa di San Pietro, ch'ella sola tira gente in questi Borghi.

2 An archaic word also spelled 'risecare' meaning to cut that which is superfluous, https://www.treccani.it/vocabolario/ricerca/risecare/ (accessed 27/10/2022).

2. Perché il Vespero, ch'è una delle due cose che si cantano ogni giorno si dice a hore 19 al presente Hora, nella quale pochi escono di casa, massime per andare in Chiesa e ben spesso assolutamente non vi è pure uno, e doppo il Vespro si chiude la Chiesa, si che pare gettata affatto la musica.
3. Perché dalle Collegiate nelle Basiliche principali in poi, poche altre tengono musica quotidiana, ma solo in certe loro feste chiamano e pagano musici, et in specie in santa Maria in Vialata, Rotonda, San Celso, Sant'Angelo, et altre, lasciando le Religioni Francescana, Dominicana, Teatina, Bernabita, et altri, che officiano con pietà e devozione, e col solo canto fermo, senz'altra musica.

In contrario si potrebbe considerare, che [1.] il levare un'uso antiquato, et inveterato dà occasione di gran querele e mormorationi, e che il dover supplire al peso di tante messe, necessita di tener Cappellani, e tenendoli con poco maggior spesa si trovano Sacerdoti, che sappino cantare, come si prattica al presente.

2. Che se bene ne'i giorni feriali non vi è che poca gente in Chiesa, nondimeno né giorni festivi e la mattina, et il giorno col Vespro ve n'è tanto numero, che non è gettata via la spesa.
3. Che levando i musici, i frati che non sanno cantare meno di canto fermo storpiarebbero il canto de Divini Offitij, e si renderebbero ridicoli, che però pare che si potrebbe prendere un temperamento di mezzo, cioè che in luogo di Sette, o otto Cappellani musici, se ne tenessero solamente quattro, che fossero Musici, e col Priore, Sagristano, e quattro novitij si havrebbe il Choro pieno, almeno di 10 Sacerdoti, e le feste si potrebbero havere quattro altri cantori con scudi duoi il mese per ciascuno.

In questa maniera la spesa di scudi 813.60 che si fa hora per i soli musicii diverrebbe solamente di 547.20 si che si avanzarebbe ogn'anno 263.40. Oltre l'avanzo fatto nell'haverli licentiati li quattro Cappellani sopranumerarij importano 384.

Et obbligando li 4 Musici à quel medesimo numero di mese che sono da celebrare, cioè di 355 l'anno, et supplendo i quattro frati, destinati al choro, ad altretante, si supplirebbe all'intiero bisogno – ma chi volesse estinguere affatto la Musica col maggiore risparmio.

Si potrebbero prendere 4 Cappellani che sapessero di Canto fermo, col dargli scudi sette il mese senz'altro, come si fa in San Gerolamo della carità, quali cantano di canto fermo, confessano, ragionano, e menano vita esemplare; con che si spenderebbero solamente l'anno 336.

Conseguentemente si avanzerebbero ogn'anno 477.60.

Discourse about Music in the Church

11 April 1660

The Church of the Holy Spirit, ordained in service of this home for invalids, for foundlings, for nuns, for spinsters, for nurses, for friars and ministers, temporal foundation of so many charitable works, which are done, is in charge of the care of souls, which is entrusted to one of the aforementioned friars, and who has a secular priest with the title of vice-curate under himself, and the care includes about 2,000 souls.

The interior of the church is quite large, with a single nave, and without transepts and besides the high altar it has 9 chapels, all similar and well-decorated, semicircular, with side entrance leading into a chapel, the church is well-supplied with precious furnishings, and any other desirable object, kept in a nice sacristy, that is more than decently adorned.

The high altar is according to old custom, set in the middle between the body of the church itself and the choir, with four pillars and columns, which support a little dome.

There is not only the physical choir, but also the human one, since, because of their rules connected to the spiritual functions, with which they have to comply, the friars also have to recite all the divine Offices in the choir every day; but considering that this house has a reduced number of friars, they are no more than 23, only 12 of them are in Rome, and having to take care of invalids, of spinsters, of nurses, of provisions, of the country estate, and of so many other things coming from Casali, Castelli, Vigne[3] and so on, for the most part they cannot be present in the choir at the fixed hours; and apart from the Prior of Church, who is never absent, they are just a few; but on feasts for the sung masses, and others during the week, except the conventual [masses], which are sung by one of them in turn; indeed they used to sing one of the conventuals a week each, but since there are plenty of extra chaplains they have relieved themselves of this burden.

As it had been done before, to keep the choir they had brought in guest Priests under the title of ordinary chaplains, and since Vespers, and sung masses were sung with polyphony, and also the lauds on solemn feasts, not only chaplains, but also lay musicians were paid a salary.

But at the time of Urban VIII of sacred memory under Commendatore Monsignor Anselmo it was considered more useful for the House that the same chaplains were musicians, and so after removing the lay musicians they have always employed chaplain choristers, although of very poor quality, and to have them ready they have board in the house, and in addition each of them is given a salary of 3 scudi and 40 baiocchi a month, but under obligation of 26 masses

[3] This could just mean things coming from farmhouses, castles and vineyards, but the capitalisation suggests instead that it refers to the Hospital's properties in Casali, Castelli (Terramo), Vigne (Terni).

a month, as the church has the obligation of 5,204[4] masses a year including low and sung masses, and the friars provide for a little part, that is for 50 low masses a year each, and sometimes up to 70, besides the masses they sing when on duty.

But in the last few years they have employed other extra chaplains up to the number of 6, even if today there are only 4, who have board and are given two scudi a month as salary, and although two confessors, that is the curate and the vice-curate, are enough for the need of the church, nevertheless, because these four (extra chaplains) are not fixed, two of them have been appointed to confessions.

Actually, during the latest Apostolic Visitation, although there were these extra chaplains, they were not mentioned, as if they were provisional, consequently I have given order to dismiss them to relieve this house of Scudi 384 a year, since they cost so much.

Today therefore, the church will stay with seven ordinary chaplain musicians, who get board and lodging in the house.

A non-priest soprano, paid monthly without board.
An organist paid monthly without board.
A vice-sacristan, who has board and salary.
A helper of sacristan, who today is a priest.
A vice-curate.
In addition, the prior of the church, and the chief sacristan, who are friars. And between them and 7 more priest friars who live in this house of Rome, busy with other matters, a lot of masses are celebrated in the church every day.
In addition, six more priests, who give their services in the hospital, and get their board there, two of them celebrate in the hospital every day and four have free Masses.
The expense for board and pay of choristers, chaplains and other salaried workers for the church, 12 in number excluding friars and extra chaplains, was estimated during the Apostolic Visitation as 1,450 scudi, but had been calculated too strictly, in my opinion this being no more than 1,131.60 scudi.

Today, therefore, it has been examined if the expense for musicians can, and is profitable to cut, or reduce. Which seems to depend on two points, that is:

1. If it is expedient to keep the choir.
2. If it is expedient to keep the music.

As to the first point. I think that to keep it two arguments can be put forward:
The first because it is in conformity with the rules of the Order at chapter 36:
The second because the church has got one.

To the contrary, it can be stated:

4 This figure seems extraordinarily high, but it works out at about fourteen Masses per day. As there were at least two each in the hospital and the nuns' chapel as well as those in the main church, with added Masses of obligation paid for in legacies or by patrons, it is probably not unreasonable.

1. That no congregation employs priests as substitutes in those convents where friars are too busy to go to the Choir;
2. That the possession (of a choir) must make the friars go if they can, but not to substitute for others. Indeed that is a bad example for all congregations, since following that example monks themselves, and others, would leave rich places and have priests as substitutes.

However, with regard to the Head of the Order, I would doubt that he would be a bad example, if he took them away to the Choir. Especially since, even if today there are a few friars, they might increase in number in time, in fact they are talking about organising some novitiate of four or six people, employing them just in the Choir and Hospital; but if the Choir were removed once and for all, it would never be formed again, because also if the number of friars had to increase, and this to keep, as the Sacred Canons state, that *Congratio sit ex tribus, sed conservatur in uno*[5] and after all I would think that the Choir had to be kept, indeed that all friars who can go there should be able to go, either to Vespers, or to Hours, or to sung mass, according to their availability connected to their tasks, and particularly the vice-sacristan.

The second point about Music has argumentation for both sides.

[1.] Against music you can say that *omne gens agit propter finem,*[6] but that the music of this church has no purpose whatsoever, since it was introduced to draw people to divine worship; but this church being (you can say) outside the city, and in an uninhabited part today and crowded with poor people, many of them cannot go to Mass even on feasts for lack of clothes, let alone at weekdays, music is completely no use, and in fact very few people attend it at weekdays; above all since there is [Santa Maria in] Traspontina, which is in a busier street, and the church of San Pietro, the only one which draws people in these suburbs.

2. Since Vespers, which are one of the two things that are sung every day, are sung at 4 p.m.,[7] a time when few people get out of home, especially to go to church and quite often no one is in (church), and after Vespers the church closes, so that music seems to be absolutely wasted.
3. Since apart from the collegiate (churches) in main basilicas, few others have daily music, but only call and pay musicians during their own feasts, and in particular in Santa Maria in Vialata, Rotonda, San Celso, Sant'Angelo, and others, omitting some Orders like the Franciscan, the Dominican, the Theatine, the Barnabite ones, and others, which celebrate with piety and devotion, and with only Gregorian chant, without other music.

5 The congregation is made up of three people, but a saviour in one.

6 Every people acts for the sake of an end (purpose).

7 In *Ore italiane,* nineteen hours after sunset would be mid-afternoon.

On the contrary it could be considered that [1] to efface an old and deep-rooted tradition can cause great complaints and grumbles, and that to have to face the burden of so many masses, means to keep chaplains, and keeping them, spending a bit more money you can find priests, who are able to sing, as it is done at present.

2. Even if at weekdays there are just a few people in the church, nevertheless on feasts and in the morning, and on the day with Vespers there is a great number, so money is not wasted.
3. Dismissing musicians, friars who can only sing Gregorian chant would spoil the singing of the Divine Office, and they would make themselves ridiculous, that anyway a compromise could be found that is to say that instead of seven or eight chaplain musicians, only four should be kept, who were musicians, and with Prior, Sacristan and four novices there would be the full chorus, of at least ten priests, and on feasts four more choristers could be employed with two scudi a month each.

In this way the expense of 813.60 scudi that is faced today just for musicians would become only of 547.20 so that 263.40 would be left every year. In addition, the money saved dismissing the four extra chaplains would reach 384 (scudi).

And requiring the 4 Musicians to perform during the same number of masses that have to be celebrated, that is 355 a year, and making the four friars, destined to the choir, be charged with as many, it would satisfy the whole need – but who would remove music completely with the greatest saving.

One could employ 4 chaplains, expert in Gregorian chant, giving them seven scudi a month, nothing more, as it is done in San Gerolamo della Carità, who sing Gregorian chant, confess, reason, and lead an exemplary life; doing that we would spend only 336 a year.

Consequently 477.60 would be saved every year.

Appendix B
Stefano Vai, 'Decreta Observanda in Ecclesia S. Spiritus circa Sacras Functiones'

Source: ASR-OSS 134, *Spedizioni e decreti, Rubricella atti, 1642–1645*, fols 129r–133r.

Minor clarifications and additions made in the copy dated 1743 (ASR OSS 1298) are included in italics in square brackets. Vai's Latin original was the point of reference for the scribe of the vernacular Rubric, given in Appendix C, and it is therefore given here in a literal transcription. The translation is by Shelagh Sneddon.

Decreta Observanda in Ecclesia S. Spiritus [in Saxia] circa Sacras Functiones

Stephanus Vaius, F. [*Pręceptor*]

Innocentii 3^{i} fundatoris nostri, ac Sanctissimi D. N. Urbani 8^{i}, nec non Sacri Concilii Tridentini inhęrendo decretis Divinum officium studiosè pariter, et Devotè, Missęque Sacrosanctum Sacrificium omni Religionis cultu, ac Veneratione nostra in ecclesia recitari, et celebrari, ex potiori parte commissi Nobis à S. Sede Apostolica muneris sedulo procuramus. Fratribus itaque dicti nostri Ordinis Sacerdotibus, et Clericis Professis iussu nostro in Ecclesię nostrę Sacrarium cum interventu Admodum R. R. Fr. Bernardini Focarii nostri Generalis Vicarii, ac Fr. Josephi de Rubeis dicte Ecclesię Prioris Superioribus Diebus congregatis quam plures Ordinationes cum [*r.* tum] Religiosum eorum statum, tum Divinum Cultum attingentes fuere confectę, quare eas ad Ecclesiasticas Functiones præcipuè pertinentes per Nos matura discussione recognitas approbavimus, et confirmavimus, ac præsentium vigore observari præcipimus, et mandamus, earumque tenorem hic duximus inserendum Videlicet.

Ad Matutinum oriente sole primò pulsetur peractaque Prima Missa fiat [*detur*] aliud signum, inter quod, et accessum fratrum, et Cappellanorum intercedat 4ª Pars Horę, ac omnibus coadunatis detur ultimum Campanulę signum pro ingressu Chori in quo omnes genuflexi submissa Voce dicant Orationem = Aperi Domine os nostrum &c. = nuper ab eodem S.^{mo}.D.N. Papa in Diurnalibus editam, Mox Priore, seu Hebdomadario surgente cæteri assurgunt, et inchoatur officium distinctè leniterque recitando, seu Canendo, et cum interpunctione in mediis Psalmorum, et Canticorum versibus in Romano Breviario novissime restituta; Conformis ordo standi, sedendi, et genuflectendi, Caput aperiendi, illud inclinandi servetur. Absint à Choro actus indecori, Ioci, colloquia, Risus; siquis post inchoatum officium advenerit genuflectens ante Altare Aliquantulum oret, postea Chorum ingressus salutet omnes, suumque petat locum, quem nullus dimittat, neque per Chorum vagetur; nec ab eo exeat inconsulto Priore; Nemo litteras, vel quid aliud legat, neque privatim officium recitet cum illud erit publicè recitandum; officio completo omnes utroque Poplite flexo, dicant Orationem = Sacrosanctę et Individuę Trinitati &c. = ac semel Pater, et Ave postmodum stantes sese [*ac se*] invicem consalutantes ordinatim à Choro discedant.

Matutinum canitur in Natali Domini et Duobus sequentibus festis in Epiphania, in Paschate Resurrectionis, ac Tribus antecedentibus, et Duobus subsequentibus Diebus, in Ascensione, in Pentecoste, et Duobus sequentibus feriis, in Assumptione B. V., et in festo omnium sanctorum. dicitur [*autem*] post Completorium Diei præcedentis Triduo Maioris Hebdomadę festo S. Marci, Dominicę 2[e] post Epiphaniam, et ferię 2[e] Pentecostes per Totam Octavam Corporis Christi, et pro Commemoratione omnium Defunctorum.

Laudes cantantur in festis omnibus de præceptu servandis, in ijs Trium Pluvialium ornatus adhibeatur, quandocumque fuerit decantatum Matutinum, et in[1] festis Consecrationis Ecclesię, et S. P. Augustini, in reliquis festis hic non expressis nullum in Laudibus adhibeatur pluviale.

Prima cum Cantu dicitur quando, et Nocturna Matutinalia fuerunt decantata; nec non in Vigilia Navitatis Domini ob solemnitatem Martirologii, et in festo S.[me] Trinitatis procanendo etiam simbolo.

Tertia canitur in omnibus festis Præceptivis Sexta, et Nona dicuntur antè, vel post conventualem missam, prout missalis Rubricę præscribunt.

Vesperarum officium dirigitur ab Hebdomadario; in solemnitatibus autem ab eo, qui Missam celebravit, quod si vesperę spectant ad consequens festum dicuntur ab eo, qui erit in Crastinum celebraturus.

Primę Vesperę cum Pluvialibus quinque celebrantur in Vigiliis Natalis, et Pentecostes, cum Tribus vero in singulis aliis festis Primę Classis S. Crucis, et S.S. Andreę [*Apostoli*], Augustini, ac Triphonis &c.

Secundas Vesperas septem Pluvialibus decorant Natalis, Pascha, et Pentecostes, quinque Epiphania, Ascensio feria 2[a] Pentecostes, Corpus [*Corporis*] Christi, Assumptio, festum omnium Sanctorum, et Ecclesię Consecratio. In aliis festis Primę, et 2[ę] Classis, ac Dominicis earumdem Classium. Item in Festis S. Crucis, et S.S. Augustini, et Triphonis, et Sociorum Tria Pluvialia; in cæteris autem festis Præceptivis, et Dominicis per Annum Unum tantummodo adhibeatur. Pro quibus Pluvialibus induendis Diaconus Hebdomadarius, seu Iunior ex [*de*] fratribus pro libito Prioris vocentur; cum autem opus erit quatuor Assistentibus, si fratrum Numerus in Choro sit parvus, addantur V. Curatus, Scolęque Magister, et in Solemnitatibus Maioribus ultra quatuor præfatos

1 Added interlineally.

Duo ex Cappellanis Hospitalis Infirmorum servitio eo tempore non detenti assumantur, quos omnes Cęremoniarius de Tono Versiculorum, Benedicamus, aliorumque rituum opportunè præmoneat.

Completorium cantatur in festis Præceptivis (Dummodo post ipsum non sint Litanię canendę), et in omnibus feriis Quadragesimę.

Litanię B. V. concinantur sabato quocumque in festo eiusdem B. V. sive ex Præcepto sive, ex Devotione servetur, et in Visitatione, et Præsentatione quando eas occurrit in Dominica celebrari. In quarum fine Litaniarum cantantur per Musicos V[*ersiculi*], et R[*esponsoria*], dicitur Oratio correspondens Antiphonę in officii Terminatione dicendę per fratrem Hebdomadarium Choralem stola semper Alba decoratum. Idem ferè servatur in Oratione quadraginta horarum post Salutationem Angelicam vespertinam; motettis namque ac Versiculis de S.^{mo} Sacramento à Musicis decantatis Hebdomadarius prædictus Orationes de eodem Sacramento, et de B. V. pariter dicat.

Missa Prima fiat Hebdomadatim à Magistro Scholę et Subsacrista (Dummodo non sit fr. Professus). In Festis vero à V. Curato, quibus aliquando legitimè impeditis præmonitus ab eis Sacrista supplere studebit.

Missas Privatas fratres, et Cappellani celebrent pro Ecclesię opportunitate à Sacrista vocati; fratres quidem alternis Hebdomadibus festisque per Annum Diebus: Cappellani vero quotidie (Una tantum Die per Hebdomadam excepta) Sacrificum iuxta Tabellam Annualis Onerum distributionis applicando.

Missę Votivę cum cantu pro Defunctis feria 2^{a}, et de Spiritu Sancto feria V^{ta}, vel alias ex Insitutione Sixti Papę 4^{i}. Item Anniversaria minus solemnia post Primam Diei, et solemniora; nec non Missę postquam S.^{mum} Sacramentum Processionaliter deferatur post Nonam celebrantur.

Missa Conventualis sine Ministris Paratis in festis, et feriis non Privilegiatis à fratre Hebdomadario canitur, in eaque per Capellanum Lectorem Epistola legitur. In Quadragesima vero, seu aliis Temporibus, occurente aliquo festo; Duę Missę Prima nempè à Cappellano consueto, et Altera ab Hebdomadario canantur.

Missa cum Ministris Paratis absque Thuris, et Abaci solemnitate fit in feriis Quadragesimę, in Sabatis quando fit de B. V. in Diebus infra Octavam Paschatis et[2] Pentecostes, in Die Octavę Corporis Christi, et Assumptionis B. V. in festis ex Devotione colendis, additis Præsentatione, et Visitatione B. V., et Commemoratione S. Pauli in quibus Scholę Magister Diaconus, et Cappellanus Consuetus Subdiaconus erunt.

Missa Solemnis celebratur in Dominicis, et festis Præceptivis additis festis Exaltationis S. Crucis, Conceptionis B. V., et S. Triphonis, nec non Diebus in quibus Oratio terminatur quadragenaria, vel Anniversaria solemnia fiunt, in iis omnibus celebrans, et Diaconus fratres Hebdomadarij; Subdiaconus vero Hospitalis Presbiter sunto.

2 Added interlineally.

Illustrissimus, et Reverendissimus Dominus celebrare consuevit Matutinum, et Tertiam Missam Natalis. Item Missas Paschatis, Pentecostes ferię V^{tę} in Cęna Domini; et festi Corporis Christi; ac Vesperas Paschatis, et Pentecostes.

Dominus Magister Domus Missam Primam, ac Vesperas Natalis Domini; ac Missam, et Vesperas Epiphanię, Dominicę Palmarum, ferię 2^{ę} Paschatis, Ascensionis, ferię 2^{ę} Pentecostes, Assumptionis et Purificationis B. V. et[3] in festis S. Augustini S. Theclę, et omnium Sanctorum, ac Matutina feriarum 4^{ę} V^{tę} et sextę in Paresceve.

Dominus Prior Ecclesię Laudes [*cantabit*] Missamque 2^{am} Natalis, et festi S. Stephani, et ferię 3^{ę} post Pascha. Itemque ferię 3^{ę} Pentecostes Dominicę 2^{ę} post Epiphaniam ferię 6^{ę} in Parasceve, festorum Consecrationis Ecclesię, et S. Marci, et quando quadragenaria exponitur Oratio ferię 4^{ę} Cinerum, et Commenorationis omnium Defunctorum. Item omnia Matutina, et Laudes, quę solemniter decantantur. Quod si Illustrissimus D[ominus] fuerit impeditus supplebit Dominus Magister Domus, quo impedito suppleat Dominus Prior, quibus omnibus impeditis functionis prædictas Uni ex fratribus Antiquioribus peragendas committunt [*committant*]. Ministros quoque quos ipsi maluerint assumant.

Parochus Ecclesię pro tempore (dummodo tamen sit frater Professus) in Sabato Sancto, et Vigilia Pentecostes Missam cum aliis functionibus sacris occurrentibus peraget.

Thurificetur hoc ordine, celebrans, Illustrissimus Dominus, Magister Domus, et fratres in eius Parte subsequentes, et absente dicto Domino Magistro Domus à Choro, Dominus Prior Ecclesię, et fratres post illum in eadem Parte subsequentes, dictoque Priore absente, Prior Hospitalis, post quem thurificentur[4] cæteri fratres in eadem parte existentes, et deinde transeatur ad fratres alterius partis, quod etiam servetur si Unus tantummodo ex dictis Privi legiatis in Choro reperiatur, eodem nempè Thurifcato, reliqui in eius parte existentes Thurficentur, antequam transitus fiat ad alteram partem, quamvis in ea [*eadem*] Tabella Chori sit apposita, omnibus vero præfatis à Choro Absentibus Thurificatio incipiat à fratre Primum Locum in Parte, quę propriè Chorus dicitur obtinente; Idemque servetur in Osculo Pacis: Duplici tamen Thuribuli ductu fratres Professi, Unico tantum Novitii, et Cappellani Thurificantur.

Concio in Dominicis Quadragesimę post evangelium, aliis Diebus peracta Missa; sed in Dominicis Palmarum, et Paschatis inter Vesperas, et Completorium, et in festo Annunciationis in qua fiat Capella Pontificia, inter Completorium, et litanias B. V. habeatur.

Organa in Missis, Vesperis, Matutinis, et Laudibus solemnibus, et Litanijs B. V. Maiora, vel Minora pro ecclesię nostrę Consuetudine pulsentur. Demptis Dominicis à Ceremoniali Episcoporum exceptis.

3 Added interlineally.

4 *thurificantur* is used consistently in 1743 in this passage.

Cantus Gregorianus, et Musicus in sacris officiis pro Temporum discretione ex præscripto Ceremoniali adhibeatur.

Processonibus quę fiunt extra ecclesiam fratres omnes etiam Choro non addicti Præsbiteri seculares, et Clerici in Domo, et Hospitali quomodolibet degentes intersint, Cantores iuxta Crucem Locum semper habeant, et initio Processionum ad Sanctum Petrum Antifona Veni Creator Spiritus &c. cum V[ers.]. *Emitte*, et oratione Deus qui corda &c., ac V[ers.]. Procedamus &c. ante Altare S.^mi^ Sacramenti hospitalis nostri, vel Ecclesię Monialium, ad Illustrissimi Domini libitum dicantur.

Communio fratrum non sacerdotum fiat in Missis, quę solemniter ab Illustrissimo Domino Præceptore, et à Domino Magistro Domus celebrantur exceptis feria 2ª Pentecostes, et festo monialium.

Defunctis fratribus officium à Priore, Missa fiat ab Hebdomadario cum ministris; Quinque Missę privatim à quolibet ex nostris Sacerdotibus celebrentur, et quinquies Nocturnum cum Laudibus à Caeteris fratribus, et sororibus recitetur, quę omnia Pietatis officia etiam fratribus extra nostrum Archihospitale decedentibus (dummodo illius habeant filiationem) atque Monialibus in nostro Monasterio decedentibus præstentur.

Ceremonię, et Ritus in functionibus prædictis, ad præscriptum Rubricarum missalis, Breviarii, et Cæremonialis exactè serventur. Quo circa Cęremoniarius Tæbellam in Sacristia Affigendam de Prioris Assensu singulo Mense; vel etiam sępius conficiat, in qua præscribat quid à singulis fratribus Cappellanis, aliisque personis, in Missa, et singulis Canonicis Horis cantandum, recitandumvè [*recitandumque*] sit, aut quęnam alia munera [*munia*] obire debeant, et ut præsentes Ordinationes facilius retineantur Priori præfato Mandamus, ut eas in huiusmodi Ecclesię sacrario affigi; Bisque in Anno publicè Legi procuret. Datum Romę ex dicto Archihospitali hac die x Maii 1644.

S. Episcopus Cyrenensis Præceptor
F. Jo: M.ª Castiglionus Secretarius

Decrees to be Observed in the Church of the Santo Spirito [in Sassia], concerning Divine Service

Stephen Vaius, Brother [*Preceptor*]

Adhering to the decrees of Innocent III our founder, and of our most holy lord Urban VIII, and also of the sacred Council of Trent, we are careful to ensure that the divine office should be recited and celebrated in our church with both attention and devotion, and also the most holy sacrifice of the mass, together with all religious worship and veneration, from the better part of the duty entrusted to us by the Holy Apostolic See. Therefore, when the brothers of our order, priests and professed clergy were gathered at our command in the sacristy of our church, with an important intervention from the reverend brothers Bernardino Focario, our Vicar General, and Joseph de Rubeis, prior of the said church, on preceding days, very many ordinances were written, touching both the status of those religious[5] and divine worship. Wherefore we have approved and confirmed those in particular that concern ecclesiastical worship, which have been accepted by us after lengthy discussion, and by the force of the present document we command and order that they should be observed, and we have resolved that their tenor should be set out here, namely:

The bell is to be rung for the first time for matins at sunrise, and when the first mass has taken place another signal is to be made, between which and the arrival of the brothers and chaplains a quarter of an hour should intervene; and when everyone has assembled, the last signal with the bell is to be given for entry to the choir, in which everyone with bent knee and lowered voice is to say the prayer 'Open, Lord, my mouth' lately published in his day-books [*diurnalibus*] by our same most holy lord Pope. Soon, when the prior or hebdomadary [*hebdomadarius*] rises, the others arise, and the office should be begun, reciting or singing clearly and gently, and with the interpunction in the middle of the verses of Psalms and Canticles very recently restored in the Roman breviary; the appropriate order of standing, sitting, genuflecting, raising the head, and inclining it is to be observed. Indecorous acts, jokes, conversations, laughter, should be absent from the choir. If anyone arrives after the office has begun, let him pray with bent knee before the altar for a little while, then, entering the choir let him greet everyone and seek his own place; no one is to dismiss him, and he should not wander about the choir, nor leave it without asking the prior. No one is to read letters or anything else, nor recite the office privately when it is to be recited publicly. When the office is complete, everyone, bending both knees, is to say the prayer = To the Most Holy and Undivided Trinity etc. = and once 'Our Father' and 'Ave Maria'. Afterwards, standing and saluting each other in turn, let them depart from the choir in order.

Matins is sung on the Lord's Nativity and the two following feasts, on Epiphany, on Easter Day and the three preceding and two following days, on Ascension Day, on Pentecost and the two following weekdays, on the Assumption of the Blessed Virgin and on the Feast of All Saints. It is said after Compline of the preceding day in the three-day period [*triduo*] of Holy Week, the Feast of St Mark, the 2nd Sunday after Epiphany and the Monday after Pentecost, for the whole octave of Corpus Domini and for the Commemoration of All Souls.

Lauds is sung on all feasts to be kept by precept. On these the embellishment of three pluvials is to be used, whenever matins has been sung, and on the feasts of the consecration of a church and of the Holy Father Augustine. On the remaining feasts not listed here no pluvial is to be used in lauds.

Prime is said with song when nocturnal matins have also been sung, and also on Christmas Eve, for the solemnity of the martyrology, and on the feast of Holy Trinity, when the creed (*simbolo*) is also sung.

5 Meaning those of the Order, living in the community.

Terce is sung on all preceptive feasts; sext and nones are said before, or after the Conventual Mass, as the Rubrics of the missal prescribe.

The office of Vespers is directed by the hebdomadary; but on feast days by him who has celebrated mass. But if the Vespers belong to a following feast, they are said by him who will be the celebrant on the morrow.

First Vespers are celebrated with five pluvials on the eves of Christmas and Pentecost; with three however on other individual feasts of the first class, of the Holy Cross and of Saints Andrew, Augustine and Triphon.

Second Vespers are adorned with seven pluvials at Christmas, Easter and Pentecost; five at Epiphany, Ascension, the Monday after Pentecost, Corpus Domini, Assumption, the feast of All Saints and the consecration of a church. On other feasts of the first and second class, and Sundays of the same classes. Item, on the feasts of the Holy Cross and of Saints Augustine and Triphon and associates: three pluvials. On other preceptive feasts, however, and on Sundays throughout the year, one pluvial only is used. For the putting on of the pluvials, the hebdomadary deacon or a junior from among the brothers are called at the prior's pleasure; but when it is necessary with four assisting. If the number of brothers in the choir is small, there may be added the vice-curate and the master of the school, and in greater feasts, beyond the four aforesaid, two from the chaplains of the hospital of the infirm who are not prevented by service at the time may be included. All of whom the ceremoniary should forewarn at the right moment about the tone [*tonus*] of the versicles, the Benedicamus and the other rites.

Compline is sung on the preceptive feasts, provided that after it there are not litanies to be sung, and on all the weekdays of Lent.

Litanies of the Blessed Virgin Mary are to be sung together on every Saturday, on the feast of the same Blessed Virgin, whether it is kept by precept or from devotion, and on the Visitation and Presentation when they happen to be celebrated on a Sunday; at the end of which litanies v[ersicles] and r[esponses] are sung by the musicians. A prayer is said corresponding to the antiphon in the termination of the office, which [the antiphon] is to be said by the hebdomadary choral brother, always adorned with a white stole. Almost the same is observed in the prayer of forty hours[6] after the angelic greeting in the evening, with motets indeed and versicles for the most holy sacrament sung by the musicians. The aforesaid hebdomadary is to say the prayers both for the same sacrament and for the Blessed Virgin.

The first weekly mass is to be celebrated by the master of the school and the sub-sacristan, provided that he is not a professed brother; but on feast days by the vice-curate. If they are legitimately prevented at any time, the sacristan, forewarned by them, will take care to fill the role.

The brothers and chaplains, called by the sacristan, may celebrate private masses for the benefit of the church: the brothers indeed in alternate weeks,

6 This refers to the 'Quarantore'.

and on feast days through the year, but the chaplains daily (one day only in the week excepted), performing the sacrifice according to the table of the annual distributions of duties.

Votive masses, with singing, for the dead [are celebrated] on Mondays, and those for the Holy Spirit on Thursdays, or at other times according to the institution of Pope Sixtus IV. Item, less solemn anniversaries [are celebrated] after the first, and more solemn, [mass] of the day; and masses are also celebrated after the most holy sacrament is carried in procession, after nones.

The conventual mass without ministers in vestments[7] is sung by the hebdomadary on the feasts and weekdays which are not privileged, and in it the epistle is read by the chaplain reader. But in Lent or at other times when some feast of two masses occurs, the first is to be sung by the usual chaplain and the other by the hebdomadary.

The mass with ministers prepared (wearing vestments) without incense and the solemnity of the abacus[8] takes place on weekdays in Lent, on Saturdays when it is for the Blessed Virgin, in the days within the octave of Easter and Pentecost, on the day of the octave of Corpus Domini and of the Assumption of the Blessed Virgin, on feasts to be kept from devotion, with the addition of the Presentation and Visitation of the Blessed Virgin and the Commemoration of St Paul, on which days the master of the school, deacon and chaplain, accustomed sub-deacon will be present.

The solemn mass is celebrated on Sundays and preceptive feasts, with the addition of the feasts of the Exaltation of the Holy Cross, the Conception of the Blessed Virgin, and St Triphon, and also on days on which the Forty-hour prayer is terminated, or solemn anniversaries take place. On all of these the celebrant, and the deacon, hebdomadary, brothers, sub-deacon, and hospital priest are to be present.

The most illustrious and reverend lord[9] has been accustomed to celebrate matins and the third mass of Christmas. Likewise, the masses of Easter, Pentecost, the Thursday of the Lord's Supper and the feast of Corpus Domini, and the Vespers of Easter and Pentecost. The lord master of the house:[10] the first mass and Vespers of Christmas; and the mass and Vespers of Epiphany, of Palm Sunday, of Easter Monday, Ascension, the Monday of Pentecost, the Assumption and Purification of the Blessed Virgin, and on the feasts of St Augustine,

7 This seems to suggest ministers not dressed in specific vestments in contrast to the next instruction that they do use vestments but not incense.

8 This word can be used for a cupboard, any kind of tablet or table as well as counting device and architectural element of a column. Its meaning here is unclear, but it seems likely to refer to a lectern such as those used for supporting large choirbooks or liturgical books with storage space below.

9 This title refers to the commendatore.

10 The master of the house is the maestro di casa or major-domo.

St Thecla and All Saints, and matins of the Wednesday, Thursday and Friday in Holy week [*Parasceue*].

The lord prior of the church [*will sing*]: lauds, and the second mass of Christmas, and of the feast of St Stephen, and of the Tuesday after Easter. Item the Tuesday after Pentecost, the second Sunday after Epiphany, Good Friday, the feasts of the consecration of a church and St Mark, and when Lenten prayer is expounded, Ash Wednesday, and the commemoration of All Souls. Item, all matins and lauds which are solemnly sung. But if the most illustrious lord[11] is prevented from being present, the lord master of the house will fill the role, and if he is prevented the lord prior is to fill the role. If they are all prevented, they entrust the aforesaid services to be performed by one of the older brothers. And they should choose the ministers whom they themselves prefer.

The current parish priest [*parochus*] of the church (provided that he is a professed brother) is to celebrate mass with the other divine services that take place on Holy Saturday, and the eve of Pentecost.

Sprinkling with incense should take place in this order: the celebrant, the most illustrious lord, the master of the house, and then the brothers on his side [of the choir]; and if the said lord master of the house is absent from the choir, the lord prior of the church and the brothers following after him on the same side; and if the said prior is absent, the prior of the hospital, after whom the other brothers on the same side should be sprinkled with incense, then crossing over to the brothers on the other side. This is to be observed even if only one of the said privileged is found in the choir: when he has been sprinkled with incense, the others on his side are to be sprinkled with incense, before going over to the other side, even if the tablet[12] of the choir is there. If all the aforesaid are absent from the choir, let the burning of incense begin with the brother who holds the first place on the side which properly is called the choir. And the same is to be observed in the Kiss of Peace, but with double leading of the thurible for the professed brothers; the novices and chaplains are sprinkled with incense once only.

The assembly [*concio*] is to be held on the Sundays of Lent after the gospel, on other days after the mass has been completed; but on Palm and Easter Sundays between Vespers and compline, and on the feast of the Annunciation, on which there is to be a/the Pontifical Chapel, it is to take place between compline and the litanies of the Blessed Virgin.

The organs: in solemn Masses, Vespers, Matins and Lauds and Litanies of the Blessed Virgin let the larger be played, or the smaller, according to the custom of our church; excepting the Sundays removed in the *Caeromoniale Episcoporum*.

11 The abbreviation D.P. in this context indicates the commendatore, not the prior, as the latter is referred to in the next line.

12 This appears to be another reference to a large lectern, perhaps meaning the same object as 'abacus' above.

Let Gregorian chant and music be used in the holy offices according to the discretion of the seasons from the prescribed ceremonial.

In processions that take place outside the church, all brothers, even those not appointed to the choir, secular priests, [*presbiteri*] and clergy living in any way in the house and hospital are to be present. The singers are always to have a place next to the cross, and at the beginning of processions to St Peter the antiphon 'Veni Creator Spiritus'[13] with verse 'Emitte'[14] and prayer 'Deus qui corda' and verse 'Procedamus'[15] are to be said before the altar of the holy sacrament of our hospital, or of the church of the nuns,[16] as it pleases the Illustrious Lord.

The communion of brothers who are not priests is to take place in the masses which are celebrated solemnly by the most illustrious lord Preceptor and by the lord master of the house, except for the Monday after Pentecost and the feast of the nuns.[17]

The office for deceased brothers is to be celebrated by the prior, the mass by the hebdomadary with ministers. Five masses are to be celebrated privately by any of our priests, and a nocturn with lauds is to be recited five times by the other brothers and sisters. All of which offices of piety are also to be provided for brothers dying outside our Arch-hospital (provided that they have an affiliation to it), and for nuns dying in our monastery.

The ceremonies and rites in the aforesaid services are to be observed exactly according to the prescription of the rubrics of the missal, breviary and Ceremonial. Concerning which the ceremoniary is to complete a table to be affixed in the sacristy, with the prior's assent, every month, or even more often, on which he is to prescribe what is to be sung or recited by each of the brothers, chaplains and other persons in the mass and at each canonical hour, or what other duties they must undertake. And so that the present ordinances may be retained more easily, we order the aforesaid prior that he should arrange for them to be affixed in the sacristy of this church, and to be read publicly twice a year. Given at Rome from the said Arch-hospital this 10th day of May 1644.

Stephen, Bishop of Cyrene, preceptor.
Brother Joseph Maria Castiglioni, secretary.

13 The musical sources are all settings of 'Veni Sancte Spiritus', but 'Veni Creator Spiritus' is referred to in the Rule.

14 'Emitte spiritum tuum et creabuntur et instaurabis faciem terrae': 'When you send your Spirit, they are created; and you renew the face of the ground.' Psalm 103:30 (Ps 104:30 NIV).

15 'God who the hearts of the faithful' and 'Let us proceed in peace'.

16 This refers to the church of Santa Tecla (St Thecla) in the nuns' cloister.

17 This refers to the feast of St Tecla, 23 September.

Appendix C
Rubrica della chiesa collegiale e parocchiale di S. Spirito in Sassia di Roma

The primary source for this documenti is ASR OSS 1299 *Chiesa di S. Spirito, Ordini e istruzioni*, a large folder of documents. The Rubrica is presented in a small booklet with neither pagination nor foliation, and is signed and dated, G. A. Bufalini, 1752. Another version exists in ASR OSS 1298 *Scritture concernenti interessi della Chiesa collegiale di S. Spirito*. The document was copied into a large folio containing numerous instructions written by the same scribe. These include Vai's 1644 Decree, along with items by Campori (1611) and Spada (1660). The presumed date of the copy of the document in OSS 1298 is 1745, which is the date on the binding of the book.

The two versions are fundamentally the same in meaning, but small differences in phrasing or word order suggest a common Latin source from which the scribes were translating for everyday use. In some places OSS 1298 is more explicit, while in others, the 1752 version is clearer. The 1752 scribe is more sparing, perhaps lazy, using more abbreviations, and leaving out some of the parenthetical information found in OSS 1298. In this transcription and translation of the 1752 Rubric, I have incorporated information that appears only in the OSS 1298 version and any variants that help to clarify meaning. To make these differences clear, I have used italics for additional words and information from OSS 1298, with longer phrases or passages that are different given in parentheses.

The many scribal abbreviations have been silently expanded, and capitalisation of Offices and titles (e.g. Te Deum) made consistent, but the original, somewhat eccentric punctuation has been kept in the transcription. Some archaisms that obscure meaning have been silently modernised, but original spellings have largely been maintained. In order for the sense of the document to be understood in English, some punctuation has been added. The translation attempts to convey the meaning clearly, rather than giving a literal rendering of the sometimes contorted original. There is, therefore, punctuation in the translation that is absent or inferred in the original.

Rubrica da osservarsi in tutto l'anno per le Feste, che accadono nella Venerabile Chiesa Collegiale, e Parrocchiale di S. Spirito in Sassia di Roma copiata dal suo originale autentico, che si conservava nella Sagrestia della medesima Chiesa dell'Anno 1644

E ridotta nel Metodo, che presentemente si osserva, secondo la Riforma fatta dalla Sacra Visita nell'Anno 1738

Tutte le Domeniche dell'anno il Matutino va detto leggendo, Laudi e Benedictus cantato, se non sia Festa Privilegiata.
[*In tutti li giorni semplici, e feriali, si recita l'officio della Beata Vergine oltre l'officio feriale.*]

Tutte le Domeniche di Quaresima officiando di Domenica, non si suona mai organo, ma si canta à cappella in coro, come non sia altrimenti notato.
[*Il primo giorno del mese non impedito si recita Vespero, Notturno, e Laudi de defonti.*]

Tutti i giorni feriali di Quaresima si dice Compieta cantata à 23 Ore; *e adesso si è introdotta à ore 20.*

Tutte le Domeniche dell'Avvento officiando di Domenica non si suona mai Organo, ma si canta à cappella in coro, come non sia altrimente notato.

Tutti li Sabbati dell'Anno si espone il Santissimo Sagramento à ore 23 con Mottetto, Litanie, Salve, o altre Secondo il tempo: Tantum ergo & *con la* Beneditione.

Nel tempo delle 40 ore si osserva quanto di sotto è notato; Doppo Terza si canta da un canonico, o Cappellano la Messa conventuale del Santo, o Feria, Concordandosi con l'officio; poi si dice Sesta, e si canta Nona, finita si canta la Messa in Organo, omnia ut in Die Corporis Cristi. Terminata la Messa si torna in Coro, e si distribuirono le parti per il Pange lingua, che si canta nella Processione, ritornata in Chiesa, due de Cappellani vanno a piedi dell'Altare Maggiore, e si aspetta sino à tanto, che il Signor Maestro di Cerimonie avvisa, che si cantino le Litanie de Santi.

Il secondo giorno delle 40 ore: Messa conventuale à cappella in Coro, e si canta da un canonico *o da un cappellano* con Ministri parati: Doppo Nona si canta in organo Messa contra Paganos, *a ut pro Pace etc.* Sine Gloria, et sine Credo, che se l'incontra in Domenica si dice il Credo.
L'introito di questa Messa ut in Domenica Sexagesimae.

Il Terzo *giorno* doppo Terzo si canta in coro la Messa Conventuale da un Cappellano, seu canonico. Doppo Nona si canta la Messa in organo, e si fà come nel primo giorno *cioè ut in die Corporis Christi*; non vi è altra differenza che le Litanie si dicono prima della Processione, avvisandone il Signor Maestro di Cerimonie.

Tutti li Sabbati dell'Anno facendosi l'officio di S. Maria in Sabbato, Risposte d'organo nella Messa cantata all'Altare della Madonna.

Quando accade giorno festivo di precetto in Sabbato, Compieta si dice bassa, perché si cantano le Litanie per la Benedizione [*per ragione della Benedizione*]

Primo Gennaio
La Santissima Circoncisione: Matutino Basso; Te Deum, Laudi cantate, Benedictus falsobordone: Messa, e Vespero in organo: e qui si osservi che nell'anno 1737 la sagra visita ridusse il canto figurato in organo in canto Gregoriano nel coro.
5. Giorno
Primo Vespero dell'Epifania in organo.
Sesto Giorno *di detta Epifania* Matutino Solenne cantato; Tutti li Gloria Patri in falsobordone, e ci tutti li finali suona l'organo: Te Deum in canto figurato, e risposte d'organo in ogni versetto; le Laudi si cantano, e un canonico e assistenti con piviali assistono come Vespero, Benedictus in falsobordone, e risponde ad ogni versetto l'organo, per dar tempo, che si incensi l'altare. L'ora di Prima si canta Martirologio, e Terza, Messa e Vespero in organo; Compieta si canta.
Domenica seconda doppo l'Epifania: Te Deum, Laudi cantate, Benedictus falsobordone; Terza si canta, Messa, e Vespero in organo, Compieta si canta.
Gennaio 17
S. Antonio Abbate: risposta d'organo alla Messa cantata senza Turificazione.
Gennaio 20
Santi Fabiano, e Sebastiano: Risposta d'organo alla Messa cantata senza Turificazione
Gennaio 25
Conversio S. Pauli: Risposte d'organo alla Messa cantata, senza Turificazione; Che si pratica solamente quando si cantan Laudi
Febbraio 2
Purificatio Beata Maria Vergine. Matutino si legge: Te Deum, Laudi cantate, Benedictus falsobordone, Terza si canta, di poi la Benedizione delle Candele, nel qual tempo si cantano in coro li versetti in canto fermo, ut in libro, e si fà la Processione, dopo la distribuzione, e per la strada *o chiesa* si canta Responsum accepit Simeon, che stà nelli libretti, finita la Processione si canta Messa, e Vespero in organo, Compieta bassa, Litanie in Organo, e Ave Regina *avanti l'altare della Madonna.*
Ceneri [*Dies Cinerum*]
Mercordì giorno delle Ceneri, Salmi graduali, Matutino della Madonna Santissima, di poi Matutino corrente, doppo Nona si canta Messa con *li ministri* Assistenti; [e] prima si fà la Benedizione *e distribuzione* delle Ceneri, doppo Messa entra la predica, che ora è dismessa per tutta la Quaresima.
Tutti li venerdì di Quaresima Matutino di Maria Vergine, e poi il corrente, Salmi penitenziali in ginocchione, doppo Nona, Messa cantata, e Predica.
Prima Domenica di Quaresima. Laudi cantate, Benedictus falsobordone, Terza si canta, Messa cantata in coro, e finita si dice la Predica, di poi si ritorno in coro à dire Sesta, e Nona.
Febbraio 24 o 25
S. Mattia Apostolo: Te Deum, Laudi cantate, Benedictus falsobordone, Terza si canta, Messa in organo del Santo à buon ora; se viene in Quaresima, dopo

Nono si canta la Messa della feria in coro, di poi la Predica, dopo la Predica, il Vespero in organo, cosi si continua tutti li giorni di Quaresima.
Marzo 9
S. Francesca Romana; risposte d'organo alla Messa della Santa: doppo Nono la Messa della feria corrente
Domenica quarta di Quaresima, Laudi cantate, Benedictus falsobordone, Terza si canta, Messa, e Vespero in organo.
Domenica di Passione: Benedictus falsobordone, Messa, e Vespero in coro à cappella.
Marzo 25
Santissima Annunziata, Benedictus falsobordone, doppo Terza Messa in organo [*si canta Terza e poi Messa in organo*]; finita si torna à dire Sesta e Nona, di poi la Messa della feria à cappella; terminata si va à cantare un' altra Messa all'Oratorio de Fratelli passato l'Ospedale; doppo della quale si torna à cantare il Vespero in organo à ore 20: si canta Compieta tutta in organo, Finito si dice la Predica, doppo si cantano le Litanie, e Ave Regina. [marginal note: Tutto l'officio Nona cantata, doppo la Messa del la feria; si va all'oratorio dove si canta la Messa della Madonna.]
Domenica Palmarum Benedictus falsobordone, Terza si canta poi *la* Messa, avanti si canta l'Asperges more Solito in coro, di poi la Benedizione delle Palme, e in coro si vien cantando in canto fermo Hosanna – Il Sanctus in canto figurato; nella distribuzione delle Palme si canta Pueri Hebreorum del Vittoria; finito, il diacono dice Procedamus in Pace, il coro risponde: in Nomine Christi Amen; e si principia la Processione, e da Cappellani si canta: Turba multa, che stà ne libretti, arrivati alla Porta della Chiesa due de cappellani cantano di dentro, l'altri che sono di fuori cantano in canto figurato: Gloria Laus & quelli di dentro cantano in canto fermo li versetti che stanno nel rituale, e si canta alternatim, sino à tanto che il Suddiacono percuote con l'asta della Croce la porta della Chiesa, la quale si apre, e si canta Ingrediente Domino: Finita la processione, comincia l'Introito: Domine P[ater]. li Kirie Eleison alla Palestina [sic] doppo l'Epistola, il suo graduale, Tratto, e versetti in canto fermo, poi il Passio da tre canonici che risposte della Turba à 4: in canto figurato del Vittoria; Finito il Passio si canta il Credo: l'Offertorio *Improperium* col Sanctus e il *suo* mottetto à sei voci all' l'elevazione. Agnus Dei al solito, post Communio: Finita la Messa, si dice Sesta e Nona, poi l'ultima Messa dal cappellano hebdomadario: Vespero à ore 20 in coro à cappella, Compieta bassa, Ave Regina e sic finis. Poi Predica, che dall'anno 1714 si è tralasciata in tutta la Quaresima.
Lunedi Santo: Matutino solo corrente, doppo Nona si canta la messa con li Assistenti parati finita si canta il Vespero more solito, à ore 23 si canta Compieta.
Martedì Santo: Matutino come sopra cosi ancora la messa. Il Passio si canta dalli tre cappellani del primo coro, dopo la Messa il Vespero al solito; Compieta ut heri.
Mercordì Santo: Matutino come sopra; Messa ut heri, la prima lezione si dice in Tono Prophetiae dall'ultimo Cappellano, l'Epistolae si canta dal Suddiacono in Tono epistole; Il Passio si canta dalli tre Cappellani del secondo coro, doppo la

Messa si canta il Vespero; Compieta à ore 20: *mezza* bassa, quale finita si canta immediatamente il Matutino solenne, senza organo perché è la Settimana Santa, i primi responsorii si cantano ne libretti, i responsorii del secondo, e terzo notturno si cantano nel libro del Vittoria, Benedictus, e Misere dell'istesso.
Giovedì Santo à ora Competente si cantano [*si recitano*] le ore basse, cioè Prima, Terza, Sesta, Nona ut in Breviario, finite si canta Messa, li Kirie in coro, prima che si cominci la Gloria suona un poco l'organo. Dopo l'Epistola si dice il graduale adagio in canto fermo per dar tempo. Doppo l'Evangelo si dice il Credo, e l'Offertorio Dextera Domini. Alla comunione generale si canta Cenatibus illis à 4 nei libretti; il post Communio in canto fermo, e poi si principia la Processione, si canta Pange lingua etc. Terminata la processione si ritorna in coro, e si dice Vespero; il celebrante intuona l'Antifona bassa. Finito il Vespero, il Celebrante intuona di nuovo Diviserunt, che è l'antifona e mentre si denudano li altari, si viene dicendo il Salmo Deus, Deus meus respice in me; finito si replica Diviserunt; Di poi suona il mezzogiorno, et in Coro dicesi l'Ave Maria in ginocchioni, e poi senza altro motivo si parte dal coro. Compieta à ore 20 *e mezza* bassa; Matutino ut in Breviario, in fine il tutto come ieri.
Venerdì Santo: à ora competente si va in coro, e diconsi tutte le ore come ieri, e poi vengono all'Altare il celebrante coll'assistenti, e l'ultimo cappellano canta la Lezione in Tono Prophetiae, al fine della quale in coro si canta il Tratto, poi il suddiacono dice l'Epistola, e à questa pure si canta in coro il Tratto. Finito li signori canonici *come pure nella Domenica della Palme* cantano il Passio di S Giovanni con le risposte della Turba in coro nel libro del Vittoria, e terminato il celebrante doppo l'orationi intuona Ecce lignam crucis, li due tenori seguono appresso, il coro risponde – Venite adoremus. Finito l'adorazione si và al *santo* sepolcro, si accendono le torcie, il celebrante riceve dalle mani del diacono il Santissimo, e in processione si dice in canto fermo Vexilla *Regis prodeunt, quale terminata,* il sacerdote seguita la funzione, ut in missali; doppo si canta il Vespero ut heri a ore 20 [*venti e mezzo*] si dice Compieta, e si canta Matutino, ut in Breviario, ut ieri; doppo le Laudi si và all'Altare del Crocifisso, e si canta Vere languores nostros, del Vittoria.
Sabato Santo à ora competente diconosi tutte le ore come ieri, e poi processionalmente si va fuori della chiesa, assistendo *il Capitolo* alla Benedizione del fuoco, si ritorna in processione per la strada fatta in chiesa, e si accende una delle *tre* candele per il Lumen Christi, sino à tanto che sono accese tutte; si canta l'Exultet, le Profezie, e poi di nuovo si va in Processione cantando Sicut Cervus. Finito si fà la Benedizione del fonte, che si fà dal canonico Curato coll'assistenenza del Capitolo; Terminata si torna processionalmente cantando le Litanie *duplicate* ut in Sabbato Santo, arrivati al Kirie si cantano in coro in canto figurato à cappella; prima che principii la Gloria suona alquanto l'organo, e campane, e poi tutto il resto in coro, il primo Alleluia doppo l'Epistola, l'intuona il Celebrante, di poi il coro risponde, due tenori dicono Confitemini & li due soprani dicono Laudate, i due Bassi, Quoniam confirmata est.
Post Sumptionem Sacramenti il Basso intuona Alleluia; il resto si canta in contrapunto, Laudate Dominum in falsobordone, finito si replica Alleluia ut supra;

di poi il Celebrante intuona Vespere autem Sabbati, il coro risponde quel che siegue, si canta la Magnificat del Morales, e risponde l'organo ad ogni versetto: Sicut erat in falsobordone, il Deo Gratias si dice unitamente coll'organo.
Compieta al solito cantata che si dice à ore 23 con l'esposizione del Santissimo Sacramento, Litanie, Regina Coeli, e Tantum ergo, e si dà la Benedizione al Popolo.
Giorno di Pasqua
Mattutino Solenne con risposte d'organo, Te Deum in canto figurato, Laudi parate come *pure* il Vespero, in luogo del Capitolo si dice, Haec Dies in canto figurato à cappella, Prima e Terza si canta, e si intuona in tuono quinto Messa in organo solenne di poi [*dopo*] *si recita* Sesta, e Nona in coro.
A ore 19: si canta Vespero *in organo e alla cattedra*, in luogo dell'Inno si canta: Haec Dies à 8: = Compieta si canta perché non vi è più la Predica solita. [*Compieta si dice bassa perché finita entra la Predica]*
Lunedi, e Martedì di Pasqua tutto come Ieri, fuor che doppo la Messa cantata, non si dice più la predica, Terminata si torna in coro à dire Sesta[1], e Nona = Vespero al solito, Compieta cantata. [*Compieta si cantano come il primo giorno*]
Tutta quest'Ottava alla Messa cantata si canta à cappella Haec dies, Victime Paschali con quel che segue in missalis.
Aprile 25
S. Marco Evangelista: risposte d'organo alla Messa parata del Santo.
Domenica in Albis Te Deum, Laudi cantate, Benedictus falsobordone: Terza cantata, Messa, e Vespero in Organo. *Compieta si canta.*
Primo Maggio
Santi Filippo, e Giacomo: Te Deum, Laudi cantate, Benedictus falsabord: Terza cantata, Messa e Vespero in organo, Compieta cantata.
Maggio 2
Festività della S. Croce, di cui ne abbiamo una insigne reliquia = Primo Vespero in organo, Compieta bassa, perché accade in giorno feriale.
Maggio 3
In venerazione della S.Croce: Te Deum, e Laudi cantate, Benedictus falsobordone; Terza cantata, e Messa e Vespero in organo, Compieta cantata.
Lunedi primo giorno delle Rogazioni; se in questo giorno accade festa doppia, o semidoppia se ne fà l'officio, e doppo Prima si canta Messa da un Cappellano, e doppo Terza si canta l'altra Messa dal Canonico ebdomadario.
Martedì Rogazioni si osserva tutto come ieri.
Mercordì Rogazioni si canta Messa del Santo da uno de Cappellani, doppo Sesta, perché è la vigilia dell'Ascenzione si canta la seconda Messa della vigilia da un altro Cappellano, e doppo *Nona* si canta Messa delle Rogazioni dal Canonico ebdomadario, e Vespero solenne si canta in organo per i primi Vesperi dell'Ascenzione.

1 OSS 1298 has a contradictory instruction. '...doppo la Messa cantata, *si dice la Predica, quale terminata*, si torna in coro à dire Sesta.'

Giovedì Ascenzione, *si canta* Matutino, e tutto si fà, e si canta come nel giorno dell'Epifania, Messa, e Vespero solenne in organo à due cori, Compieta cantata.
Maggio 17
Primo Vespero in organo per la Dedicazione della nostra chiesa [18 Maggio]
Dedicazione: – *doppio di prima classe, cum ottava* – Matutino basso, Te Deum in canto figurato con risposta d'organo ad ogni versetto; Laudi parate alla catedra, il tutto si fà come nel giorno dell'Epifania.
Si osservi che la processione del Capitolo famiglia di Casa, e Zitelle del Conservatorio alla Basilica di S. Pietro è stata abolita dalla Sacra Visita nell'anno 1738. =
Vigilia della Pentecoste. Doppo Nona dal Canonico Curato si fa la benedizione del fonte con l'assistenza del capitolo, e si osserva il medesimo modo, che nel Sabbato Santo, ubi à missali; nella processione si canta il mottetto: Sicut cervus, Litanie ut in Sabbato Sancto; Messa in coro con risposta di organo, e sei Profezie, e primo Vespero solenne in organo e alla cattedra.
Pentecoste. Matutino cantato, e tutto si fà come nel giorno di Pasqua. Se viene il Papa e si esponga il Santissimo sacramento nel Lunedi seguente come era solito. Messa e Vespero in organo ordinario, Compieta bassa, et poi mattutino per lunedì si legge.
Lunedi à ora competente senza astanti e senza musica si espone il Santissimo sagramento, finita la Processione Papale e generale si va in coro, e si dice l'ora di Prima bassa, Terza si canta, Messa in organo, ma breve per esser tardi, doppo *la quale* si ritorna in coro à dir Sesta e Nona. Vespero solenne per la festa della Chiesa, Compieta e Mattutino basso per il giorno seguente di poi all'Ave Maria si canta il Tantum ergo o in canto fermo, o figurato in organo, e si dà la Benedizione al popolo. Alla processione delle zitelle, che si và à S. Pietro il giorno di Martedì i musici di S. Pietro favoriscono, e portano motetti da cantare per strada: nel ritorno si canta il Te Deum che stà ne libretti. Arrivati in Chiesa l'organista suona l'organo sino à tanto che si è data la dote alla zitelle di poi si và in coro, e si dice Prima bassa, Terza si canta, doppo Messa solenne à quatto cori, finita si dice Sesta, e Nona=Vespero solenne à Quattro cori, Tantum ergo da musici del primo coro, Benedizione e Compieta bassa, detto Martedì solenne, come il Lunedi. [*Martedì si va processionalmente con le nostre zitelle alla Basilica di S. Pietro, e per strada si cantano le Litanie di tutti li Santi, Te Deum & ed il Primo Capitolo di S. Petro benedice la nostra famiglia con l'ostensione delle tre più insigni reliquie, di poi si ritorna cantando alla nostra chiesa, dove arrivati l'organista suona l'organo sino à tanto che Monsignore commendatore abbia data la dote alle zitelle, e doppo si dice Prima bassa...*
Si osservi, che dal Pontificato di Benedetto XIII sino al presente, li pontefici, col sacro Collegio non sono più venuti processionalmente alla nostra chiesa, e che dall'anno 1738 è stata sospesa la processione delle nostre zitelle à S. Pietro e però in questo triduo il tutto si costuma, come nella Pasqua di Resurrezione; nel secondo giorno però della Pentecoste solennizza con la musica la quale è stata levata dalla Sacra Visita Apostolica sino dal primo Novembre dell'anno 1737,

e si è introdotto il canto gregoriano nella Pentecosta però si appara da festaroli tutta la chiesa come prima]
Mercordì Quattro Tempora della Pentecoste tutto l'officio và detto basso, doppo Nona si canta Messa con li assistenti, la prima lezione si canta in Tuono Prophetiae, dall'ultimo Cappellano, Vespero al solito in coro, Compieta bassa.
Giovedì Matutino ut heri, Messa si canta apparata doppo Terza, e và come ieri tutto.
Venerdì doppo Nona si canta Messa in coro ut in missali con ministri parati.
Sabbato ut supra, le Profezie diconsi da cappellani una per uno.
[*Mercordi quattro Tempora della Pentecoste Matutino di dice basso, e doppo Nona si canta Messa con li ministri assistenti come parimente in tutti li giorni di questa Ottava privileggiata e nel sabato dopo la Pentecoste, e due giorni susseguenti si espone il santissimo sacramento le 40 hore nelle quali si deve osservare l'istruzione che si rinuova in ogni Ponteficato per questa solennità.*]
Domenica della Santissima Trinità: Te Deum, Laudi cantate, Benedictus falsobordone: Prima si canta, cosi anco il Martirologio per il simbolo *di S. Atanasio* Quicumque, Terza cantata, Messa e Vespero in organo Compieta cantata.
Mercordì primo Vespero in organo *et alla cattedra* per il Corpus Domini, Compieta, e Salve bassa poi Matutino basso per la Mattina seguente, che dura per tutta detta ottava solamente.
Giovedì Corpus Domini: Quando la processione Papale di S. Pietro stà à S. Giacomo Scossacavalli, *la nostra chiesa* cominicia à suonare, di poi si entra in coro e si dice Prima, Terza e Sesta bassa, Nona si canta.
L'inno và cantato sopra l'Inno della Madonna [*sopra il tuono della Madonna*] = il Salmo Mirabilia si canta nel Tono del libro corale. Messa in organo, *quale* finita si distribuiscono le parti del Pange lingua, e si comincia la processione, quando si trova à piedi dell'Ospedale, dove vi stà un Altare [*l'altare preparato*] à posta, si dà la benedizione a Castello [*il quale corrisponde col sparo del cannone*], doppo spara, e si viene cantando il Tantum ergo, si ritorna per l'Ospedale, et all'Altare si posa, e si ritorna di nuovo à cantare il Tantum ergo, e dalli soprani il versetto Panem de Coelo, e si dà la Benedizione all'Infermi [*si entra cantando come prima nell'ospedale ed il celebrante colloca il santissimo su l'altare di mezzo e cantato di nuovo il Tantum ergo e si dà la benedizione*]; Di qui si và alle monache, e zitelle, e si fà il medesimo nella chiesa di S. Tecla; Alla porta del conservatorio si dà parimente la Benedizione cantando prima le zitelle il Tantum ergo: si ritorna in chiesa cantandosi medesimamente il Tantum ergo e con il versetto da soprani Ut supra, detta l'orazione, e data la benedizione si espone il Santissimo Sacramento sino all'ultima Messa, e poi si ripone. Vespero in organo, Compieta, e Salve bassa, Mattutino per la Mattina, finito si canta in canto fermo da cappellani il Tantum ergo e Genitori e Panem de coelo, e si dà la Benedizione al Popolo con risposta dell'organo, e cosi si fà in tutta l'ottava in cui si deve cantare la Messa con Ministri parati e Turificazione.
Venerdì à ora competente si và in coro à dire Prima, e Terza bassa, Messa come ne giorni festivi, doppo Sesta, e Nona, di poi si dà la Benedizione come ieri, Vespero al solito, e Compieta e Matutino per il Sabato. [*Venerdì à ora competente*

si dice Prima e Terza bassa, la Messa si è recitata per il passato in canto come ne giorni feriali ma per l'avvenire si lascia ad libitum del Capitolo di cantarla con ministri parati e risposte d'organo in tutta questa Ottava, in cui su l'altare vi sta esposto il santissimo sacramento. Doppo la Messa cantata si recita Sesta, e Nona, di poi si da la Benedizione col Tantum ergo e semplice risposta d'organo come ieri. Vespro si canta in coro al solito, si recita Compieta, Matutino e Laudi per il sabato seguente.]

Sabato tutto come ieri, Vespero, e Compieta al solito, e si suona per questo giorno solo à ore 21: Doppo finito *il tutto* si cantano le Litanie, Salve, e Tantum ergo in organo, e si dà la Benedizione sul tardi.

Domenica infra octavam Corporis Christi, ut heri, Terza si canta, Messa, e Vespero in organo, [*si canta però Terza, Messa e Vespro in Organo*] Compieta, e Matutino bassa, tutto và come ieri.

Lunedì, Martedì, e Mercordì tutto come ieri. [*Lunedì, martedì Mercordì tutto si fà come nell'altri giorni feriali di questa Ottava, eccettuata la Messa cantata, che si potrebbe fare con ministri parati e risposta d'organo senza però la Turificazione, se cosi piacerà come si è detto di sopra al nostro Capitolo.*]

Giovedì ottava del Corpus Domini, Prima et Terza bassa, *si canta* Messa in organo *con ministri parati,* di poi Sesta e Nona e Benedizione ut Supra. Vespero *si canta* in organo *et alla catedra,* Compieta bassa, Salve cantata, poi si principia la processione per la chiesa, e si canta il Pange Lingua, il versetto da soprani, e poi la Benedizione al popolo col suono dell'organo, questa è tutta la funzione dell'ottava del Corpus Domini.

Giugno 24

S. Giovanni Battista: Te Deum, Laudi cantate, Benedictus falsobordone:, Messa e Vespero in organo, Compieta si canta, e l'inni si cantano sopra il Tuono Deus tuorum militum.

Giugno 28

Vigilia di S. Pietro e Paolo; si cantano due Messe una che è di San Leone, e l'altra doppo Nona che è della vigilia *de SS. Apostoli* e primo Vespero solenne *in organo et alla catedra.*

Giugno 29

SS Pietro e Paolo: Te Deum, Laudi cantate, Benedictus falsobordone: Terza cantata, Messa solenne, e Vespero in organo, Compieta cantata, Salve al solito. [*Si osservi, che la Santità di Nostro Signore Benedetto Papa XIV nell'anno 1744 con suo Breve à decretato, che in avvenire si celebri la Festa di detti SS Apostoli speciali protettori di Roma con maggiore solennità, e che per tutta l'Ottava vi sia cappella nelle primarie basiliche et altre chiese dedicate in onore di sudetti Gloriosi Apostoli con l'assistenza del sagro collegio ò pure di altro Ordine della Prelatura secondo la distribitione de giorni de detta Ottava resasi in perpetuum privilegiata.*]

Giugno 30

Commemorazione di S. Paolo *Apostolo,* Messa apparata e risposta d'organo alla Messa.

Luglio 2
Visitatio Beata Maria Vergine. Te Deum, Laudi cantate, Benedictus falsobordone: Compieta bassa, risposte d'organo alla Messa, le Litanie doppo Compieta, solo al secondo Vespero si viene in Domenica.
Luglio 15
Messa in organo per S. Camillo
Luglio 22
Risposte d'organo alla Messa apparata S. Maria Madalena senza turificazione.
Luglio 25
S. Giacomo Apostolo: Te Deum, Laudi cantate, Benedictus falsobordone: Terza cantata, Messa, e Vespero in organo, Compieta cantata.
Luglio 26
S. Anna: Te Deum, Laudi cantate, e Terza, Messa, e Vespero in organo, Compieta cantata. [*Si osservi che la Santità di Nostro Signore Benedetto Papa XIV con suo Breve speciale dell'anno 1743 à concesso Privilegio alla nostra chiesa et Archiospedale di celebrare la Messa et Offcio sub Ritu Duplici del Beato Camillo de Lellis nel giorno de 15 luglio in perpetuum, coll'espositione della reliquia ex ossibus di detto Beato che si conserva in detta nostra chiesa, et altra in detto nostro Archiospedale.*]
Primo Agosto
S. Pietro in Vincula, risposta d'organo alla Messa cantata senza turificazione
Agosto 5
Madre Santissima della Neve, Te Deum Laudi cantate, Benedictus falsobordone: Terza cantata; Messa con Turificazione, e Vespero senz'organo, Litanie doppo Compieta bassa in secondo Vespero.
Agosto 9
SS. Ciriaco & Marco: e vigilia di S. Lorenzo, doppo Terza si canta in coro la Messa dei Santi Martiri e doppo nona quella della vigilia.
Agosto 10
San Lorenzo: Te Deum, Laudi cantate, Benedictus falsobordone: Terza si canta, Messa e Vespero in organo, e Compieta cantata.
Agosto 14
Vigilia dell'Assunta Titolare della nostra Chiesa, doppo Terza si dice la Messa cantata dell'ottava di S. Lorenzo, e doppo Nona quella della vigilia = Primo Vespero in organo solenne, Compieta bassa.
Agosto 15
Assunzione di Maria Vergine: Mattutino solenne cantato, ut in die Epiphaniae, Messa, e Vespero à due cori, *col Panegirico in onore dell'Assuntione di Maria Vergine doppo l'Evangelo della Messa, con l'assistenza del Prelato e Capitolo.* Compieta bassa, e poi Litanie e Salve in organo, per esser festa Titolare di S. Maria in Sassia.
Agosto 16
S. Giacinto: Risposta d'organo alla messa cantata in onore di S. Rocco per il culto Immemorabile

Agosto 22
Ottava dell'Assunta, Te Deum, Laudi cantate, Benedictus falsobordone: Terza cantata, e risposta di Organo alla Messa cantata *e turificatione.*
Agosto 25
S. Bartolomeo Apostolo: Te Deum, Laudi *e Terza* cantate, Benedictus falsobordone: Messa, e Vespero in organo, Compieta cantata *come in tutti l'altri giorni festivi di Precetto.*
Agosto 27
Primo Vespero di S. Agostino Protettore della nostra religione; si canta in organo, et alla catedra con ministri con Piviale, e se ne fà l'ottava per indulto speciale. &
Agosto 28
S. Agostino si fà con ottava, Te Deum in canto figurato [*canto fermo*] con risposta d'organo ad ogni versetto, Laudi cantate apparate, tutti le Gloria Patri in falsobordone: In fine si fà tutto come nell'Epifania, Messa, e Vespero alquanto solenne. [*si cantano le Laudi apparate e l'Hora di Terza con la Messa solenne e Vespro in organo, et alla catedra*]
Agosto 29
Decollatio S. Giovanni Battistae: Risposte di organo alla Messa cantata senza turificazione.
Settembre 8
Natività di Maria Vergine, Te Deum, Laudi cantate, Benedictus falsobordone: Terza si canta, Messa e Vespero in organo, Compieta bassa, Litanie, Salve cantate in organo.
Domenica infra octavam Nativitatis si fà tutto come nel giorno della Natività di Maria Vergine.
Settembre 13
Primo Vespero in organo per la Santissima Croce [*per l'Esaltazione dello santissimo Croce di nostro Signore Gesu Christo di cui ne abbiamo una insigne Reliquia donata con altre alla nostra chiesa da Sisto Papa Quarto di Sancta Memoria*].
Settembre14
Santissima Croce, di cui abbiamo un'insigna reliquia: Te Deum, Laudi cantate, Benedictus falsobordone: Terza cantata, Messa, e Vespero in organo, di poi Compieta bassa, ma se viene in Domenica si canta.
Settembre 21
S. Matteo Apostolo. Te Deum, Laudi cantate, Benedictus falsobordone: Terza cantata, Messa, e Vespero in organo, Compieta cantata.
Settembre 29
S. Michele Arcangelo, Te Deum, Laudi cantate, Benedictus falsobordone: Terza si canta Messa, e Vespero in organo, Compieta cantata.
Ottobre 2
SS. Angelorum Custodum: Te Deum, Laudi cantate, Benedictus falsobordone: Terza si canta, Messa in organo con turificazione, Vespero in coro à cappella. *Compieta bassa perché è giorno feriale.*

Ottobre 4
S. Francesco: Messa parata con sue risposte d'organo senza turificazione [*si canta la Messa parata con sole risposte di organo*].
Ottobre 18
S. Luca Evangelista; risposta d'organo alla Messa cantata, Benedictus, falsobordone:
Ottobre 28
Santi Simone, e Giuda Apostoli, Te Deum, Laudi *e Terza* cantate, Benedictus falsobordone: Messa e Vespero in organo, Compieta cantata
Ottobre 31
Vigilia omnium sanctorum: Primo Vespero Solenne
Primo novembre
Festum Omnium Sanctorum: Matutino si canta come il giorno dell'Epifania, Messa, e Vespero a due cori, finito subito si canta il Vespero de morti, e poi Compieta, finalmente Matutino basso, e tutto letto infra octavam, si canta Prima, si seguita come si è detto nell'Epifania
Novembre 2
Officio de Morti solenne nella prima Aurora si suona à ore undici, finito dicesi Prima, e Terza doppo si canta Messa dell'Ottava da un Cappellano, doppo si và sotto la chiesa à cantare la Messa de Morti, che presentemente si canta dal Parroco all'Altare Privilegiato doppo le Laudi de Defunti Solenne, al fine della quale si ritorna in chiesa, e si da tempo, che si possino celebrare le messe, e poi all'ora solita Vespero consueto alla sua ora, e tempo. [*Si canta in coro l'Officio de Morti della prima Aurora, doppo di cui si canta dal canonico curato la prima Messa de Requiem all'altare privilegiato, et immediatamente si canta da un cappellano la messa dell'Ottava di tutti i santi, e poi all'hora solita si dice Sesta e Nona e si canta la Messa solenne de morti all'altare maggiore.*]
Novembre 3
Doppo Terza cantasi la Messa solita ut infra octavam da un cappellano, poi Sesta, e Nona all'ora solita con la Messa solenne omnium Praeceptorum defunctorum.
Novembre 4
S. Carlo. Risposta d'organo alla Messa cantata, senza turificazione
Novembre 5
Doppo Terza Messa cantata omnium Sanctorum da un cappellano, all'ora solita Sesta, e Nona, e poi Messa solenne Omnium canonicorum mortuorum [*la messa solenne per tutti li nostri Religiosi defunti*].
Novembre 9
Primo Vespero per li Santi Trifone, Respicio & de quali abbiamo li corpi sotto l'Altare maggiore, solenne alla catedra nelle Laudi, e Vesperi seguenti.
Novembre 10
SS.Trifone & Te Deum, Laudi cantate, Benedictus falsobordone: Lect: 1: Noct: de script: 2 ª noct: 2 ª Lect: Sanctorum ut in Mense, 2 ª et 3 ª in Com:plurim: Mart: quotiescumque, terzo noct: Hom: ut in festo SS. Joannis, et Paulis 26 Junii Attendite à fermento Phariseorum, Messa, e Vespero in organo, Gloria

e Credo: Compieta bassa. [*al Matutino basso le lezioni del primo notturno per scriptura occurrente, del secondo notturno la prima de SS. Martiri in die, la seconda e Terza un in Comune plurioruim Martyrium quotiescumque, terzo notturno = homilia ut in festo SS. Ioannis, et Pauli 26 junii: attendite fermento Phariseorum.*

Novembre 11

S. Martino: Risposta d'organo alla Messa cantata, senza turificazione [*Si canta la Messa con risposta di organo e ministri parati alla medesima*].

Novembre 21

Presentatio Beata Maria Vergine: Te Deum, Laudi cantate, Benedictus falsobordone: Terza si canta, e alla Messa risposta d'organo, e se fosse Domenica, Litanie cantate al secondo Vespero solamente, Compieta bassa in giorno feriale, cantata in giorno festivo, non però mai si canta quando si cantano doppo le Litanie. [*Te Deum, Laudi, e Terza cantate et alla messa parata con risposta di organo, e Turificazione, e se fosse Domenica si cantano le Litanie della Madonna al secondo Vespro solamente, recitandosi Compieta in giorno feriale, e si canta in giorno festive, non però mai quando dopo Compieta si devono cantare le Litanie.*]

Novembre 22

S. Cecilia *Vergine e Martire*: Messa cantata in organo, Te Deum, Laudi cantate, Benedictus falsobordone: Terza si canta e Vespero in coro à cappella, Compieta bassa.

Novembre 25

S. Catarina Vergine e Martire: risposte d'organo alla Messa cantata senza turificazione.

Novembre 29 *Vigilia di S. Andrea Apostolo*

Quando si dice il Vespro de' Morti, la Compieta si dice sempre bassa. Vigilia di S. Andrea Apostolo, Primo Vespero in organo perché abbiamo il braccio destro di detto Santo Apostolo.

Novembre 30

S. Andrea Apostolo: Te Deum, Laudi cantate, Benedictus falsobordone: Terza cantata, Messa e Vespero in organo, Compieta si canta.

Dicembre 8

Santissima Concezione: Te Deum, Laudi cantate, Benedictus falsobordone: Terza cantata, Messa e Vespero in organo, Compieta bassa, Litanie & in organo. *Domenica prima dell'Avvento al solito.*

Domenica prima dell'Avvento: Mattutino letto, Laudi cantate, Benedictus falsobordone: Terza al solito cantata, Messa, e Vespero in organo, Compieta si canta.

Dicembre 13

S. Lucia: Risposta d'organo alla Messa cantata solenne con turificazione.

Dicembre 15

Ottava di Maria Santissima Concetta, accadendo le quattro tempora doppo Terza Messa dell'Ottava, e doppo Nona della Vigilia.

Dicembre 21

S. Tommaso Apostolo: Te Deum, Laudi cantate, Benedictus falsobordone: Terza si canta, Messa e Vespero in organo, Compieta si canta.
Dicembre 24 e 25
Vigilia del Santissimo Natale, Matutino feriale, Laudi cantate doppie, Benedictus falsobordone. Prima si canta, il Martirologio solenne con Piviale dal Parroco, e due cappellani assistenti e con l'assistenza del Capitolo con due candelabri con incensazione del Testo del libro.
Finito l'annunzio del Santissimo Natale il cappellano ebdomadario siegue il restante del Martirologio in Tono Prophetiae; Terza e Sesta bassa, Nona cantata, Messa apparata, e si canta in coro à cappella.
Primo Vespero solenne in organo.
Mattutino della Notte à ore Otto, ed ora à ore 9 perché non vi è più la Musica, ma il canto Gregoriano, e tutto và cantato, Invitatorio, Inni, in questa notte alla catedra e responsori in canto figurato, l'intonazione de Salmi si fà in organo dal cappellano ebdomadario, e in tutti li salmi, il Gloria Patri si cantano in falsobordone, Te Deum cantato in canto figurato, e in tanto si incensa l'Altare, al fine del quale entra la Messa cantata solenne, e finita si cantano le Laudi parate, e cantate con risposta di organo, e Antifone in contrapunto pure in organo: Inno in canto figurato, Benedictus in falsobordone; Prima si canta in coro, cosi anco il Martirologio, Terminata prima, si canta la seconda Messa con risposte d'organo in coro. Finalmente à ora competente si canta Terza, Messa solennemente in organo à due cori, Vespero al solito, Compieta cantata.
Dicembre 26
S. Stefano. Matutino solenne cantate, tutto come nell'Epifania, compieta cantata.
Dicembre 27
S. Giovanni Apostolo et Evangelista come ieri Solenne, cioè Matutino etc. cantata.
Dicembre 28
SS. Innocenti. Matutino basso, Laudi cantate, Benedictus falsobordone: Terza si canta, Messa e Vespero in organo, Compieta cantata.
Dicembre 31
S. Silvestro. Te Deum, Laudi cantate, Terza cantata, Messa e Vespero in organo, Compieta cantata.

Deo Gratias
Die Primae Januarii 1752
Asperuetur in sacrario nostrae Ecclesie et observetur ab omnibus vista presentem statem.
G. A. Bufalini S. Spiritus praeceptore

Rubric to be observed throughout the year for the feasts which happen in the venerable collegiate and parish church of S. Spirito in Sassia in Rome copied from its authentic original which has been kept in the sacristy of the same church since the year 1644

And reduced to the method that is observed at present according to the reform made by the Apostolic Visitation of the year 1738.[2]

All Sundays of the year if it is not a privileged feast, Matins are said reading, Lauds and Benedictus sung.

[*In all simple and ferial days, the office of the Blessed Virgin is recited in addition to the ferial office.*]

On all Sundays of Lent, for the Sunday Offices unless it is otherwise noted, the organ is never played but the choir sings a cappella.

[*The first day of the month, nothing should prevent the recitation of Vespers, Nocturnes and Lauds for the dead.*]

All the ferial days of Lent, one sings Compline at 23 hours; and now it is introduced at 20 hours.[3]

On all the Sundays of Advent, the Sunday Offices are sung a cappella in the choir and the organ is never played unless it is otherwise noted.

All Saturdays of the year the Holy Sacrament is exposed at 23 hours with motets, Litanies, Salve, or others, according to the season, Tantum ergo and the Benediction

At the time of the forty-hours devotion one observes that which is noted below: After Terce, the conventual Mass of the saint or ferial [Mass] is sung by a canon or chaplain, according with the Office, then Sext is said and Nones is sung. When Nones is finished, the Organ Mass is sung, all as in the day of Corpus Domini. After Mass is ended, one returns to the choir and the parts for the Pange Lingua are distributed which is sung in the procession. Having returned to the church two of the chaplains come on foot to the High Altar and wait there until the Master of ceremonies advises, then the Litany of the Saints is sung.

The second day of the forty hours: Conventual Mass à cappella in the choir, sung by a canon *or chaplain* with embellished Ministers:[4] After Nones an organ

2 The Apostolic Visitation started in December 1737 with decrees issued at various times thereafter.

3 This is clearly a change from earlier versions presumably since 1738. Times are given in *Ore italiane* – a twenty-four-hour clock in which time was calculated from sunset. From the mid-seventeenth century the Angelus marking twenty-four hours was rung about half an hour after sunset. Compline at twenty-three hours would have been just before sunset.

4 This relates to Vai's instructions regarding the correct number of pluvials to be worn for various feast days.

mass against paganism is sung without Gloria and Credo, but if it happens on Sunday the Credo is said.
The introit for this Mass as in Sexagesima Sunday.

The third day: After Terce the conventual Mass is sung in the choir by a chaplain or canon. After Nones, the organ mass is sung, and one does the same as on the first day, *that is as for Corpus Domini*. There is no difference other than the Litanies are said before the procession at the sign from the Master of Ceremonies.

All the Saturdays of the year, the Saturday Office of St Mary is done, organ responses to the sung Mass at the altar of the Madonna.

When a feast day falls by obligation on a Saturday, low Compline is said because the Litanies are sung for the Benediction [*because of the Benediction*].
January first

Holy Circumcision: Low Matins; Te Deum, sung Lauds, Benedictus falsobordone. Mass and Vespers with organ. Here it is observed that since the Apostolic Visitation in 1737, the polyphony with organ has been reduced to Gregorian chant in the choir.
5th day [5 January]
First Vespers of Epiphany with organ.
Sixth day *of said Epiphany*
Solemn sung Matins, all the Gloria Patri in falsobordone, and at all the finals (cadences) the organ plays. Te Deum in polyphony, and organ responses to every verse. Lauds is sung, and a canon or assistant with pluvials assists as at Vespers; Benedictus in falsobordone and organ responses with every verse to give time to incense the altar. The Hour of Prime is sung, Martyriology and Terce (sung), Mass and Vespers with organ; Compline is sung.
Second Sunday after Epiphany: Te Deum, sung Lauds, Benedictus in falsobordone, sung Terce, Mass and Vespers with organ, Compline is sung.
January 17
St Anthony Abbot: Organ response to the sung Mass without incense.[5]
January 20
Saints Fabian and Sebastian: Organ response to the sung Mass without incense.
January 25
Conversion of St. Paul: Organ response[6] to the sung Mass without incense; as one does only when Lauds is sung.[7]
February 2

[5] In OSS 1298 the explicit direction 'senza turificazione' is missing, using instead the vaguer *messa cantata parata*. The days that follow, instead of spelling out 'without thurification' are simply '*come sopra*' – 'as above'.

[6] The description of alternatim performance with the organ is inconsistent, using both singular and plural forms of 'response'.

[7] This last phrase is missing in OSS 1298.

Purification of the Blessed Virgin Mary: Matins is read. Te Deum and Lauds sung, Benedictus falsobordone, Terce is sung then the blessing of the candles at which time versetti are sung in plainchant in the choir, 'on the book'[8] and one does the procession after the distribution [of the candles]. On the streets *or in the church* Responsum accepit Simeon is sung, which is in the booklets. The procession finished, Mass is sung and Vespers with organ, low Compline, Litanies with organ, and Ave Regina *in front of the altar of the Madonna.*
Ash Wednesday
Ash Wednesday, Psalms from the gradual, Matins of the most holy Madonna then the current Matins. After Nones, Mass is sung with ministers assisting and before [Mass] the blessing *and distribution* of the Ashes is done, after Mass, the sermon, which is now dispensed with for all of Lent.[9]
All the Fridays of Lent, Matins of the Virgin Mary and then the current, penitential Psalms on the knees. After Nones, sung Mass and sermon.
First Sunday of Lent, sung Lauds, Benedictus falsobordone, sung Terce, sung Mass in the choir, when finished the sermon is said, then one returns to the choir to say Sext and Nones.
February 24 or 25
St Matthew the Apostle: Te Deum, sung Lauds, Benedictus falsobordone, sung Terce, Organ Mass of the saint at the correct time. If it falls during Lent, after Nones the ferial Mass is sung in the choir, then the sermon, after which, organ Vespers. It continues this way all the days of Lent.
March 9
St Francesca Romana: Organ responses to the Mass of the saint. After Nones the current ferial Mass.
Fourth Sunday of Lent. Sung Lauds, Benedictus falsobordone, sung Terce, Mass and Vespers with organ.
Passion Sunday: Benedictus falsobordone, Mass and Vespers a cappella in the choir.[10]
March 25
Most Holy Annunciation: Benedictus falsobordone, after Terce, Mass with organ [*Terce is sung, then organ Mass*]; when finished return to say Sext and Nones and then the ferial Mass a cappella; when finished, one goes to sing another Mass at the oratorio of the brothers past the hospital; after which one returns to sing Vespers with organ at 20 hours. Compline is also sung with organ; when finished, the sermon is said, then one sings the Litanies and Ave Regina. [marginal note: all offices, Nones sung, after the ferial Mass one goes to the oratorio where the Mass of the Madonna is sung.]
Palm Sunday: Benedictus falsobordone, sung Terce then Mass. Before [the Mass] Asperges is sung in the usual way in the choir, then the blessing of the

8 'ut in libro' indicates improvised counterpoint on the given chant verse.

9 The last phrase is missing in OSS 1298.

10 OSS 1298 does not state it should be a cappella.

palms, and the choir comes singing in plainchant Hosanna. The Sanctus in polyphony, at the distribution of the palms Pueri Hebreorum by Victoria is sung; when finished, the deacon says Procedamus in Pace, the choir responds in Nomine Christi – Amen and the procession begins and the chaplains sing Turba multa which is in the booklets. Arriving at the door of the church two of the chaplains sing from inside while the others who are outside sing in polyphony Gloria Laus[11] and those who are inside sing in plainchant the verses that are in the ritual, and they sing in alternatim until the sub-deacon strikes the door of the church with the rod of the cross, the door opens and Ingrediente Domino is sung. The procession ended, the introit begins Domine P[ater] then Kyrie Eleison 'alla Palestrina'[12] after the Epistle, its gradual, Tract and versetti in plainchant, then the Passion by three canons[13] and the responds of the crowd in 4 voices in polyphony by Victoria. The Passion finished, the Credo is sung, the Offertory *Improperium* with Sanctus and the [*its*] motet for 6 voices at the elevation. Agnus Dei as usual, post Communion. The Mass finished, Sext and Nones are said. Then the last Mass by the hebdomadary. Vespers at 20 hours a cappella in the choir, low Compline, Ave Regina and so it ends. Then the sermon that since 1714 is omitted for all of Lent.

Holy Monday: only the current Matins, after Nones, the Mass is sung with attendants wearing vestments. When finished Vespers is sung as usual, at 23 hours Compline is sung.

Holy Tuesday: Matins as above and also the Mass. The Passion is sung by three chaplains of the first choir, after the Mass, Vespers as usual, Compline as yesterday.

Holy Wednesday: Matins as above; Mass as yesterday, the first lesson is said in the Tono prophetiae by the last chaplain, the Epistle is sung by the sub-deacon in the Tono epistole; the Passion is sung by the three chaplains of the second choir, after Mass, Vespers is sung, Compline at 20 hours, *semi* low because when finished Solemn Matins is immediately sung without organ because it is Holy week. The first responses are sung in the booklets, the responses of the second and third nocturnes are sung from the book by Victoria, Benedictus and Miserere of the same.

Holy Thursday at appropriate times the low Offices are sung [*recited*], that is Prime, Terce, Sext and Nones as in the breviary, when finished Mass is sung. The Kyrie in the choir, before the Gloria starts the organ is played a little. After the Epistle, the gradual is recited slowly in plainchant to give time. After the Evangelist the Credo is said, and the Offertory Dextera Domini. At the general communion Cenatibus illis in four voices in the booklets is sung. The post-Communion in plainchant and then the procession begins, singing Pange lingua etc. The procession ended one returns to the choir and says Vespers, the

11 The hymn 'Gloria, laus et honor' which has a response between each verse.

12 In the style of Palestrina or perhaps by Palestrina.

13 The number of canons is not in OSS 1298.

celebrant intones the antiphon quietly. Vespers ended the celebrants intones again Diviserunt which is the antiphon, and while the altars are stripped, one comes reciting the psalm Deus, Deus meus respice in me, when [the psalm is] finished Diviserunt is repeated. Then midday is sounded and the Ave Maria is recited kneeling in the choir, and then without other motive one leaves the choir. Compline at 20 hours and semi-low, Matins as in the breviary, at the end, everything as yesterday.

Holy Friday. At the appropriate time one goes to the choir and says all the Hours as yesterday, then the celebrant comes to the altar with assistants and the last chaplain sings the lesson in the tono prophetiae, at the end of which one sings the Tract in the choir. Finished the gentlemen canons (as usual on Palm Sunday) sing the Passion of St John with the 'turba' responses in the choir in the book by Victoria. Once ended, after the prayers the celebrant intones Ecce lignam crucis, the two tenors follow after the choir respond Venite adoremus. The adoration ended, one goes to the *holy* sepulchre, the torches are lit, the celebrant receives the sacrament from the hands of the deacon and in the procession Vexilla Regis prodeunt is recited in plainchant. This ended, the priest follows the function as in the missal. Afterwards, Vespers is sung as yesterday. At 20 hours [*twenty and a half hours*], Compline is said and Matins is sung as in the breviary, as yesterday. After Lauds one goes to the altar of the Crucifix and sings Vere languores nostros by Victoria.

Holy Saturday. At an appropriate hour one says all the Hours as yesterday and then one goes in procession outside the church, assisting the Chapter at the Benediction of the fire [light]. One returns in procession to the church and one of the three candles is lit for the Lumen Christi, after which all are lit and the Exultet and the Prophecy are sung. Then one goes again in procession singing Sicut cervus. When finished the font is blessed which is done by the Canon Curate with the assistance of the Chapter. When ended one returns in procession singing the Litany for Holy Saturday. On reaching the Kyrie one sings in the choir in polyphony a cappella. Before the beginning of the Gloria the organ is played somewhat and bells are rung, and then the rest [of the mass] in the choir. The celebrant intones the first Alleluia after the Epistle and then the choir responds, two tenors chant Confitemini and two sopranos chant Laudate, two basses Quoniam confirmata est.

After taking the sacrament, the bass intones Alleluia, the rest is sung in counterpoint, Laudate Dominum in falsobordone, finishing with a repeat of Alleluia as above, then the Celebrant intones Vespere autem Sabbati, the choir responds to that which follows. The Magnificat of Morales is sung and the organ responds for every verse. Sicut erat in falsobordone, the Deo gratia is said [chanted] in unison with organ.

Compline as usual sung because at 23 hours with the exposition of the most Holy Sacrament, Litanies, Regina Coeli, and Tantum ergo and the blessing is given to the people.

Easter day:

Solemn Matins with organ responses, Te Deum in polyphony, Lauds embellished the same as Vespers, in place of the Capitolo, Haec dies in polyphony a cappella, Prime and Terce sung and a solemn organ Mass in the fifth tone is played, then Sext and Nones *are recited* in the choir.
At 19 hours: Vespers is sung *with organ in catedra*, in place of the hymn Haec dies is sung in 8 voices. Compline is sung because there is no longer the usual sermon [*Low Compline is said because at the end there is the sermon*].
Monday and Tuesday of Easter all as for yesterday, except that after the sung Mass, one no longer gives a sermon. When finished return to the choir to say Sext and Nones = Vespers as usual, Compline sung [*Compline is sung as for the first day*].
All of this octave at the sung Mass, Haec dies, Victime paschali is sung a cappella with that which follows in the missal.
April 25
St Mark the Evangelist: organ responses to the Mass embellished for the saint.
Domenica in Albis, Te Deum, Lauds sung, Benedictus falsobordone: Terce sung, Mass and Vespers with organ. *Compline is sung.*
May first
Saints Phillip and James: Te Deum, sung Lauds, Benedictus falsobordone, Terce sung, Mass and Vespers with organ, sung Compline.
May 2
Feast of the Holy Cross of which we have a holy relic = First Vespers with organ, low Compline because it falls on a ferial day.
May 3
[*In veneration of the*] Holy Cross: Te Deum and Lauds sung, Benedictus falsobordone, Terce sung and Mass and Vespers with organ. Compline sung.
Monday, first day of Rogation; if a double feast or semi-double feast falls on this day one does its office, and after Prime Mass is sung by a chaplain and after Terce another Mass is sung by the hebdomadary Canon.
Rogation Tuesday everything is observed yesterday.
Rogation Wednesday: Mass of the saint is sung by one of the chaplains. After Sext because it is the vigil of Ascension the second Mass of the vigil is sung by another chaplain, and after that the Mass of the Rogation is sung by the hebdomadary Canon and Solemn Vespers are sung with organ for the first Vespers of Ascension.
Ascension Thursday: Matins and everything is done and sung as on the day of Epiphany. Solemn Mass and Vespers with organ with two choirs, sung Compline.
May 17
First Vespers with organ for the dedication of our church [18 May].

Dedication: – *double of the first class with octave* – low Matins, Te Deum in polyphony with organ response to every verse, Lauds celebrated from the cathedra[14], the whole is done as for the day of Epiphany.
[Note that the procession of the Chapter of the whole house, and spinsters of the Conservatory to the Basilica of St Peters was abolished by the Apostolic Visitation in 1738.]
Vigil of Pentecost: After Nones the blessing of the font is done by the singer-Curate with the assistance of the Chapter, and in the same manner observed on Holy Saturday, all in the missal. In the procession the motet Sicut cervus is sung. Litanies as on Holy Saturday; Mass in the choir with organ responses and six Prophecies, and solemn first Vespers with organ and from the cathedra.
Pentecost: sung Matins and all is done as at Easter. If the pope comes, the most Holy Sacrament is exposed on the Monday following as usual. Ordinary Mass and Vespers with organ, low Compline and then Matins for the Monday are read.
Monday at an appropriate hour without onlookers and without music the Holy Sacrament is exposed. When the papal and general procession is finished one goes to the choir and says the Hours of low Prime, Terce and one sings Mass with the organ, a short one for being late, after which one returns to the choir and says Sext and Nones. Solemn Vespers for the feast day of the church, Compline and low Matins for the following day and then at the Ave Maria the Tantum ergo is sung in cantus firmus or polyphony with organ and the blessing is given to the people. At the procession of the maidens that goes to St Peter's on the Tuesday the musicians of St Peter's choose and take motets to sing in the street. On the return the Te Deum is sung as it is in the libretti. When they arrive in church, the organist plays the organ until all the dowries are given to the maidens and then one goes into the choir and says low Prime. Terce is sung, and after [Terce] the solemn Mass in four choirs. When it is finished, Sext is said, and Nones. Solemn Vespers in four choirs, Tantum ergo from the musicians of the first choir, Benediction and low Compline. Said on solemn Tuesday as for Monday. [*Tuesday one goes in procession with our maidens to the Basilica of St Peter and on the streets the Litany of the Saints, Te Deum etc is sung, and the first Chapter of St Peter's blesses our family with the monstrances of the three very distinguished relics, and then one returns singing to our church, where on arrival the organist plays until Monsignor the commendatore has given dowries to all the maidens, and afterwards one says low Prime...*[15] *It is observed that since the pontificate of Benedict XIII*[16] *until the present, the pope with the Sacred*

[14] The term cathedra refers to the ceremonial throne, traditionally used by a bishop, but also by senior clergy such as an abbot in a monastic setting. This seems to infer that the Offices in cathedra were led by one of the senior members of the Order.

[15] The remainder of the directive is identical in the two sources up to the additional material concerning the procession which only appears in OSS 1298.

[16] Pope Benedict XIII Orsini (r. 1724–1730).

College no longer come in procession to our church, and from the year 1738 the procession of our maidens to St Peter's has been suspended, but in this triduo all is as customary for Easter; therefore on the second day of Pentecost solemnised with music, the music has been removed by the Sacred Apostolic Visitation since the first of November 1737 and Gregorian chant introduced, however the whole church is decorated by the master of ceremonies as before.]

Wednesday fourth day of Pentecost all the Offices are low, said. After Nones, Mass is sung with attendants, the first lesson is sung in *Tono prophetiae* by the last chaplain, Vespers as usual in the choir, low Compline.

Thursday: Matins as yesterday, sung Mass with appropriate embellishment after Terce and everything as yesterday.

Friday: After Nones, Mass is sung in the choir, as in the missal with ministers appropriately dressed. Saturday as above, the Prophecies said by the chaplains one by one.

[*Wednesday fourth day of Pentecost, Matins is said low and after Nones Mass is sung with ministers assisting, the same as all the days of this privileged octave and on the Saturday after Pentecost and the two subsequent days, the most holy sacrament is exposed for 40 hours, during which is observed the instructions that are renewed in each pontificate for this solemnity*].

Sunday of Holy Trinity: Te Deum, Lauds sung, Benedictus falsobordone. Prime sung and also the martyrology for the Creed Quicumque.[17] Terce sung, Mass and Vespers with organ, Compline sung.

Wednesday first Vespers with organ for Corpus Domini, Compline and Salve low then low Matins for the following morning, which continues for the whole octave.

Thursday Corpus Domini: When the papal procession from St Peter's is at St Giacomo Scossacavalli, *our church* starts to play then one enters in the choir and says Prime, Terce and low Sext, Nones is sung.

The hymn is sung on *the tone of the* Hymn of the Madonna = the Psalm Mirabilia is sung in the tone of the choir book, Mass with organ, when finished the parts of the Pange lingua are distributed and the procession begins. When the foot of the hospital is reached where there is an Altar placed, the blessing is given to the castle, [*which responds by firing the cannons*] after firing, one comes singing the Tantum ergo, and returns to the hospital, pausing at the altar and once more singing the Tantum ergo and with the versetto Panem de Coelo from the sopranos, and the blessing is given to the patients. [*one enters the hospital singing as before, and the celebrant places the Sacrament on the altar in the middle and the Tantum ergo is sung again and the benediction given.*] From there one goes to the nuns and maidens and one does the same at the church of St Tecla. At the door of the conservatory the same blessing is given, the maidens first singing the Tantum ergo, one then returns to the church sing-

17 This reference to the Athanasian Creed, 'Quicumque Vult', is explicit in OSS 1298, but assumed knowledge in 1752.

ing the Tantum ergo in the same way with the versetto from the sopranos as above, prayers are said and the blessing given, the Holy sacrament is exposed until the last Mass and then one retires. Vespers with organ, low Compline and Salve, Matins for the morning. When finished the chaplains sing the Tantum ergo and Genitori and Panem de coelo in plainchant and the blessing is given to the people with organ responses. So it is done for the whole octave in which one must sing the Mass with ministers in embellished vestments and incense.[18]
Friday at the appropriate hour go to the choir to say Prime, low Terce, mass as on feast days, after Sext and Nones then the blessing is given again as yesterday. Vespers as usual and Compline and Matins for Saturday. [*Friday at an appropriate hour Prime and Terce are said, low, the Mass that in the past was recited in chant as for ferial days but for the future is left to the choice of the Chapter to sing it with ministers in vestments with organ responses for the whole Octave in which the holy sacrament is exposed on the altar. After the sung Mass, Sext and Nones are recited and then the Benediction with Tantum ergo and simple organ responses as yesterday. Vespers is sung in the choir as usual, Compline, Matins and Lauds for the following Saturday recited.*]
Saturday everything as yesterday. Vespers and Compline as usual and for this day only it is sounded at 21 hours.[19] When finished the Litanies are sung, Salve and Tantum ergo with organ and the blessing is given to aged.
Sunday Octave of Corpus Domini: as yesterday. Sung Terce, Mass and Vespers with organ, low Compline and Matins. Everything as yesterday.
Monday, Tuesday and Wednesday all as yesterday. [*Monday, Tuesday, Wednesday all is done as for other ferial days of this Octave, except the sung Mass that could be done with ministers in vestments and organ responses without incense however, if it will please our Chapter as it is said above.*]
Thursday octave of Corpus Domini: low Prime and Terce, *sung* Mass with organ *and ministers in vestments* then Sext and Nones, Benediction as above. Vespers *sung* with organ, *led from the cathedra,* low Compline, sung Salve then the procession to the church begins and the Pange Lingua is sung, the versetto by the sopranos, and the blessing of the people with organ playing. This is all the business of the octave of Corpus Domini.
June 24
St John the Baptist: Te Deum, sung Lauds, Benedictus falsobordone. Mass and Vespers with organ, Compline sung and the hymn sung on the tone Deus tuorum militum.
June 28
Vigil of Sts Peter and Paul: Two masses are sung, of which one is St Leo, and the other after Nones that is for the vigil *of the holy Apostles* and solemn first Vespers *with organ and from the chair.*

18 Although OSS 1298 outlines the same procession and rituals, there are fewer details regarding the plainchant for the final part of the day.

19 Presumably this means the bell that marks the start of Vespers is sounded at that time.

June 29
Sts Peter and Paul: Te Deum, sung Lauds, Benedictus falsobordone. Terce is sung, solemn Mass and Vespers with organ, sung Compline, Salve as usual. [*It is observed that His holiness our Lord Pope Benedict XIV in the year 1744 decreed in his Breve that in future the feast of said holy Apostles, special protectors of Rome, be celebrated with major solemnity and that for the whole Octave it would be celebrated in the primary basilicas and other churches dedicated in honour of abovesaid glorious apostles with the assistance of sacred College or further of other orders of prelates according to the distribution of days of said Octave, privileged in perpetuity.*]
June 30
Commemoration of St Paul *Apostle*: embellished Mass and organ response to the Mass
July 2
Visitation of the Blessed Virgin Mary: Te Deum, sung Lauds, Benedictus falsobordone, low Compline, organ responses to the Mass, Litanies after Compline, but only after second Vespers if it falls on Sunday.
July 15
Organ mass for St Camillo.[20]
July 22
Organ responses to the mass embellished for St Mary Magdalene without incense.
July 25
St James the Apostle: Te Deum, sung Lauds, Benedictus falsobordone. Sung Terce, Mass and Vespers with organ, sung Compline.
July 26
St Anne. Te Deum, sung Lauds and Terce, Mass and Vespers with organ, sung Compline. [*It is observed that His Holiness our pope Benedict XIV ceded a privilege to our church and arch-hospital to celebrate under a double rite the Mass and Office of the Blessed Camillo de Lellis on 15 July in perpetuum with the exposure of the relics of the bones of said Blessed that are kept in our church and the other in our arch-hospital.*]
August first
St Peter in chains. Organ response to the sung mass without incense.
August 5
Holy Mother of the Snow. Te Deum, sung Lauds, Benedictus falsobordone, sung Terce, Mass with incense and Vespers without organ, Litanies after low Compline in second Vespers.
August 9
Sts Cyriac & Martyrs and vigil of St Lawrence. After Terce the mass of the holy martyrs is sung in the choir and after Nones that of the vigil.
August 10

[20] This feast is missing in OSS 1298.

St Lawrence. Te Deum, sung Lauds, Benedictus falsobordone, Terce is sung Mass and Vespers with organ and sung Compline.
August 14
Vigil of the Assumption, titular of our church. After Terce the Mass of the octave of St Lawrence is sung and after Nones that of the vigil. Solemn first Vespers with organ, low Compline.
August 15
Assumption of the Virgin Mary. Solemn sung Matins as for Epiphany. Mass and Vespers for two choirs, *with the panegyric in honour of the Assumption of the Virgin Mary after the Evangelist of the Mass, with the assistance of the Prelate and Chapter,* low Compline and then Litanies and Salve with organ as it is the titular feast of St Mary in Sassia.
August 16.
St Giacinto: Organ response to the mass sung in honour of St Rock for immemorial worship.
August 22
Octave of the Assumption. Te Deum, sung Lauds, Benedictus falsobordone, sung Terce and organ response to the sung mass *with incense.*
August 25
St Bartholomew the Apostle. Sung Te Deum, Lauds, *and Terce* Benedictus falsobordone, Mass and Vespers with organ, sung Compline *as for all other feasts of precept.*
August 27
First Vespers of St Augustine Protector of our Order is sung with organ and in from the cathedra with ministers wearing pluvials, and it is done thus at the Octave for special indulgences etc.
August 28
St Augustine is done with its Octave, Te Deum in polyphony [*plainchant*] with organ responses to every verse. Embellished sung Lauds, all the Gloria Patri in falsobordone. In fact everything is done as for Epiphany. Mass and Vespers equally solemn. [*Embellished Lauds and the hour of Terce with Solemn Mass and Vespers are sung with organ led from the cathedra*]
August 29
Beheading of John the Baptist: Organ responses to the mass without incense.
September 8
Nativity of the Virgin Mary: Te Deum, sung Lauds, Benedictus falsobordone. Terce is sung, Mass and Vespers [sung] with organ, low Compline, Litanies and Salve sung with organ.
Sunday Octave of the Nativity everything is done the same as the day of the nativity of the Virgin Mary.
September 13
First Vespers with organ for the most Holy Cross [*for the exaltation of the most holy cross of our Lord Jesus Christ of which we have a precious relic donated with others by Pope Sixtus IV of blessed memory*].
September 14

Holy Cross of which we have a precious relic. Te Deum, sung Lauds, Benedictus falsobordone. Terce is sung, Mass and Vespers with organ and then low Compline but if it falls on Sunday it is sung.

September 21

St Matthew the Apostle. Te Deum, sung Lauds, Benedictus falsobordone. Sung Terce, Mass and Vespers with organ, sung Compline.

September 29

St Michael Archangel. Te Deum, sung Lauds, Benedictus falsobordone. Terce is sung, Mass and Vespers [sung] with organ, sung Compline.

October 2

Holy Guardian Angels: Te Deum, sung Lauds, Benedictus falsobordone. Terce is sung, Mass with organ and incense. Vespers in the choir a cappella. *Low Compline because it is a ferial day.*

October 4

St Francis. Embellished Mass with its organ responses without incense. [*Embellished Mass is sung only with its organ responses.*]

October 18

St Luke the evangelist. Organ response to the sung mass, Benedictus falsobordone.[21]

October 28

Sts Simon and Jude Apostles. Te Deum, sung Lauds, Benedictus falsobordone *and Terce.* Mass and Vespers with organ, sung Compline.

October 31

Vigil of All Saints. Solemn first Vespers.

First November

Feast of All Saints: Sung Matins the same as the day of Epiphany. Mass and Vespers for two choirs. Vespers for the dead is sung immediately after and then Compline, finally low Matins, and all as read for the Octave, Prime is sung then it follows as for Epiphany.

November 2

Solemn Office of the dead, at first light of dawn [the bell] is sounded at 11 hours,[22] when finished Prime and Terce are said, afterwards a chaplain sings the Mass of the Octave, afterwards one goes under the church to sing the Mass of the dead which presently is sung by the parish priest at the chosen altar. Afterwards solemn Lauds for the dead at the end of which one returns to church and if there is time, one can celebrate Mass and then at the usual hour Vespers customary to the time and season. [*The Office of the dead is sung in the choir at first light, after which the first Requiem Mass is sung by the curate-canon at the privileged altar, and immediately the Mass of the Octave of All Saints is sung by a chaplain and then at the usual hour Sext and Nones are said and the solemn Mass of the dead is sung at the high altar*]

21 OSS 1298 is fundamentally the same, but noted 'as for the day above'.

22 *In Ore italiane*: this means eleven hours after sunset, thus around 6:30 am.

November 3[23]
After Terce the usual Mass of the octave is sung by a chaplain, then Sext and Nones at the usual hour with the solemn Mass for all dead preceptors.
November 4
St Charles: organ response to the sung Mass without incense.
November 5
After Terce a Mass for All Saints is sung by a chaplain, at the usual hour, Sext and Nones and then solemn Mass for all of the dead canons. [*Solemn Mass for all the dead of our Order.*]
November 9
Solemn first Vespers in the nave for Saints Tryphon and Respicius etc. whose bodies we have under the high altar.[24] Lauds and Vespers following.
November 10
Saints Tryphon etc. Te Deum, sung Lauds, Benedictus falsobordone. [*At low Matins the Lessons of the first Nocturne as for the current scripture, of the second Nocturne, the first [Lesson] of the holy martyrs of the day, the second and third [Lesson] from the Common of the Saints, starting quotiescumque, the third Nocturne, from the homily for the feast of Saints John and Paul 26 June, 'beware the leaven of the pharisees.'*] Mass and Vespers with organ, Gloria and Credo. Low Compline.[25]
November 11
St Martin: Organ response to the sung mass without incense.
November 21
Presentation of the Blessed Virgin Mary: Te Deum, sung Lauds, Benedictus falsobordone. Terce is sung and at Mass responses from the organ and if it is a Sunday, Litanies sung only at second Vespers, low Compline on a ferial day, sung on feast day, nevertheless never sung when the Litanies are sung afterwards. *Te Deum, Lauds and Terce sung and at the embellished Mass with organ responses and incense, and if it is a Sunday the Litany of the Madonna is sung only at second Vespers, Compline is recited for a ferial day, sung for a festive day but never when the Litanies must be sung after Compline.*
November 22
St Cecilia *virgin and martyr*. Sung Mass with organ, Te Deum, sung Lauds, Benedictus falsobordone. Terce sung and Vespers in the choir a cappella, low Compline.

23 OSS 1298 adds a long digression about the singing of a solemn Requiem Mass for the most recent commendatore who did not die in the house but was commendatore at the time of his death, in the same way that a Requiem Mass is sung for Monsignor Zosino Valignani who died in his home town of Chieti during the time he was commendatore.

24 That is, the relics of Saints Tryphon, Repicius and Nympha that were preserved at Santo Spirito.

25 The scribal abbreviations in this instruction have been untangled with reference to OSS 1298 which is more comprehensible.

November 25
St Catherine Virgin and Martyr. Organ responses to sung mass without incense.
November 29 *Vigil of S. Andrew the Apostle*
When the Vespers of the dead are said, Compline is always low. Vigil of St Andrew the Apostle. First Vespers with organ because we have the right arm of said Holy Apostle.[26]
November 30
St Andrew the Apostle: Te Deum, sung Lauds, Benedictus falsobordone. Terce sung, Mass and Vespers with organ, Compline sung.
December 8
Holy Conception: Te Deum, sung Lauds, Benedictus falsobordone. Terce sung, Mass and Vespers with organ, low Compline, Litanies etc. with organ. *First Sunday of Advent as usual.*
First Sunday of Advent: read Matins, sung Lauds, Benedictus falsobordone. Terce sung as usual, Mass and Vespers with organ, Compline is sung.
December 13
St Lucy. Organ response to solemn sung mass with incense.
December 15
Octave of the Holy Conception of Mary, falling on the fourth Ember Day, after Terce, Mass of the Octave, and after Nones [the Mass] of the vigil.[27]
December 21
St Thomas the Apostle. Te Deum, sung Lauds, Benedictus falsobordone. Terce is sung, Mass and Vespers with organ, Compline is sung.
December 24 and 25[28]
Vigil of the most Holy Nativity. Ferial Matins, double Lauds sung, Benedictus falsobordone. Prime is sung, the solemn Martyrology with vestments of the parish priest and two assistant chaplains and with assistance of the Chapter with two candelabra with censing of the text of the book.
At the end of the announcement of the Holy Nativity the hebdomadary chaplain follows with the remainder of the martyrology in tono prophetiae. Low Terce and Sext, sung Nones, Embellished mass sung in the choir à cappella.
Solemn first Vespers with organ.
Matins of the night at 8 hours and at 9 hours because there is no longer music but Gregorian chant.[29] All is sung, Invitation, Hymns, for this night from the cathedra with responses in polyphony. The intonation of the psalms is done by the hebdomadary with organ and in all the Psalms the Gloria Patri is sung in falsobordone. Te Deum sung in polyphony while the altar is incensed, after

[26] OSS 1298 adds that the relic was donated by Pope Sixtus IV.

[27] This feast is missing in OSS 1298.

[28] OSS 1298 lacks a lot of the detail and runs together the two following feasts with that of Christmas.

[29] In other words, there is no longer polyphony. This seems to be immediately contradicted in the passage that follows.

which the solemn sung Mass starts. When finished embellished Lauds are sung with organ responses and antiphons in counterpoint also with organ. Hymns in polyphony, Benedictus in falsobordone. Prime is sung in the choir so also the Martyrology, after Prime the second Mass is sung in the choir with organ responses. Finally at an appropriate hour Terce is sung. Solemn Mass with organ for two choirs, Vespers as usual, sung Compline.

December 26

St Stephen. Solemn sung Matins, all as for Epiphany, sung Compline.

December 27

St John Apostle and Evangelist. As yesterday, that is Matins etc. sung.

December 28

Holy innocents. Low Matins, sung Lauds, Benedictus falsobordone. Terce is sung, Mass and Vespers with organ, sung Compline.

December 31

St Silvester. Te Deum, sung Lauds, sung Terce Mass and Vespers with organ sung Compline.

Thanks be to God

On the first day of January 1752

It will be displayed in the sacristy of our church and observed by all present.

G. A. Bufalini Praeceptor of Santo Spirito.

Bibliography

Primary documentary sources in manuscript

GB-Lwl London, Wellcome library

EPB 46633/B *Relatione del modo; che si tiene da Religione di S. Spirito nel governo dell'Archihospitale Apostolico di Santo Spirito in Sassia di Roma, et dell'ordine, che vi osserva nella cura de gli'Infermi, et esposti scritta da fra Domenico Borgarucci Religioso, et secretario del medesimo ordine*, 1623.

I-Ras, Archivio di Stato di Roma, Fondo Ospedale di Santo Spirito (ASR OSS)

OSS 29 *Inventari* 1582
OSS 47 Spada, *Stato della Casa dell'Archiospedale di Santo Spirito di Roma, 1661*
OSS 50 *Bolle dei precettori* 1575–1785
OSS 72 *Martirologio* (Liber annualium)
OSS 78 *Stefano Vai corrispondenze*
OSS 118 *Spedizioni e decreti, Rubricella atti* 1565–1572
OSS 130–132 *Spedizioni e decreti, Rubricella atti* 1606–1630
OSS 134 *Spedizioni e decreti, Rubricella atti* 1642–1645
OSS 137–138 *Spedizioni e decreti, Rubricella atti* 1657–1668
OSS 231, 237, 240 *Istromenti: Atti del notaio*
OSS 300 *Instromentum* 1618
OSS 306–307 *Instromentum* 1624–1625
OSS 901 *Sacra visita, Atti diversi relazione* 1592–1734
OSS 1083 *Beni Urbani*
OSS 1894–1995 *Ospedale di S. Spirito copie di mandati* 1555–1700
OSS 1296 *Chiesa di S. Spirito, Scritture varie*
OSS 1298 *Chiesa di S. Spirito, Scritture concernenti interessi della Chiesa collegiale di S. Spirito*
OSS 1299 *Chiesa di S. Spirito, Ordini e istruzioni*
OSS 1301 *Archiconfraternità di S. Spirito, atti diversi*
OSS 2816 *Libro mastro giornale* 1618
OSS 2820 *Libro mastro giornale* 1622
OSS 3098 *Buste miscellanee, Documenti storici, sec XV seguenti, Visite apostoliche 1592–1844*

I-Rla Biblioteca Lancisiana

Ms 342 *Epistolario di Bernardino Cirillo,* letter 142 fol. 58
Ms 338 *Epistolario di Bernardino Cirillo,* letter 11, fol. 31v

I-Rn Biblioteca Nazionale di Roma

Ms Vittorio Emmanuele 721 *Notizie e Statistiche di Roma sotto il Pontificato di Clemente VIII*
I-Rvic Archivio diocesano di Roma (Archivio storico del vicariato di Roma)
Stato del Anime Santo Spirito in Sassia, 1626

V-CVbav Biblioteca Apostolica Vaticana

Ottob Lat 2473 ff179–204 *Relatione della fabrica e casa di S. Spirito di Roma* (1571)
Barb Lat 4315 f157r–157v Mancini, *Dell'origine et nobilita del ballo,* available at https://digi.vatlib.it/view/MSS_Barb.lat.4315

V-CVaav Archivio Apostolico Vaticano

Misc. Arm IV–V/3 *Bolle indulti, decreti et indulgenze per diverse confraternite e congregazioni pie*
Misc. Arm IV–V/7 *Editto della sacra visita apostolica sopra le musiche, Editto sulle feste*
Misc. Arm IV–V/9 *Bolle et editti per ammalati in campagna, ospedali di Roma e fuori, ospizii di Roma per li poveri mendicanti et altri miserabili*
Misc. Arm VII/77 *Stato temporale delle chiese di Roma fatto nel pontificato di Urbano VIII l'anno 1625*
Misc. Arm VIII /112 (1649) *Chiesa di S. Spirito canonici regolari*
Misc. Arm VII/ 113 *Acti Sacrae Visitationis Apostolicae S.d. N Urbani VIII pars 3a continent collegia hospitalia etc ecclesias simplices*

Music manuscripts

(Select list of items specifically mentioned)

D-Rp Bishöfliche Zentralbibliothek, Regensburg, Sammlung Proske-Haberl

BH 6001 *Missae Antonii Cifrae*
BH 6002 [Masses and motets]

BH 6003 *Messe diversi e mottetti*
BH 6004 [Latin motets and one mass]
BH 6005 [Latin motets]
BH 6006 [Latin motets]
BH 6007 *Motetti di Palestrina a cinque voci... copiata da me Fra Paolo Troiano...* 1625
BH 6008 [Latin motets]
BH 6009 [Masses and Latin motets copied by Domenico Aniboni 1603]
BH 6257 Anon, *Christus resurgans*

I-Rc, Biblioteca Casanatense, Rome

Ms 5371 Felice Anerio, *Dixit dominus*
Ms 5376 Anselmi, *Cum complerentur*
Ms 5411 Carpani, *Angeles ad pastores*
Ms 5375 Zoilo, *Hec ist Virgo*

I-Rsc, Biblioteca del Conservatorio di Santa Cecilia, Rome

G.MS. 082 Beretta, *Salmodia* 1688
G.MS. 0148 Carpani, *Exulta filia zion*
G.MSS. 796–805 *Motetti per le processioni*

I-TrFeininger, Trento, Biblioteca del Castello di Buonconsiglio, Feininger collection

FP 130/1–3 Anon, *Ad inflammanda apostolorum*
FP 121/1–10 Anon, *Veni Sancte Spiritus*

Printed Primary Sources

Benoist, F, P. et al, *Rome dans sa grandeur: vues, monuments anciens et modernes*, vol. 2, (Paris, 1870)

Breviarium secundum usum Ordinis Sancti Johannis Hierosolymitani (Lyon, 1518)

Breviarum Romanum ex Decreto Sacrosancti Concilii Tridentini Restitutum (Venice, 1568); https://archive.org/details/breviarium-romanum-1568

Castiglione, Sabba di, *Ricordi di Frate Sabba di Castiglione* (Bartolomeo Bonardo da Parma, 1549)

Caeremoniale Episcoporum (Rome, 1600); https://archive.org/details/caeremonialeepiscoporum1600

D.B [Dux Bragantiae = John IV of Portugal], *Difesa della musica moderna contro la falsa opinione del Vescovo C. F.*, etc. (c 1650) GB-Lbl 557*.d.26

Da Luca, Pietro. *Regole della vita spirituale et secreta theologia* (Bologna, 1526). https://archive.org/details/bub_gb_IhdAsrE1syoC/mode/2up

——, *L'arte del ben pensare e contemplare la passione del nostro signor Jesu Christo* (Bologna, 1532); https://archive.org/details/bub_gb_caNojQ5oaMMC

De Silvestris, Florido (ed.), *Directorium Chori ad usum Omnium Ecclesiarum, Cathedralium & Collegiatarum* (Rome, Andrea Fei, 1642)

Dragondelli. *Trattato del Sacro Ordine di S. Spirito detto in Sassia ... del Rev. Fra Pietro Saunier.* (Rome, Giacomo Dragondelli, 1662); https://archive.org/details/bub_gb_WwOtrQSTNXIC

Facultates, Et Priuilegia Concessa Ven. Archihospitalis S. Spiritus in Saxia (Rome, Ex Typographia Reverendae Apostolicae, 1606). GB-En Crawford B. 87 (23)

Fiaschi, Cesare, *Trattato dell'imbrigliare, manegiare et ferrare cavalli...* (Bologna, 1556), book 2, p. 88; https://archive.org/details/hin-wel-all-00000629-001

Lettere Volgari di diversi nobilissimi huomini et eccellentisimi ingegni, scritte in diverse materie, vol. 3 (Venice, Aldo Manuzio, 1564); https://archive.org/details/delleletterevolg00manu/page/114/mode/2up

Mace, Thomas. *Music's Monument* 1676; https://s9.imslp.org/files/imglnks/usimg/6/62/IMSLP93639-PMLP193185-Mace,_Thomas_-_Musick's_Monument.pdf

Mattioli, Pietro Andrea (ed.), *Petri Andreae Matthioli Senensis... Commentarii Denuo Aucti in Libros Sex Pedacii Dioscoridis Anazarbei De Medica Materia...* (Lyon, Apud Gabrielem Coterium, 1563); https://archive.org/details/ARes18410

Missale Romanum Ex Decreto Sacrosancti Concilii Tridentini Restitutum. Apud Ioannem Variscum, & haeredes, 1570; https://archive.org/details/bub_gb_adC-aRGza70C

Negri, Giulio, *Istoria degli scrittori fiorentini* (Ferrara, Bernardino Pomatelli, 1722); https://archive.org/details/bub_gb_G7SV8dn6B2UC

Notificatione [Archiospedale di Santo Spirito] (Rome, Stamperia della Reverenda Camera Apostolica, 1681); GB-En Crawford B. 29 (111)

Panciroli, Ottavio, *I Tesori nascosti nell'alma città di Roma* (Rome, Luigi Zanetti, 1600); https://archive.org/details/itesorinascostin00panc/page/n3/mode/2up

Regole da Osservarsi nel sacro ed apostolico Archiospedale di Santo Spirito in Sassia di Roma (Rome, Niccolò e Marco Pagliarini, 1751); https://archive.org/details/regoledaosservar00ospe

Regole per bene operare al servitio de' poveri infermi nell'hospedale di San Spirito in Sassia (Rome, J. Fei, 1671)

Ristretto Generale di tutti gl'infermi, projetti, e famiglia nel ... Archiospedale di S. Spirito in Sassia di Roma per lo scorso anno MDCCLXIII (Rome, M. Pagliarini 1764)

Sanudo, Marino, *I diarii di Marino Sanuto: (MCCCCXCVI-MDXXXIII) dall' autografo Marciano ital. cl. VII codd* (Padua, 1890); https://onlinebooks.library.upenn.edu/webbin/metabook?id=sanudodiary; https://archive.org/details/idiariidimarino00sanugoog/page/n243/mode/2up

Saulnier, Petrus, *De Capite Sacri Ordinis Sancti Spiritus Dissertatio. In Qua Ortus, Progressusque Ordinis Totius, Ac Speciatim Romanæ Domus Amplitudo, Prærogatiuum Jus, & Oeconomia Disseruntur* (Lyon, 1649)

Sommario delle indulgenze concesse nuovamente da N. S. Papa Paolo Quinto (Rome, Stamperia della Reverenda Camera Apostolica, 1609)

Spada, Virgilio. *Notificazione sopra li dieci capitoli di avvertimenti di Monsignor Spada per li novizi dell'ordine dei canonici regolari di S. Spirito* (Rome, 1815)

Statuta Ordinis Domus Hospitalis Hierusalem (Rome, Blado, 1586)

Totti, Pompilio et al., *Ritratto di Roma Antica: nel quale sono figurati i principali tempij, teatri, anfiteatri, cerchi, naumachie, archi trionfali, curie, basiliche, colonne, ordine del trionfo, dignità militari, e civili, riti, ceremonie, medaglie, & altre cose notabili* (Rome, Andrea Fei, 1627)

——, *Ritratto di Roma moderna* (Rome, Mascardi, 1638)

Zacchia, Paolo, *De' mali hipchondriaci libri due di Paolo Zacchia medico romano* (Rome, Pietro Antonio Facciotti, 1639); https://archive.org/details/bub_gb_5SdwlEStS4oC/page/n119/mode/2up

——, *Il Vitto quaresimale di Paulo Zacchia medico romano* (Rome, Pietro Antonio Facciotti, 1636); https://archive.org/details/bub_gb_5FJb1F5jZKkC/mode/2up

Music

Allegri, Gregorio, *Motecta Binis, Ternis... Vocibus* (Rome, Luca Antonio Soldi, 1621)

Cifra, Antonio, *Missarum Liber Primus* (Rome, Luca Antonio Soldi, 1619)

——, *Missarum Liber Secundum* (Rome, Luca Antonio Soldi, 1621)

——, *Motecta Ex Sacris Cantionibus Que Binis, Ternis, Quaternis Vocibus Concinuntur, Liber Quartus* (Rome, Luca Antonio Soldi, 1619)

——, *Psalmi Septem Qui in Vesperis Ad Concentus...* (Rome, Luca Antonio Soldi, 1619)

——, *Scherzi e Arie* (Rome, Luca Antonio Soldi, 1623)

Durante, Ottavio, *Arie Devote* (Rome, Simone Verovio, 1608)

Frescobaldi, Girolamo, *Il Primo Libro di Capricci fatti sopra diversi soggetti et arie in partitura* (Rome, Luca Antonio Soldi, 1624)

——, *Il Secondo Libro di Toccate, Canzone, Versi d'hinni, Magnificat, Gagliarde, Corrente et altre partite d'intavolatura di cimbalo et organo* (Rome, Niccolo Borbone, 1627)

Kapsberger, Girolamo. *Libro quarto di Villanelle a una e più voci* (Rome, Luca Antonio Soldi, 1623)
——, *Poematia et carmina composita a Maffaeo Barberino Olim S.R.E. Card. nunc autem Urbano Octavo P.O.M, Musicis modis aptata a Hieronymo Kapsberger nobili Germano Volumen Primum* (Rome, Luca Antonio Soldi, 1624)
Orgas, Annibale, *Sacrarum Cantionem* (Rome, Luca Antonio Soldi, 1619)
Rontani, Raffaele, *Le Varie Musiche* (Rome, Luca Antonio Soldi, 1619)
Soriano, *Passio Secundum Mattaeum* (Rome, Luca Antonio Soldi, 1619)
Ugolini, Vincenzo, *Motecta Et Missae Octonis Et Duodenis Vocibus Cum Basso Ad Organum, Liber Secundus* (Rome, Luca Antonio Soldi, 1622)
Veneri, Gregorio, *Sacrarum Cantionum* (Rome, Luca Antonio Soldi, 1621)
Vitali, Filippo, *L'aretusa* (Rome, Luca Antonio Soldi, 1620)

Secondary Sources (Books, Articles, Theses, Webpages, Music)

Abbate, Carolyn, 'Music: Drastic or Gnostic?, *Critical inquiry*, 30 (2004), 505–536; doi:https://doi.org/10.1086/421160
Akombo, David Otieno, *Music and Healing across Cultures* (Ames, IA, 2006)
Allegra, Antonio, 'La Cappella musicale di S. Spirito in Saxia di Roma: Appunti storici (1551–1737)', *Note d'Archivio*, 17 (1940), 26–38
Annibaldi, Claudio, 'Palestrina and Frescobaldi: Discovering a Missing Link', *Music & Letters*, 79:3 (1998), 329–345
Anon 'Cirillo, Bernardino', *Dizionario biografico degli italiani*, vol. 25 (Treccani, 1981)
Antolini, Bianca Maria, Arnaldo Morello and Vera Vita Spagnuolo (eds), *La Musica a Roma attraverso le fonti d'archivio* (Lucca, 1994)
Aquinas, Thomas. *Summa Theologica*, trans. The Fathers of the English Dominican Province (Cincinnati, OH, 1947); https://www.ccel.org/a/aquinas/summa/home.html
Arikha, Noga, *Passions and Tempers: A History of the Humours* (New York, 2007)
Aristotle, *On Sense and the Sensible*, trans. J.I. Beare, MIT, The Internet Classics Archive; http://classics.mit.edu/Aristotle/sense.html
——, *Physics* trans. R. P. Hardie and R. K. Gaye, MIT, *The Internet Classics Archive*
Ariès, Philippe et al, *A History of Private Life* (Cambridge, MA, 1989)
Asiedu, F. B. A., 'The Song of Songs and the Ascent of the Soul: Ambrose, Augustine, and the Language of Mysticism', *Vigiliae Christianae*, 55 (2001), 299–317.
Augustine, *The Rule of Saint Augustine with Commentary by Hugh of St. Victor*, trans. Dom Aloysius Smith, Chaucer House Scholars (n.p., n.d)
Augustine, St., *Confessions*, trans. R.S. Pine-Coffin (London, 1961)
Austern, Linda Phyllis, '"No Pill's Gonna Cure My Ill": Gender, Erotic Melancholy and Traditions of Musical Healing in the Modern West', in Penelope

Gouk (ed.), *Musical Healing in Cultural Contexts* (Aldershot, 2000), pp. 113–136

Balboni, Michael and John Peteet (eds), *Spirituality and Religion within the Culture of Medicine: From Evidence to Practice* (New York, 2017); https://doi.org/10.1093/med/9780190272432.001.0001

Banchieri, Adriano, *L'organo Suonarino* (1611) Facsimile edition, ed. Giulio Cattin (The Netherlands, 1969)

Barbieri, Patrizio, 'Musica, Tipografi E Librai a Roma: Tecnologia Di Stampa E Integrazioni Biografiche 1583–1833', *Ricercare,* VII (1995), 47–85

——, 'Music Printers and Booksellers in Rome 1583–1600, with New Documents on Coattino, Diani, Donangeli, Tornieri and Franzini', *Recercare,* XVI (2004), 69–112

——, 'Music-Selling in Seventeenth-Century Rome: Three New Inventories from Franzini's Bookshops, 1621, 1633, 1686', *Recercare,* XXIII (2011), 131–171

——, 'Music Printing and Selling in Rome: New Findings on Palestrina, Kerle and Guidotti, 1554–1574', *Recercare,* XXXII (2020), 35–55

Barker, Andrew, *Greek Musical Writings.* Cambridge readings in the Literature of Music, 2 vols (Cambridge, 1989)

Barker, Naomi J., 'Frescobaldi at the Ospedale Di Santo Spirito: Evidence of a Portfolio Career in Seventeenth-Century Rome', *Early Music,* 49:3 (2021) 395–412; doi:https://doi.org/10.1093/em/caab044

——, 'Mottos and Metaphors: Towards an Interpretation of the Emblems in Frescobaldi's *Primo Libro d'Arie musicali*', *Journal of Seventeenth-century music,* vol. 25, 2019 [online]

Barker, Sheila, 'Poussin, Plague, and Early Modern Medicine', *The Art Bulletin,* 86:4 (2004), 569–689

Barry, Jonathan and Colin Jones, *Medicine and Charity before the Welfare State* (London and New York, 1991)

Becker, Judith, 'Anthropological Perspectives on Music and Emotion', in Patrik N. Juslin and John A. Sloboda (eds), *Music and Emotion* (Oxford, 2001), pp. 135–160

Bennett, Peter, 'Hearing King David in Early Modern France', *Journal of the American Musicological Society,* 69:1 (2016), 47–109

Bentivenga, Giuseppe, *Effusione dello Spirito Santo e doni carismatici: La testimonianza di Sant'Agostino* (Rome, 1995)

Bertoglio, Chiara. 'Cats, Bulls and Donkeys: Bernardino Cirillo on 16th-Century Church Music', *Early Music,* XLV:4 (2017), 559–572; doi:10.1093/em/cax081

——, *Reforming Music: Music and the Religious Reformations of the Sixteenth Century* (Berlin, 2017)

Bianchi, Eric, 'Bad Latin, Bad Manners: Giovanni Battista Doni, Marin Mersenne and Literary Style in Seventeenth-Century Music Theory', *Music & Letters,* 92:2 (2015), 167–184

——, 'Scholars, Friends, Plagiarists,' *Journal of the American Musicological Society*, 70:1 (2017), 61–128

Biller, Peter and Joseph Ziegler (eds), *Religion and Medicine in the Middle Ages*, York Studies in Medieval Theology (York, 2001)

Bizzotto, Renata, *L'ospedale di S. Spirito: rilievo dell'architettura* (Rome, 2001)

Black, Christopher, *Italian Confraternities in the Sixteenth Century* (Cambridge, 1989)

Blackburn, Bonnie J., 'For Whom Do the Singers Sing?,' *Early Music*, 25:4 (1997), 593–609

Blackburn, Bonnie J. and Edward Lowinsky, 'Luigi Zenobi's Letter on the Perfect Musician,' *Studi Musicali*, 22 (1993), 61–114

Blazey, David Anthony, 'The Litany in Seventeenth-Century Italy,' 2 vols (unpublished PhD thesis, Durham University, 1990)

Boethius, A.M.S., *Fundamentals of Music*, trans. Calvin M. Bower and Claude V. Palisca (New Haven, CT and London, 1989)

Boillet, Elise, 'Vernacular Sermons on the Psalms Printed in Sixteenth-Century Italy: An Interface between Oral and Written Cultures,' in Stefano Dall'Aglio, Brian Richardson and Massimo Rosprocher (eds), *Voices and Texts in Early Modern Italian Society* (London and New York, 2017), pp. 200–211

Bowers, Barbara S, *The Medieval Hospital and Medical Practice*. Avista Studies in the History of Medieval Technology, Science and Art (Aldershot, 2007)

Boynton, Susan, 'Prayer as Liturgical Performance in Eleventh- and Twelfth-Century Monastic Psalters,' *Speculum*, 82 (2007), 896–931

Brennecke, Wilfried, 'Kerle, Jacobus De,' *Grove Music Online* (Oxford, 2001); doi:10.1093/gmo/9781561592630.article.14911

Brevaglieri, Sabina, 'Science, Books and Censorship in the Academy of the Lincei: Johannes Faber as Cultural Mediator,' in Maria Pia Donato and Jill Kraye (eds), *Conflicting Duties: Science, Medicine and Religion in Rome, 1550–1750* (London and Turin, 2009), pp. 133–157

Brodman, James W., 'Religion and Discipline in the Hospitals of Thirteenth-Century France,' in Barbara S. Bowers (ed.), *The Medieval Hospital and Medical Practice* (Aldershot, 2007), pp. 123–131

Brodman, James William, *Charity and Religion in Medieval Europe* (Washington DC, 2009)

Bross, Louise Smith, 'The Church of Santo Spirito in Sassia : A Study in the Development of Art, Architecture and Patronage in Counter Reformation Rome' (unpublished PhD dissertation, University of Chicago, 1994)

Brown, Howard Mayer and Richard Sherr, 'Carpentras,' *Grove Music Online* (Oxford, 2019); doi:10.1093/gmo/9781561592630.article.04995

Burke, Peter, 'Is There a Cultural History of Emotions?,' in Penelope Gouk and Helen Hills (eds), *Representing Emotions: New Connections in the Histories of Art, Music and Medicine* (Aldershot, 2005), pp. 35–47

Burnett, Charles, 'European Knowledge of Arabic Texts Referring to Music: Some New Material,' *Early Music History*, 12 (1993), 1–17

——, '"Spiritual Medicine": Music and Healing in Islam and Its Influence in the West', in Penelope Gouk (ed.), *Musical Healing in Cultural Contexts* (Aldershot, 2000), pp. 85–91

Burnett, Charles, Michael Fend and Penelope Gouk, *The Second Sense: Studies in Hearing and Musical Judgement from Antiquity to the Seventeenth Century*. Warburg Institute surveys and texts 22 (London, 1991)

Burton, Robert, *The Anatomy of Melancholy (1628)* ed. Holbrook Jackson (New York, 2001)

Burton-Christie, Douglas, 'Early Monasticism', in Amy Hollywood and Patricia Z. Beckman (eds), *Cambridge Companion to Christian Mysticism* (Cambridge, 2012), pp. 37–58

Calcagno, Mauro, *From Madrigal to Opera: Monteverdi's Staging of the Self* (Berkeley, CA, 2012)

Camiz, Franca Trinchieri, 'Musical Performance and Healing in Renaissance Rome Revealed by Texts and Images', in Katherine A. McIver (ed.), *Art and Music in the Early Modern Period: Essays in Honor of Franca Trinchieri Camiz* (New York and London, 2016)

Camporesi, Piero, *The Fear of Hell: Images of Damnation and Salvation in Early Modern Europe*, trans. Linda Byatt ([Milan, 1987] Cambridge, 1990)

Canezza, Alessandro and G. Spano, *Gli Arcispedali di Roma nella vita cittadina, nella storia e nell'arte* (Rome, 1933)

Cantus: A Database for Latin Ecclesiastical Chant; < https://cantus.uwaterloo.ca/ >

Caraci, Maria, 'Cannicciari, Pompeo'; < https://www.treccani.it/enciclopedia/pompeo-cannicciari_%28Dizionario-Biografico%29/

Caravale, Giorgio, 'Private and Public Devotion in Late Renaissance Italy: The Role of Church Censorship', in Maya Corry, Marco Faini and Alessia Meneghin (eds), *Domestic Devotions in Early Modern Italy* (Leiden, 2019), pp. 389–407

Carlson, Jeffrey, 'The Past, Present and Future of Flood Control in Rome', *Engineering Rome*, 2022; < https://engineeringrome.org/ >

Carruthers, Mary, *The Book of Memory: A Study of Memory in Medieval Culture* (Cambridge, 2008)

Casimiri, Rafaele, 'Il disperso archivio musicale di Santo Spirito in Saxia', *Note d'Archivio*, XV (1938), 140–144

Catholic Encyclopedia, The, New Advent, 2021; https://www.newadvent.org/cathen/

Cavallo, Sandra, 'The Motivations of Benefactors: An Overview of Approaches to the Study of Charity', in Jonathan Barry and Colin Jones (eds), *Medicine and Charity before the Welfare State* (London and New York, 1991), pp. 46–62

Cavallo, Sandra and Tessa Storey, *Healthy Living in Late Renaissance Italy* (Oxford, 2013)

Chadwick, Anthony, *Missa Tridentina: The Reform of the Roman Mass Liturgy in the Sixteenth Century*; <https://civitas-dei.eu/Mass_of_St_Pius_V.pdf.>

Chiaramida, Michele, *Manuale di canto fermo: modelli e consuetudini nella prassi didattica tra xvi e xviii secolo* (Lucca, 2020)
Chiu, Remi, 'Music, Pestilence and Two Settings of "O Beate Sebastiane"', *Early Music History*, 31 (2012), 153–188
——, *Plague and Music in the Renaissance* (Cambridge, (1st 2017) 2020)
——, 'Singing on the Street and in the Home in Times of Pestilence: Lessons from the 1576–78 Plague of Milan', in Maya Corry, Marco Faini and Alessia Meneghin (eds), *Domestic Devotions in Early Modern Italy* (Leiden, 2019), pp. 27–44
Chojnacka, Monica, 'Women, Charity and Community in Early Modern Venice: The Casa Delle Zitelle', *Renaissance Quarterly*, 51:1 (1998), 68–91
'Choral Wiki'; <http://ChoralWiki (cpdl.org)>
Cicero, *De Oratore*, trans. E. W. Sutton, Loeb Classical Library (Princeton, 1976 (1st 1942))
Cipolla, Carlo M., *Public Health and the Medical Profession in the Renaissance* (Cambridge, 1976)
Clark, Leah R., *Courtly Mediators* (Cambridge, 2023)
Classen, Constance, *Worlds of Sense: Exploring the Senses in History and across Cultures* (New York and London, 1993)
Cobussen, Marcel, *Thresholds: Rethinking Spirituality through Music* (Aldershot, 2008)
Colonna, Flavia, *L'ospedale di Santo Spirito a Roma: Lo sviluppo dell'assistenza e le trasformazioni architettonico-funzionali*, Gradus: Studi di storia dell'architettura e restauro (Rome, 2009)
Conforti, Maria et al, 'Ospedale, accademie, esperimenti: Giovanni Maria Lancisi e l'ospedale di Santo Spirito in Sassia', *Medic*, 15 (2007), 31–38
Connolly, Thomas, *Mourning into Joy: Music, Raphael, and Saint Cecilia* (Princeton, 1994)
Corry, Maya, Marco Faini and Alessia Meneghin (eds), *Domestic Devotions in Early Modern Italy* (Leiden, 2019)
Courtenay, Lynn T., 'The Hospital of Notre Dame De Fontanilles at Tonnerre: Medicine as Misericordia', in Barbara S. Bowers (ed.), *The Medieval Hospital and Medical Practice* (Aldershot, 2007), pp. 77–106
Crook, David, 'Proper to the Day: Calendrical Ordering in Post-Tridentine Motet Books', in Esperanza Rodríguez-Garcìa and Daniele Filippi, *Mapping the Motet in the Post-Tridentine Era* (New York and London, 2019), pp. 16–35
Curti, Danilo and Fabrizio Leondelli (eds), *La biblioteca musicale Laurence Feininger* (Trento, 1985)
Daboo, Jerry, *Ritual, Rapture and Remorse: A Study of Tarantism and 'Pizzica' in Salento* (Bern, 2010)
Dall'Aglio, Stefano, Brian Richardson and Massimo Rosprocher (eds), *Voices and Texts in Early Modern Italian Society* (New York and London, 2017)

Darbellay, Etienne, 'L'énigme de La première édition (1624) Des *Caprices* De Girolamo Frescobaldi', *Canadian University Music Review*, 3 (1982), 123–157

Davies, Matthew and Andrew Prescott (eds), *London and the Kingdom: Essays in Honour of Caroline M. Barron*, Harlaxton Medieval Studies XVI (Donington, 2008)

De Angelis, Pietro, *Musica e musicisti nell'Arcispedale di Santo Spirito in Saxia dal quattrocentro all'ottocento*, Collana di Studi Storici sull'Ospedale di Santo Spirito in Saxia e sugli ospedali romani (Rome, 1950)

——, *L'arciconfraternita di Santo Spirito in Saxia*, Collana di Studi Storici sull'Ospedale di Santo Spirito in Saxia e sugli ospedali romani (Rome, 1950)

——, *La chiesa di Santo Spirito in Saxia*, Collana di Studi Storici sull'Ospedale di Santo Spirito in Saxia e sugli ospedali romani (Rome, 1952)

——, *Giovanni Faber, linceo, primario in Santo Spirito in Saxia 1598–1629: Il microscopio*, Collana di Studi Storici sull'Ospedale di Santo Spirito in Saxia e sugli ospedali romani (Rome, 1953)

——, *L'ospedale Apostolico di Santo Spirito in Saxia nella mente e nel cuore dei papi*, Collana di Studi Storici sull'Ospedale di Santo Spirito in Saxia e sugli ospedali romani, 16, (Rome, 1956)

——, *L'ospedale di S. Spirito dalle origini al 1500* (2 vols), Collana di Studi Storici sull'Ospedale di Santo Spirito in Saxia e sugli ospedali romani (Rome, 1960–1962)

——, *L'architetto e gli affreschi di Santo Spirito in Saxia*, Collana di Studi Storici sull'Ospedale di Santo Spirito in Saxia e sugli ospedali romani (Rome, 1961)

——, *Guido Di Montpellier, Innocenzo III e la fondazione dell'Ospedale Apostolico di Santo Spirito in Santa Maria in Saxia*, Collana di Studi Storici sull'Ospedale di Santo Spirito in Saxia e sugli ospedali romani 22 (Rome, 1962)

de Beer, E. S. and Roy Strong (eds), *The Diary of John Evelyn*, Everyman's library ([Oxford,1959] Oxford 2006)

De Lucca, Valeria and Christine Jeanneret, 'Exploring the Soundscape of Early Modern Rome through Uberti's *Contrasto Musico*', in Valeria De Lucca and Christine Jeanneret (eds), *The Grand Theater of the World: Music, Space and the Performance of Identity in Early Modern Rome* (Abingdon, 2020), pp. 11–30

—— (eds), *The Grand Theater of the World: Music, Space, and the Performance of Identity in Early Modern Rome* (Abingdon, 2020)

De Martino, Ernesto, *La terra del rimorso* (Milan, 2015, 1st edition 1961)

De Renzi, Silvia, '"A Fountain for the Thirsty" and a Bank for the Pope: Charity, Conflicts, and Medical Careers at the Hospital of Santo Spirito in Seventeenth-Century Rome', in Jon Arrizabalaga, Andrew Cunningham and Ole Peter Grell (eds), *Healthcare and Poor Relief in Counter-Reformation Europe* (London, 1999), pp. 99–130

——, 'Medical Competence, Anatomy and the Polity in Seventeenth-Century Rome', *Renaissance studies*, 21:4 (2007), 551–567

——, 'A Career in Manuscripts: Genres and Purposes of a Physicians Writings in Rome, 1600–1630', *Italian studies*, 66:2 (2011), 234–248

de Vries, Lyke and Leen Spruit, 'Paracelsus and Roman Censorship – Johannes Faber's 1616 Report in Context', *Intellectual History Review*, 28:2 (2018), 225–254; doi:DOI: 10.1080/17496977.2017.1361060

de Waard, Cornelius, *Correspondence Du P. Marin Mersenne, religieux minime*, vol. 9 (Paris, 1965)

Dell'Antonio, Andrew, *Listening as Spiritual Practice in Early Modern Italy* (Berkeley and Los Angeles, CA, 2011)

Della Libera, Luca, 'Repertori ed organici vocali-strumentali nella Basilica di Santa Maria Maggiore a Roma, 1557–1624', *Studi musicali*, XXXIX (2000), 3–58

di Falco, Anna, *Francesco Borromini, Virgilio Spada e la costruzione della Casa dei Filipini. Contributi per la storia costruttiva dell'oratorio a seguito dei lavori di restauro e di alcune fonti inedite*, Miscellanea della Società romana di storia patria LXII (Rome, 2015)

Diruta, Girolamo, *Il Transilvano (1593, 1609). A Facsimile Edition with Introduction*, edited by Edward J. Soehnlen and Murray C. Bradshaw (Buren, 1983)

Dixon, Graham, 'The Origins of the Roman "Colossal Baroque"', *Proceedings of the Royal Musical Association*, 106 (1979–1980), 115–128

Dixon, Thomas, *From Passions to Emotions: The Creation of a Secular Psychological Category* (Cambridge, 2003)

Dobszay, Laszlo, 'Concerning a Chronology for Chant', in Sean Gallagher et al (eds), *Western Plainchant in the First Millennium: Studies in the Medieval Liturgy and Its Music* (Aldershot, 2003)

Donato, Maria Pia and Jill Kraye (eds), *Conflicting Duties: Science, Medicine and Religion in Rome, 1550–1750* (London and Turin, 2009)

Duffin, Jacalyn, 'Questioning Medicine in Seventeenth-Century Rome: The Consultations of Paolo Zacchia', *CBMH / BCHM*, 28 (2011), 149–170

——, *Medical Miracles: Doctors, Saints, and Healing in the Modern World* (Oxford, 2009)

Duggan, Mary Kay, *Italian Music Incunabula: Printers and Type* (Berkeley and Los Angeles, CA, 1991); http://ark.cdlib.org/ark:/13030/ft409nb31c/

Durante, Castore, *Il Tesoro della Sanità*, ed. Elena Camillo (Milan, 1982)

Durling, Richard J, 'A Chronological Census of Renaissance Editions and Translations of Galen', *Journal of the Warburg and Courtauld Institutes*, 3-4 (1961), 230–305

Dyer, Joseph, 'The Desert, the City and Psalmody in the Late Fourth Century', in Sean Gallagher et al (eds), *Western Plainchant in the First Millennium: Studies in the Medieval Liturgy and Its Music* (Aldershot, 2003), pp. 11–43

——, 'The Singing of Psalms in the Early-Medieval Office', *Speculum*, 64:3 (1989), 535–578

——, 'Tropis Semper Variantibus: Compositional Strategies in the Offertories of Old Roman Chant', *Early Music History*, 17 (1998), 1–60

Eco, Umberto, *The Aesthetics of Thomas Aquinas*, trans. Hugh Bredin ([Milan, 1970] n.p., 1988)

Elmer, Peter (ed.), *The Healing Arts: Health, Disease and Society in Europe 1500–1800* (Manchester and Milton Keynes, 2004)

Erlmann, Veit, *Hearing Cultures: Essays on Sound, Listening, and Modernity* (Oxford, 2004)

Eternal Word Television Network; / Church Councils. <https://www.ewtn.com/catholicism/library/thirteenth-session-of-the-council-of-trent-14792022.>

Everist, Mark (ed.), *The Cambridge Companion to Medieval Music* (Cambridge, 2011)

Farndell, Arthur (ed.), *On the Nature of Love: Ficino on Plato's Symposium* (London, 2016)

Fassler, Margot E., 'The Office of the Cantor in Early Western Monastic Rules and Customaries: A Preliminary Investigation', *Early Music History*, 5 (1985), 29–51

Fastiggi, Robert, 'The Contributions of the Council of Trent to the Catholic reformation', *Perichoresis*, 18:6 (2020), 3–20

Feininger, Lorenzo, 'Membra disjecta reperta', *Acta Societatis Universalis Sanctae Ceciliae*, 3 (Trento, 1964)

——, 'Membra disjecta conjuncta', *Acta Societatis Universalis Sanctae Ceciliae*, 4 (Trento, 1966)

Fenlon, Iain, 'Music and Domestic Devotion in the Age of Reform', in Maya Corry, Marco Faini and Alessia Meneghin (eds), *Domestic Devotions in Early Modern Italy* (Leiden, 2019), pp. 89–114

Ficino, Marsilio, *The Letters of Marsilio Ficino*, vol. 1, trans. from the Latin by members of the Language department of the School of Economics (London, 1975)

——, *Three Books on Life*, trans. and ed. Carol V. Kaske and John R. Clark, Medieval and Renaissance Texts and Studies (Tempe, AZ, 1989)

——, *On the Nature of Love: Ficino on Plato's 'Symposium'*, trans. Arthur Farndell (London, 2016)

——, *Commentary on Plotinus Ennead III, Part 2 and Ennead IV*, vol. 5, ed. Stephen Gersh (Cambridge, MA, 2018)

Filippi, Daniele V., 'Earthly Music, Interior Hearing and Celestial Harmonies: Philipe De Monte's First Book of Spiritual Madrigals (1581)', *Journal of the Alamire Foundation*, 3 (2011), 208–234

——, '"Ask the Jesuits to Send Verses from Rome": The Society's Networks and the European Dissemination of Devotional Music', in Robert Aleksander Maryks (ed.), *Exploring Jesuit Distinctiveness: Interdisciplinary Perspectives on Ways of Proceeding within the Society of Jesus* (Leiden, 2016), pp. 62-80; http://www.jstor.org/stable/10.1163/j.ctt1w76ttq.9

——, '*Catechismum Modulans Docebat:* Teaching the Doctrine through Singing', in Daniele V. Filippi and Michael Noone (eds), *Listening to Early Modern Catholicism* (Leiden, 2017), pp. 129–148

Filippi, Daniele V. and Michael Noone (eds), *Listening to Early Modern Catholicism: Perspectives from Musicology*, Intersections: interdisciplinary studies in early modern culture 49 (Leiden, 2017)
Finocchiaro, Giuseppe, *Il Museo di curiosità di Virgilio Spada: Una raccolta romana del seicento* (Rome, 1999)
Fosi, Irene, 'The Hospital as a Space of Conversion: Roman Examples from the Seventeenth Century', in Giuseppe Marcocci (ed.), *Space and Conversion in a Global Perspective*, Intersections 5 (Leiden, 2015), pp. 154–174
Franchi, Saverio, 'Stampatori ed editori musicali a Roma dal 1550 al 1608: Vicende e osservazioni', *Recercare*, XI (1999), 5–50
Franchi, Saverio and Orietta Sartori, 'Luca Antonio Soldi', *Dizionario Biografico degli Italiani* vol. 98 (Trecani, 2018)
——, *Annali della stampa musicale romana dei secoli xvi – xviii.* 2 vols (Rome, 2006–2012)
Frigo, Alberto, 'Can One Speak of Painting If One Cannot Hold a Brush? Giulio Mancini, Medicine, and the Birth of the Connoisseur', *Journal of the History of Ideas*, 73:3 (2012), 417–436
Froberger, Johann Jacob, *Neue Ausgabe Sämtlicher Clavier- Und Orgelwerke*, ed. Siegbert Rampe, vol. 2 (Kassel, 1995)
Fry, Timothy OSB, *The Rule of St. Benedict in English* (Collegeville, MI, 1982)
Gage, Frances, 'Exercise for Mind and Body: Giulio Mancini, Collecting, and the Beholding of Landscape Painting in the Seventeenth Century', *Renaissance Quarterly*, 61:4 (2008), 1167–1207
——, *Painting as Medicine in Early Modern Rome: Giulio Mancini and the Efficacy of Art.* (University Park, PA, 2016)
Gallagher, Sean et al (eds), *Western Plainchant in the First Millennium: Studies in the Medieval Liturgy and Its Music* (Aldershot, 2003)
Gaukroger, Stephen, (ed.), *The Soft Underbelly of Reason: The Passions in the Seventeenth Century* (London, 1998)
Geertz, Clifford, *The Interpretation of Cultures* (New York, 1973)
Gemienweiser, Siegfried, 'Cannicciari, Pompeo', *Grove Music Online* (Oxford, 2001)
Gentilcore, David, 'Methods and Approaches in the Social History of the Counter-Reformation in Italy', *Social History*, 17:1 (1992), 73–98
Gersh, Stephen, *Concord in Discourse: Harmonics and Semiotics in Late Classical and Early Medieval Platonism* (Berlin and New York, 1996)
Gigli, Giacinto, *Diario Di Roma*, ed. Manlio Barberito (Rome, 1994)
Glixon, Jonathan, *Honoring God and the City: Music at Venetian Confraternities, 1260–1807* (Oxford, 2003)
Golding, Rosemary, *Music and Moral Management in the Nineteenth-Century English Lunatic Asylum*, Mental Health in Historical Perspective (London, 2021)
Gouk, Penelope, *Musical Healing in Cultural Contexts* (Aldershot, 2000)
——, 'Music, Melancholy, and Medical Spirits in Early Modern Thought', in Peregrine Horden (ed.), *Music as Medicine* (Aldershot, 2000), pp. 173–194

——, 'Sister Disciplines? Music and Medicine in Historical Perspective', in Penelope Gouk (ed.), *Musical Healing in Cultural Contexts* (Aldershot, 2000), pp. 171–197

——, 'Raising Spirits and Restoring Souls: Early Modern Medical Explanations for Music's Effects', in Veit Erlmann (ed.), *Hearing Cultures: Essays on Sound, Listening and Modernity* (Oxford and New York, 2004), pp. 87–105

——, 'Harmony, Health, and Healing: Music's Role in Early Modern Paracelsian Thought', in Margaret Pelling and Scott Mandelbrote (eds), *The Practice of Reform in Health, Medicine and Science 1500–2000* (Aldershot, 2005), pp. 23–42

Gouk, Penelope, and Helen Hills (eds), *Representing Emotions: New Connections in the Histories of Art, Music, and Medicine* (Aldershot, 2005)

Gouk, Penelope et al (eds), *The Routledge Companion to Music, Mind and Wellbeing* (New York, 2018)

Gowland, Angus, 'The Problem of Early Modern Melancholy', *Past & Present*, 191 (2006), 77–120

Gozzi, Marco, 'Italy to 1300', in Mark Everist (ed.), *The Cambridge Companion to Medieval Music* (Cambridge, 2011), pp. 121–135

——, 'Liturgical Music and Liturgical Experience in Early Modern Italy', in Daniele V. Filippi and Michael Noone (eds), *Listening to Early Modern Catholicism* (Leiden, 2017), pp. 55–78

Grampp, Florian Bassani, 'On a Roman Polychoral Performance in August 1665', *Early Music*, 36:3 (2008), 415–433

Grant, Roger Matthew, *Beating Time and Measuring Music in the Early Modern Era* (Oxford, 2014)

Gross, Daniel M., *The Secret History of Emotion: From Aristotle's Rhetoric to Modern Brain Science* (Chicago, IL, 2006)

Guido, Massimiliano, 'Counterpoint in the Fingers. A Practical Approach to Girolamo Diruta's *Breve & facile regola di contrapunto*", *PhilomusicaOnline*, 11:1 (2012), 63–76; http://riviste.paviauniversitypress.it/index.php/phi/article/view/1452

—— (ed.), *Studies in Historical Improvisation: From Cantare Super Librum to Partimenti* (Abingdon, 2017)

Guido, Massimiliano and Peter Schubert, "Unpacking the Box in Frescobaldi's Ricercari of 1615", *Music Theory Online: Journal of the Society for Music Theory*, 20:2 (2014); <https://mtosmt.org/issues/mto.14.20.2/mto.14.20.2.guido_schubert.html.>

Haar, James, 'Festa, Costanzo', *Grove Music Online* (Oxford, 2001); doi:10.1093/gmo/9781561592630.article.09554

Haberl, Dieter, *Bischöfliche Zentralbibliothek Regensburg, Thematischer Katalog der Musikhandscriften, 7 Bibliothek Franz Xaver Haberl Manuskripte Bh6001 Bis Bh6949*, Kataloge Bayerischer Musiksammlungen, Herausgegeben von der Bayerischen Staatsbibliothek, vol. 14/7–8 (Munich, 2000)

Hall, James, *Hall's Dictionary of Signs and Symbols in Art* (London, 1974)

Hammond, Frederick, *Girolamo Frescobaldi* (Cambridge, MA, 1983)

——, *Music and Spectacle in Baroque Rome: Barberini Patronage under Urban VII.* (New Haven, CT and London, 1994)

——, *Girolamo Frescobaldi: An Extended Biography* (online, 2017–2020; <https://girolamofrescobaldi.com/.>

Harkins, Paul W. and Walther Riese (eds), *Galen on the Passions and Errors of the Soul* (Columbus, OH, 1963)

Harmon, Roger, '*Musica Laetitae Comes* and Vermeer's Music Lesson', *Oud Holland*, 113:3 (1999), 161–166

Harper, John, 'Frescobaldi's Early *Inganni* and Their Background', *Proceedings of the Royal Musical Association*, 105 (1978), 1–12

——, *The Forms and Orders of Western Liturgy from the Tenth Century to the Eighteenth Century* (Oxford, 1991)

Haug, Judith I., 'Medical Knowledge in 'Alī Ufukī's Musical Notebook (Mid-17th-Century)', *Intellectual History of the Islamicate World*, 6 (2018), 117–143

Henderson, John, *The Renaissance Hospital: Healing the Body and Healing the Soul* (New Haven, CT and London, 2006)

Hildebrand, Stephen M., *Basil of Caesarea*, The Early Christian Fathers (Abingdon, 2018)

Hiley, David, *Gregorian Chant* (Cambridge, 2009)

Holford-Strevens, Leofranc, 'The Harmonious Pulse', *The Classical Quarterly*, 43:2 (1993), 475–479

——, 'Fa Mi La So La: The Erotic Implications of Solmization Syllables', in Bonnie J. Blackburn and Laurie Stras (eds), *Eroticism in Early Modern Music* (Aldershot, 2015), pp. 43–58

Hollywood, Amy, 'Song Experience, and the Book in Benedictine Monasticism', in Amy Hollywood and Patricia Z. Beckman (eds), *The Cambridge Companion to Christian Mysticism* (Cambridge, 2012), pp. 37–58

Hollywood, Amy and Patricia Z. Beckman (eds), *The Cambridge Companion to Christian Mysticism* (Cambridge, 2012)

Honisch, Erika Supria, 'Hearing the Body of Christ in Early Modern Prague', *Early Music History*, 38 (2019), 58–105; doi:doi:10.1017/S0261127919000032

Horden, Peregrine (ed.), *Music as Medicine: The History of Music Therapy since Antiquity* (Aldershot, 2000)

——, 'Religion as Medicine: Music in Medieval Hospitals', in Peter Biller and Joseph Ziegler (eds), *Religion and Medicine in the Middle Ages*, York Studies in Medieval Theology (York, 2001), pp. 135–154

——, 'The Earliest Hospitals in Byzantium, Western Europe, and Islam', *The Journal of Interdisciplinary History*, 35:3 (2005), 361–389

——, 'A Non-Natural Environment: Medicine without Doctors and the Medieval European Hospital', in Barbara S. Bowers (ed.), *The Medieval Hospital and Medical Practice* (Aldershot, 2007), pp. 133–145

Horrigan, B., 'Therese Schroeder-Sheker Music Thanatology and Spiritual Care for the Dying', *Alternative therapies in health and medicine*, 7 (2001), 6–77

Horstmanshoff, Manfred, Helen King and Claus Zittel (eds), *Blood, Sweat and Tears: The Changing Concepts of Physiology from Antiquity into Early Modern Europe*, Intersections 25 (Leiden and Boston, 2012)

Howe, Eunice D., *The Hospital of Santo Spirito and Pope Sixtus IV*, Outstanding Dissertations in the Fine Arts (New York and London, 1978)

——, *Art and Culture at the Sistine Court: Platina's 'Life of Sixtus IV' and the Frescoes of the Hospital of Santo Spirito* (Vatican City, 2005)

——, '"Architecture for 'Divine Hymns": The Organ of Antonio da Sangallo the Younger for the Church of Santo Spirito in Sassia', in Katherine A. McIver (ed.), *Art and Music in the Early Modern Period: Essays in Honor of Franca Trinchieri Camiz* (London and New York, 2016)

Howes, David, *A Cultural History of the Senses in the Modern Age* (London, 2014)

Irwin, Joyce L., 'The Mystical Music of Jean Gerson', *Early Music History: Studies in Medieval and Early Modern Music*, 1 (1981), 187–201

Jackson, Donald F., 'Greek Medicine in the Fifteenth Century', *Early Science and Medicine*, 17:4 (2012), 378–390

Jackson, Stanley W., *Melancholia and Depression: From Hippocratic Times to Modern Times* (New Haven, CT and London, 1986)

James, Jamie, *The Music of the Spheres: Music, Science and the Natural Order of the Universe* (London, 1993)

Jansen, Katherine L., Joanna Drell and Frances Andrews (eds), *Medieval Italy: Texts in Translation* (Philadelphia, PA, 2010)

Jeffery, Peter, 'Monastic Reading and the Emerging Roman Chant Repertory', in Sean Gallagher et al (eds), *Western Plainchant in the First Millennium: Studies in the Medieval Liturgy and Its Music* (Aldershot, 2003)

Juslin, Patrik N., 'Communicating Emotion in Music Performance: A Review and Theoretical Framework', in Patrik N. Juslin and John A. Sloboda (eds), *Music and Emotion: Theory and Research* (Oxford, 2001), pp. 309–337

Juslin, Patrik N. and John A. Sloboda (eds), *Music and Emotion: Theory and Research* (Oxford, 2001)

Juslin, Patrik N. and Renee Timmers, 'Expression and Communication of Emotion in Music Performance', in Patrik N. Juslin and John Sloboda (eds), *Handbook of Music and Emotion: Theory, Research, Application* (Oxford, 2010), pp. 453–492

Jütte, Robert *A History of the Senses from Antiquity to Cyberspace*, trans. James Lynn (Cambridge, 2005)

Katinis, Teodoro, 'A Humanist Confronts the Plague: Ficino's Consilio contro la Pestilentia', *MLN*, 125:1 (2010), 72–83

Kelsey, Morton T., *Healing and Christianity: In Ancient Thought and Modern Times* (New York and London, 1973)

Kendrick, Robert, 'Orality and Sacred Music in Early Modern Italy', in Stefano Dall'Aglio, Brian Richardson and Massimo Rosprocher (eds), *Voices and Texts in Early Modern Italian Society* (London and New York, 2017), pp. 229–240

Kerr, Fergus, *Thomas Aquinas: A Very Short Introduction* (Oxford, 2009)
Keyvanian, Carla, *Hospitals and Urbanism in Rome, 1200–1500*, Brill's Studies in Intellectual History, vol. 252 (Leiden, 2015)
——, 'Paduan Humanism in Sistine Rome: The Hospital of Santo Spirito in Sassia', unpublished conference paper, *Early Modern Rome IV*, 11–13 November 2021
Kirby, Dom Mark Daniel, OSB, 'The Psalmody of the Divine Office: A Path to Holiness for the Apostolic Religious', *Sacred Music*, 138:1 (2011), 7–18
Kostylo, Joanna, 'Contested Devotions: Space, Identities and Religious Dissent in the Apothecary's Home', in Maya Corry, Marco Faini and Alessia Meneghin (eds), *Domestic Devotions in Early Modern Italy* (Leiden, 2018), pp. 409–435
Kurtzman, Jeffrey, 'Motets, Vespers, Antiphons and the Performance of the Post-Tridentine Liturgy in Italy', in Esperanza Rodríguez-Garcìa and Daniele Filippi (eds), *Mapping the Motet in the Post-Tridentine Era* (Abingdon, 2019), pp. 36–56
Kurtzman, Jeffrey and Anne Schnoebelen, 'A Catalogue of Motets, Mass, Office and Holy Week Music Printed in Italy, 1516–1770'; <https://sscm-jscm.org/instrumenta/instrumenta-volumes/instrumenta-volume-2/>
Le Mee, Katherine, *The Benedictine Gift to Music* (New York, 2003)
Leli, Letizia (ed.), *Vivere la Misericordia nel trecento: le miniature del Liber Regulae dell'ospedale romano di Santo Spirito in Sassia* (Rome, 2018)
Lincoln, Harry B., 'Zoilo, Annibale', *Grove Music Online* (Oxford, 2001); doi:10.1093/gmo/9781561592630.article.31017
——, 'Zoilo, Cesare', *Grove Music Online* (Oxford, 2001); doi:10.1093/gmo/9781561592630.article.31018
Lionnet, Jean, 'La musique a Saint-Louis des Français de Rome au XVII° siècle', *Note d'Archivio* III (1985) supplement
Lockwood, Lewis H., 'Vincenzo Ruffo and Musical Reform after the Council of Trent', *The Musical Quarterly*, 43:3 (1957), 342–371
—— (ed.), *Giovanni Pierluigi Da Palestrina, Pope Marcellus Mass*, Norton Critical Scores (New York, 1975)
Lockwood, Lewis, Noel O'Regan and Jessie-Ann Owens, 'Palestrina [Prenestino] Giovanni Pierluigi da ['Giannetto']', *Grove Music Online*, (Oxford, 2001)
Lockwood, Lewis and Noel O'Regan, 'Animuccia, Giovanni', *Grove Music Online* (Oxford, 2001); doi:10.1093/gmo/9781561592630.article.00955
Lombard, Jean, *Platone e la medicina*, trans. M. A. Raggi ([Paris, 1999] Forlì, 2016)
Luccichenti, Furio, 'Luca Blasi (C.1545–1608): Profilo di un organaro', *L'Organo*, XIX (1981), 113–131
Lumbroso, Matizia Maroni and Antonio Martini, *Le confraternite romane nelle lore chiese* (Rome, 1963)
Lunelli, Clemente, *I manoscritti polifonici della biblioteca musicale L. Feininger* (Trento, 1994)

Lynch, Tosca A.C. and Eleanora Rocconi (eds), *A Companion to Greek and Roman Music* (Oxford, 2020)

M.B., *La Chiesa di S. Maria Annunziata in Borgo, l'arciconfraternita di S. Spirito, l'opera pia di S Michele Arcangelo* (Rome, 1973)

Macey, Patrick, *Bonfire Songs: Savanarola's Musical Legacy* (Oxford, 1998)

Macklin, Christopher, 'Plague, Performance and the Elusive History of the *Stella Celi Extirpavit*', *Early Music History*, 29 (2010), 1–31

Maconie, Robin, 'Musical Acoustics in the Age of Vitruvius', *Musical Times*, 146:1890 (2005), 75–82

Marcase, Donald Earl, 'Adriano Banchieri: L'organo Suonarino: Transcription, Translation and Commentary' (unpublished PhD dissertation, Indiana University, 1970)

Marcocci, Giuseppe, Aliocha Maldavsky and Wietse de Boer (eds), *Space and Conversion in Global Perspective*, Intersections vol. 35 (Leiden, 2015)

Marder, Tod A., 'Vitruvius and the Architectural Treatise in Early Modern Europe', in Alina Payne (ed.), *Companions to the History of Architecture, Volume I, Renaissance and Baroque Architecture* (Oxford, 2017)

Martin, Gregory, *Roma Sancta* (1581), ed. George Bruner Parks (Rome, 1969)

Martin, Michael, *Thesaurus Precum Latinarum*; <https://www.preces-latinae.org/index.htm>

Martini, Stefano. *Il senso dell'udito nel Corpus Aristotelicum*, European University Studies, Series XX (Bern, 2011)

Marucchi Andrea (ed.), *Giulio Mancini: Considerazioni Sulla Pittura* (Rome, 1956–1957)

Mattei-Gentili, Guido, '"Membra disjecta" dell'archivio musicale di Santo Spirito in Saxia', *Nova et vetera*, XVI (1937), 5–81

Matthieson, Thomas, *Apollo's Lyre: Greek Music and Music Theory in Antiquity and the Middle Ages* (London and Lincoln, NE, 1999)

McClary, Susan, *Desire and Pleasure in Seventeenth Century Music* (Berkeley and Los Angeles, CA, 2012)

McClellan, Randall, *The Healing Forces of Music: History, Theory and Practice* (New York, 1988)

McIver, Katherine A. (ed.), *Art and Music in the Early Modern Period: Essays in Honor of Franca Trinchieri Camiz* (New York and London, 2016)

McKinney, Timothy R., 'Hearing in the Sixth Sense', *The Musical Quarterly*, 82:3–4 (1998), 517–536

McKinnon, James W., *Music in Early Christian Literature* (Cambridge, 1987)

——, 'Desert Monasticism and the Later Fourth-Century Psalmodic Movement', *Music and Letters*, 75:4 (1994), 505–521

McNeely, Ian F., 'The Renaissance Academies between Science and the Humanities', *Configurations*, 17:3 (2009), 227–258

Mellela, Patrizia, 'Vita musicale e arte organaria a Santo Spirito in Sassia nel cinquecento: note e documenti', in Bianca Maria Antolini, Arnaldo Morello and Vera Vita Spagnuolo (eds), *La musica a Roma attraverso le fonti d'archivio* (Lucca, 1994), pp. 507–519

Meloncelli, Raoul, 'Musica nell'arcispedale di Santo Spirito', *Il Veltro*, XLVI: 1–4 (2002), 263–277

Mercuriale, Girolamo, *De Arte Gymnastica. The Art of Gymnastics*, ed. Concetta Pennuto, trans. Vivian Nutton (Florence, 2008)

Messbarger, Rebecca, Christopher Johns and Philip Gavitt (eds), *Benedict XIV and the Enlightenment: Art, Science, and Spirituality* (Toronto, 2016), ProQuest ebook central

Middleton, Joyce Irene, 'Rhetorical Listening: When the Eye Defers to the Ear for Civic Discourse', *The English Journal*, 101:1 (2011), 105–107

Miller, Clement A. (ed), *Hieronymus Cardanus (1501–1576): Writings on Music*. American Institute of Musicology, 1973

Miller, Timothy S., *The Birth of the Hospital in the Byzantine Empire* (Baltimore and London, 1997)

Modrak, Deborah K. W., *Aristotle: The Power of Perception* (Chicago, 1989)

Monson, Craig, 'The Council of Trent Revisited', *Journal of the American Musicological Society*, 55:1 (2002), 1–37

Morelli, Arnaldo. *Teatro della vista e dell'udito: la musica e i suoi luoghi nell'età moderna* (Lucca, 2017)

——, 'Un amico di Frescobaldi: Lelio Guidiccioni, uomo di lettere, connoisseur d'arte e di musica', in Benno Boccadoro and Georges Starobinski (eds), *A Fresco: Mélanges offerts au Professeur Etienne Darbellay* (Bern, 2013) pp. 51–67

Moroni, Gaetano, 'Commendatore di Santo Spirito', *Dizionario di erudizione storico-ecclesiastica*, vol. XV (Venice, 1842); <https://archive.org/details/volume-15/page/73/mode/2up.>

Murray, Peter, *The Architecture of the Italian Renaissance* (London, 1963)

Nichols, Stephen G. Andreas Kablitz and Alison Calhoun (eds), *Rethinking the Medieval Senses: Heritage, Fascinations, Frames* (Baltimore, 2008)

O'Malley, J. W., *Trent and all that: Renaming Catholicism in the Early Modern Era* (Cambridge, MA, 2000)

——, 'Early Modern Catholicism: The State of Research', in Daniele V. Fillipi and Michael Noone (eds), *Listening to Early Modern Catholicism: Perspectives from Musicology*, Intersections: Interdisciplinary Studies in Early Modern Culture 49 (Leiden, 2017), pp. 21–34

O'Regan, Noel, 'Sacred Polychoral Music in Rome 1575–1621' (unpublished D.Phil thesis, University of Oxford, 1988)

——, 'Blessed with the Holy Father's Entertainment' Roman Ceremonial Music as Experienced by the Irish Earls in Rome 1608', *Irish Musical Studies*, 2 (1993), 41–57

——, 'Music at the Archconfraternity of San Rocco in the late Sixteenth Century', in Bianca Maria Antolini, Arnaldo Morelli and Vera Vita Spagnuolo (eds), *La musica a Roma attraverso le fonti d'archivio* (Lucca, 1994), pp. 521–552

——, *Institutional Patronage in Post-Tridentine Rome: Music at Santissima Trinita Dei Pellegrini 1550–1650*, Royal Musical Association Monographs 7 (London, 1995)

——, 'Music in the Liturgy of San Pietro in Vaticano During the Reign of Paul V (1605–1621): A Preliminary Survey of the Liturgical Diary (Part 1) of Andrea Amici', *Recercare*, 11 (1999), 119–151

——, 'Music at Roman "Ospedali" in the Sixteenth Century', *Il Veltro*, XLVI:1–4 (2002), 251–260

——, 'Music at Roman Confraternities to 1650: The Current State of Research', *Analecta Musicologica*, 45 (2011), 132–158

——, 'Music, Memory, and Faith: How Did Singing in Latin and the Vernacular Influence What People Knew About Their Faith in Early Modern Rome?', *The Italianist*, 34:3 (2014), 437–448

——, 'Palestrina's Mid-Life Compositional Summary: The Three Motet Books of 1569–75', in Esperanza Rodrìguez-Garcìa and Daniele V. Filippi (eds), *Mapping the Motet in the Post-Tridentine Era* (Abingdon, 2019), pp. 102–122

Page, Christopher, *The Christian West and Its Singers: The First Thousand Years* (New Haven, CT and London, 2010)

Palisca, Claude V., *Humanism in Italian Renaissance Musical Thought* (New Haven, CT and London, 1985)

——, *Studies in the History of Italian Music and Music Theory* (Oxford, 1994)

——, 'Bernardino Da Cirillo's Critique of Polyphonic Church Music of 1549: Its Background and Resonance', in Jessie Ann Owens and M. A. Cummings (eds), *Music in Renaissance Cities and Courts: Studies in Honor of Lewis Lockwood* (Warren MI, 1997), pp. 282–292

——, 'The Humanist Reaction to Polyphony', in Claude V. Palisca (ed.), *Music and Ideas in the Sixteenth and Seventeenth Centuries* (Champaign IL, 2006); https://doi.org/10.5406/j.ctt1xcmq8

Palma, Angelo, *L'ospedale di Santo Spirito in Saxia* (Padua, 1994)

Paster, Gail Kern, Katherine Rowe and Mary Floyd-Wilson (eds), *Reading the Early Modern Passions: Essays in the Cultural History of Emotion* (Philadelphia, PA, 2004)

Pavanello, Agnese, 'The Elevation as Liturgical Climax in Gesture and Sound: Milanese Elevation Motets in Context', *Journal of the Alamire Foundation*, 9 (2017), 33–60

Pelosi, Francesco, *Plato on Music, Soul and Body*, trans. Sophie Henderson (Cambridge, 2010)

Pender, Stephen, 'Medicine and the Senses: Physicians, Sensation and the Soul', in Herman Roodenburg (ed.), *A Cultural History of the Senses in the Renaissance* (London and New York, 2014), pp. 127–147

Pennuto, Concetta, 'Pulsations du corps en medicine: sentre et mesurer par la musique', *Histoire, médecine et santé*, 11 (2017) ; doi:https://doi.org/10.4000/hms.1095

Pesic, Peter, *Music and the Making of Modern Science.* (Cambridge, MA, 2014)

Piccialuti, Maura, *La carità come metodo di governo: istituzioni caritative a Roma dal pontificato dii Innocenzo XII a quello di Benedetto XIV* (Turin, 1994)

Piejus, Anne, 'Artistic Revival and Conquest of the Soul in Early Modern Rome', in Daniele V. Fillipi and Michael Noone (eds), *Listening to Early Modern Catholicism: Perspectives from Musicology*, Intersections: Interdisciplinary Studies in Early Modern Culture 49 (Leiden, 2017), pp. 149–172

——, 'The Roman Motet (1550–1600): A Collective Issue? New Attributions and Reflections on Authorship in the Light of a New Document', *Early Music History*, 40 (2022), 253–293

Pillsbury, Edmund, 'Jacopo Zucchi in S. Spirito in Sassia', *The Burlington Magazine*, 116:857 (1974), 434–444

Pine-Coffin, R.S. (ed. and trans.), *Saint Augustine: Confessions* (London, 1961)

Plato, *Republic*, trans. Robin Waterfield (Oxford, 1994)

——, *Timaeus*, trans. Desmond Lee and Thomas Kjeller Johansen (London, 1965)

Porterfield, Amanda, *Healing in the History of Christianity* (Oxford, 2005)

Presciutti, Diana Bullen, 'Dead Infants, Cruel Mothers and Heroic Popes: The Visual Rhetoric of Foundling Care at the Hospital of Santo Spirito Rome', *Renaissance Quarterly*, 64:3 (2011), 752–799

——, *Visual Cultures of Foundling Care in Renaissance Italy* (Abingdon, 2018)

Prins, Jacomien, 'The Music of the Pulse in Marsilio Ficino's Timaeus Commentary', in Manfred Horstmanshoff, Helen King and Claus Zittel (eds), *Blood, Sweat and Tears: The Changing Concepts of Physiology from Antiquity into Early Modern Europe*, Intersections 25 (Leiden and Boston, 2012)

——, 'Girolamo Cardano and Julius Caesar Scaliger in Debate About Nature's Musical Secrets', *Journal of the history of ideas*, 78:2 (2017), 169–189

——, 'Girolamo Cardano on Music as a Remedy "For the Troubles That Result from the Misery of Human Misfortune"', in Penelope Gouk et al (eds), *The Routledge Companion to Music, Mind and Wellbeing* (New York, 2018)

Printed Sacred Music Database – Printed Sacred Music in Europe 1500–1800, Fondazione Giorgio Cini, Institute of Musicology, Fribourg; Swiss RISM Office Bern; Swiss National Science Foundation; <http://www.printed-sacred-music.org. 2021>

Provenza, Antonietta, 'Music and Medicine', in Tosca A.C. Lynch and Eleanora Rocconi (eds), *A Companion to Greek and Roman Music* (Oxford, 2020)

Pruett, Lilian P., 'Porta, Costanzo', *Grove Music Online* (Oxford, 2001); doi:10.1093/gmo/9781561592630.article.22134

Pseudo-Cicero, *Ad Herrenium*, trans. Henry Caplan, Loeb Classical Library (Cambridge MA, [1954] 1989)

Pullan, Brian, 'Catholics, Protestants, and the Poor in Early Modern Europe', *The Journal of Interdisciplinary History*, 35:3 (2005), 441–456

Quintillian, *The Orator's Education (Institutio Oratoria)*, trans. Donald A. Russell, Loeb Classical Library (Cambridge, MA, 2001)

Rawcliffe, Carol, 'Christ the Physician Walks the Wards: Celestial Therapeutics in the Medieval Hospital', in Matthew Davies and Andrew Prescott (eds), *London and the Kingdom: Essays in Honour of Caroline M. Barron*, Harlaxton Medieval Studies (Donington, 2008), pp. 78–97

Redondi, Pietro, *Galileo Heretic* (Princeton, NJ, 1987)

Restaino, Angelo.,'Il *Liber annualium* e la memoria cultuale dell'ordine', in Letizia Leli (ed.), *Vivere la misericordia nel trecento: le miniature del Liber Regulae dell'ospedale romano di Santo Spirito in Sassia* (Rome, 2018), pp. 129–131

Rietbergen, Peter, *Power and Religion In Baroque Rome: Barberini Cultural Policies* (Leiden, 2006); http://www.jstor.org/stable/10.1163/j.ctt1w76twr.14

Risse, Guenter B., *Mending Bodies, Saving Souls: A History of Hospitals* (Oxford, 1999)

Roberts, Holly J., 'Ecstatic Devotion: Musical Rapture and Erotic Death in Seventeenth- and Eighteenth-Century Iconography, Operas, and Oratorios' (unpublished PhD dissertation, University of Oregon, 2020)

Roche, Jerome, 'Cifra, Antonio', *Grove Music Online* (Oxford, 2001)

Rodríguez-Garcìa, Esperanza and Filippi Daniele (eds), *Mapping the Motet in the Post-Tridentine Era* (Abingdon, 2019)

Roodenberg, Herman (ed), *A Cultural History of the Senses in the Renaissance* (London & New York, 2014)

Rosenfeld, Sophia, 'On Being Heard: A Case for Paying Attention to the Historical Ear', *The American Historical Review*, 116:2 (2011), 316–334

Rosenwein, Barbara H., *Generations of Feeling: A History of Emotions 600–1700* (Cambridge, 2016)

Rostirolla, Giancarlo, 'L'archivio musicale della chiesa annessa all'Ospedale di Santo Spirito', *Il Veltro*, XLVI: 1–4 (2002), 279–343

——, *Musica e musicisti nella basilica di San Pietro: cinque secoli di storia della Cappella Giulia* (Vatican City, 2014)

Rostirolla, Giancarlo, Livia Martinoli Santini and Candida Santoro (eds), *Musica, medicina, cronache di corte al tempo di Arcangelo Corelli: Il diario di G. A. Francesco Massonetti, 1659–1729* (Rome, 2021)

Rostirolla, Giancarlo, Danilo Zardin and Oscar Mischiati (eds), *La lauda spirituale tra cinque e seicento: poesie e canti devozionali nell'Italia della controriforma* (Rome, 2001)

Rota, Daniele, *I Gesuiti e le tarantole* (Lucca, 2012)

Rowland, Ingrid D., 'Vitruvius and His Influence', in Roger B. Ulrich and Caroline K. Quenemoen (eds), *A Companion to Roman Architecture* (Oxford, 2014), pp. 412–425

Rubin, Miri, 'Imagining Medieval Hospitals: Considerations on the Cultural Meaning of Institutional Change', in Jonathan Barry and Colin Jones (eds), *Medicine and Charity before the Welfare State* (London and New York, 1991), pp. 14–25

Schafer, R. Murray, *The Soundscape: Our Sonic Environment and the Tuning of the World* (Rochester VT, 1993)

Schaff, Philip, *St. Basil: Letters and Select Works*, Series 2, vol 8; https://ccel.org/ccel/schaff/npnf208/npnf208.vi.ii.iii.html

Schwarz, Michael, 'Bodies of Transcendence: The Spirit of Affect in Giotto and Piero', in Penelope Gouk and Helen Hills (eds), *Representing Emotions: New Connections in the Histories of Art, Music and Medicine* (Aldershot, 2005), pp. 69–87

Sella, Domenico, *Italy in the Seventeenth Century*, Longman History of Italy (Abingdon, [1997] 2014)

Sherr, Richard, 'Competence and Incompetence in the Papal Choir in the Age of Palestrina', *Early Music*, XXII:4 (1994), 606–630; doi:https://doi.org/10.1093/earlyj/XXII.4.606

Siegel, Rudolph E., *Galen on Sense Perception: His Doctrines, Observations and Experiments on Vision, Hearing, Smell, Taste, Touch and Pain, and Their Historical Sources* (Basel, 1970)

Siraisi, Nancy G., 'The Music of Pulse in the Writings of Italian Academic Physicians (Fourteenth and Fifteenth Centuries)', *Speculum*, 50:3 (1975), 689–710

——, *Medieval and Early Renaissance Medicine: An Introduction to Knowledge and Practice* (Chicago, IL, 1990)

——, 'Anatomizing the Past: Physicians and History in Renaissance Culture', *Renaissance Quarterly*, 53:1 (2000), 1–30

——, 'History, Antiquarianism, and Medicine: The Case of Girolamo Mercuriale', *Journal of the History of Ideas*, 64:2 (2003), 231–251

——, 'Medicine, 1450–1620, and the History of Science', *Isis*, 103:3 (2012), 491–514

Smith, Dom Aloyisius (trans.), *The Rule of St. Augustine with Commentary by Hugh of St. Victor* (n.p., n.d.)

Smith, Bruce R., 'Listening to the Wild Blue Yonder: The Challenges of Acoustic Ecology', in Veit Erlmann (ed.), *Hearing Cultures: Essays on Sound, Listening and Modernity* (Oxford, 2004), pp. 21–41

——, *The Key of Green: Passion and Perception in Renaissance Culture* (Chicago, IL, 2009)

Smith, J. A., 'First-Century Christian Singing and Its Relationship to Contemporary Jewish Religious Song', *Music & Letters*, 75:1 (1994), 1–5

——, 'The Ancient Synagogue, the Early Church and Singing', *Music & Letters*, 65:1 (1984), 1–16

Smith, Mark M., *Sensory History* (Oxford, 2007)

Spitzer, Michael, *A History of Emotion in Western Music: A Thousand Years from Chant to Pop* (Oxford, 2020)

Stevenson, Robert, 'Victoria, Tomás Luis De', *Grove Music Online* (Oxford, 2001); doi:10.1093/gmo/9781561592630.article.29298

Stevenson, Robert and Alejandro Enrique Planchart, 'Morales, Cristóbal De', *Grove Music Online* (Oxford, 2001); doi:10.1093/gmo/9781561592630.article.19078

Stoltzfus, Philip, *Theology as Performance: Music, Aesthetics and God in Modern Theology* (London, 2006)

Storey, Tessa, '*La villanella della gravidanza:* Singing Medical Knowledge in Early Modern Rome', unpublished conference paper *Early Modern Rome IV*, 11–13 November 2021

Storey, Tessa and Sandra Cavallo, *Healthy Living in Late-Renaissance Italy* (Oxford, 2013)

——, *Conserving Health in Early Modern Culture: Bodies and Environments in Italy and England* (Manchester, 2017)

Surdacki, Marian, 'Il "conservatorio" e la "scuola dei putti" nell'Ospedale di Santo Spirito nei secoli xvii e xviii', *Il Veltro*, XLV: 5–6 (2001), 253–267

Talbot, Michael, '*Ore Italiane:* The Reckoning of the Time of Day in Pre-Napoleonic Italy', *Italian Studies*, 40:1 (1985), 51–62

Tomasetti, Stefano, 'Stefano Vai', *Dizionario Biografico degli Italiani*, vol. 97, 2020; https://www.treccani.it/enciclopedia/stefano-vai_%28Dizionario-Biografico%29/ 20/04/2021

Tonkovitch, Jennifer, 'Two Studies for the "Gesu" and a "Quarantore" Design by Bernini', *Burlington Magazine*, 140:1138 (1998), 34–37

Trucchi, Francesco (ed.), *Poesie Italiane inedite di dugento autori* (Prato, 1846)

Uberti, Grazio, *Contrasto Musico*, ed. Giancarlo Rostirolla (Lucca, 1991)

Ulrich, Roger B. and Caroline K. Quenemoen (eds), *A Companion to Roman Architecture* (Oxford, 2014)

Valone, Carolyn, 'Pentecost: Image and Experience in Late Sixteenth-Century Rome', *Sixteenth Century Journal*, 24:4 (1993), 801–828

Van Deusen, Nancy and Luisa Giudice (eds), *Performing Ecstasies: Music, Dance, and Ritual in the Mediterranean*, Claremont Cultural Studies (Ottawa, 2005)

Van Orden, Kate, *Music, Discipline and Arms in Early Modern France* (Chicago, IL, 2005)

Varwig, Bettina, *Music in the Flesh: An Early Modern Musical Physiology* (Chicago, IL, 2023)

Veldhorst, Natascha, 'Pharmacy for Body and Soul: Dutch Songbooks in the Seventeenth Century', *Early Music History*, 27 (2008), 217–285

Vickers, Brian, *In Defence of Rhetoric* (Oxford, 1988)

Vidal, Fernando, 'Miracles, Science, and Testimony in Post-Tridentine Saint-Making', *Science in Context*, 20:3 (2007), 481–508

——, 'Modernising the Miraculous Body in Prospero Lambertini's *De servorum Dei*', in Rebecca Messbarger, Christopher Johns and Philip Gavitt (eds), *Benedict XIV and the Enlightenment: Art, Science, and Spirituality* (Toronto, 2016), pp. 151–174

Vitruvius, *The Ten Books on Architecture*, trans. and ed. Morris Hicky Morgan (New York, 1960)

Vocabolario della Crusca (1612); http://www.lessicografia.it/

Voss, Angela, 'Marsilio Ficino, the Second Orpheus', in Peregrine Horden (ed.), *Music as Medicine: The History of Music Therapy since Antiquity* (Aldershot, 2000), pp. 154–172

Walden, Daniel K.S., 'Frozen Music: Music and Architecture in Vitruvius' De Architectura', *Greek and Roman Musical Studies*, 2 (2014), 124–145; doi:10.1163/22129758-12341255

Walker, D. P., *Spiritual and Demonic Magic from Ficino to Campanella* (Philadelphia, PA, 2000)

Wegman, Rob, 'Music as Heard: Listeners and Listening in Late-Medieval and Early Modern Europe (1300–1600)', *The Musical Quarterly*, 82:3–4 (1998), 3–4

Weill, Marc S., 'The Devotion of the Forty Hours and Roman Baroque Illusions', *Journal of the Warburg and Courtauld Institutes*, 37 (1974), 218–248; doi:https://doi.org/10.2307/750841

West, Martin, 'Music Therapy in Antiquity', in Peregrine Horden (ed.), *Music as Medicine: The History of Music Therapy since Antiquity* (Aldershot, 2000), pp. 51–68

West, Martin L., *Ancient Greek Music* (Oxford, 1992)

White, Michael, *Galileo Antichrist* (London, 2007)

Williamson, Beth, 'Sensory Experience in Medieval Devotion: Sound and Vision, Invisibility and Silence', *Speculum*, 88:1 (2013), 1–43; doi:doi:10.1017/S00387134

Wilson, Blake, *Music and Merchants: The Laudesi Companies of Republican Florence* (Oxford, 1992)

Zarlino, Gioseffo, *The Art of Counterpoint: Part Three of Le Istitutione Harmoniche, 1588*, trans. Guy A. Marco and Claude V. Palisca (New Haven, CT, 1968)

Index

Music in Society and Culture

Volumes already published

History in Mighty Sounds:
Musical Constructions of German National Identity, 1848–1914
Barbara Eichner

Music and Ultra-Modernism in France: A Fragile Consensus, 1913–1939
Barbara L. Kelly

The Idea of Art Music in a Commercial World, 1800–1930
Edited by Christina Bashford and Roberta Montemorra Marvin

Nation and Classical Music: From Handel to Copland
Matthew Riley and Anthony D. Smith

Musical Debate and Political Culture in France, 1700–1830
R. J. Arnold

Performing Propaganda:
Musical Life and Culture in Paris during the First World War
Rachel Moore

Musical Journeys:
Performing Migration in Twentieth-Century Music
Florian Scheding

Béla Bartók in Italy:
The Politics of Myth-Making
Nicolò Palazzetti

The Creative Labor of Music Patronage in Interwar France
Louis K. Epstein

America in the French Imaginary, 1789–1914:
Music, Revolution and Race
Edited by Diana R. Hallman and César A. Leal

Music, Nature and Divine Knowledge in England, 1650–1750:
Between the Rational and the Mystical
Tom Dixon

Printed and bound by CPI Group (UK) Ltd, Croydon, CR0 4YY
26/03/2024
14476337-0001